2004
YEAR BOOK OF
DERMATOLOGY
AND
DERMATOLOGIC
SURGERY™

The 2004 Year Book Series

Year Book of Allergy, Asthma, and Clinical Immunology™: Drs Rosenwasser, Boguniewicz, Milgrom, Routes, and Spahn

Year Book of Anesthesiology and Pain Management™: Drs Chestnut, Abram, Black, Lang, Roizen, Trankina, and Wood

Year Book of Cardiology®: Drs Gersh, Cheitlin, Graham, Kaplan, Sundt, and Waldo

Year Book of Critical Care Medicine®: Drs Dellinger, Parrillo, Balk, Bekes, Dries, and Roberts

Year Book of Dentistry®: Drs Zakariasen, Boghosian, Burgess, Hatcher, Horswell, McIntyre, and Zakariasen

Year Book of Dermatology and Dermatologic Surgery™: Drs Thiers and Lang

Year Book of Diagnostic Radiology®: Drs Osborn, Birdwell, Dalinka, Gardiner, Groskin, Levy, Maynard, and Oestreich

Year Book of Emergency Medicine®: Drs Burdick, Cone, Cydulka, Hamilton, Handly, and Quintana

Year Book of Endocrinology®: Drs Mazzaferri, Becker, Kannan, Kennedy, Kreisberg, Meikle, Molitch, Osei, Poehlman, and Rogol

Year Book of Family Practice®: Drs Bowman, Apgar, Dexter, Miser, Neill, and Scherger

Year Book of Gastroenterology™: Drs Lichtenstein, Dempsey, Ginsberg, Katzka, Kochman, Morris, Nunes, Reddy, Rosato, and Stein

Year Book of Hand Surgery®: Drs Berger and Ladd

Year Book of Medicine®: Drs Barkin, Frishman, Klahr, Loehrer, Mazzaferri, Phillips, Pillinger, and Snydman

Year Book of Neonatal and Perinatal Medicine®: Drs Fanaroff, Maisels, and Stevenson

Year Book of Neurology and Neurosurgery®: Drs Gibbs and Verma

Year Book of Nuclear Medicine®: Drs Coleman, Blaufox, Royal, Strauss, and Zubal

Year Book of Obstetrics, Gynecology, and Women's Health®: Drs Mishell, Kirschbaum, and Miller

Year Book of Oncology®: Drs Loehrer, Arceci, Glatstein, Gordon, Morrow, Schiller, and Thigpen

Year Book of Ophthalmology®: Drs Rapuano, Cohen, Eagle, Grossman, Myers, Nelson, Penne, Regillo, Sergott, Shields, and Tipperman

Year Book of Orthopedics®: Drs Morrey, Beauchamp, Peterson, Swiontkowski, Trigg, and Yaszemski

Year Book of Otolaryngology-Head and Neck Surgery®: Drs Paparella, Keefe, and Otto

2004

The Year Book of DERMATOLOGY AND DERMATOLOGIC SURGERY™

Editor-in-Chief
Bruce H. Thiers, MD
Professor and Chair, Department of Dermatology, Medical University of South Carolina, Charleston, South Carolina

Associate Editor
Pearon G. Lang, Jr, MD
Professor of Dermatology, Pathology, Otolaryngology, and Communicative Sciences, Medical University of South Carolina, Charleston, South Carolina

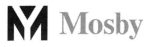

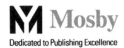

Dedicated to Publishing Excellence

Vice President, Continuity Publishing: Timothy M. Griswold
Senior Manager, Continuity Production: Idelle L. Winer
Developmental Editor: Ali Gavenda
Senior Issue Manager: Pat Costigan
Composition Specialist: Betty Dockins
Senior Illustrations and Permissions Coordinator: Chidi M. Nwaseki

Printed in the United States of America
Composition by Thomas Technology Solutions, Inc.
Printing/binding by Sheridan Books, Inc.

Editorial Office:
Elsevier
300 East
170 South Independence Mall West
Philadelphia, PA 19106-3399

International Standard Serial Number: 0093-3619
International Standard Book Number: 0-323-02082-8

Contributors

Margaret M. Boyle, BS
Research Associate, Dermatoepidemiology Unit, Brown University, Rhode Island

Thomas L. Diepgen, MD
Professor, Department of Social Medicine, Occupational and Environmental Dermatology, University of Heidelberg, Heidelberg, Germany

Alan B. Fleischer, Jr, MD
Department of Dermatology, Wake Forest University School of Medicine, Winston-Salem, North Carolina

Gillian M. P. Galbraith, MD
Professor of Biomedical Sciences, University of Las Vegas School of Dental Medicine, Las Vegas, Nevada

C. William Hanke, MD, MPH
Medical Director, Laser and Skin Surgery Center of Indiana, Carmel; Clinical Professor of Otolaryngology-Head and Neck Surgery, Indiana University School of Medicine, Indianapolis, Indiana

John C. Maize, MD
Clinical Professor and Chairman Emeritus, Department of Dermatology, Medical University of South Carolina, Charleston, South Carolina

Sharon Raimer, MD
Professor of Dermatology and Pediatrics; Chair, Department of Dermatology, University of Texas Medical Branch, Galveston, Texas

Martin A. Weinstock, MD, PhD
Professor of Dermatology and Community Health, Brown University; Chief of Dermatology, VA Medical Center; Director, Pigmented Lesion Unit and Photomedicine, Rhode Island Hospital, Providence, Rhode Island

Elke Weisshaar, MD
Consultant, Department of Social Medicine, Occupational and Environmental Dermatology, University of Heidelberg, Heidelberg, Germany

Table of Contents

Journals Represented

Mosby and its editors survey approximately 500 journals for its abstract and commentary publications. From these journals, the editors select the articles to be abstracted. Journals represented in this YEAR BOOK are listed below.

Acta Dermato-Venereologica
Allergy
American Journal of Clinical Nutrition
American Journal of Clinical Pathology
American Journal of Dermatopathology
American Journal of Human Genetics
American Journal of Medicine
American Journal of Ophthalmology
American Journal of Pathology
American Journal of Surgery
Annals of Internal Medicine
Annals of Rheumatic Diseases
Annals of Surgery
Annals of Surgical Oncology
Archives of Dermatology
Archives of Neurology
Archives of Pediatrics and Adolescent Medicine
Archives of Surgery
Arthritis and Rheumatism
Blood
British Journal of Cancer
British Journal of Dermatology
British Journal of Plastic Surgery
British Medical Journal
Cancer
Cancer Research
Clinical Infectious Diseases
Comprehensive Psychiatry
Dermatologic Surgery
Dermatology
European Journal of Vascular and Endovascular Surgery
Experimental Dermatology
Gastroenterology
Human Pathology
International Journal of Cancer
Journal of Allergy and Clinical Immunology
Journal of Bone and Joint Surgery (American Volume)
Journal of Clinical Epidemiology
Journal of Clinical Investigation
Journal of Clinical Oncology
Journal of Clinical Psychiatry
Journal of Clinical Rheumatology
Journal of Cutaneous Pathology
Journal of Immunology
Journal of Investigative Dermatology
Journal of Reproductive Medicine
Journal of the American Academy of Dermatology

Journal of the American College of Surgeons
Journal of the American Medical Association
Journal of the National Cancer Institute
Lancet
Medicine
Nature
Nature Genetics
Nature Medicine
New England Journal of Medicine
Pediatric Dermatology
Pediatrics
Plastic and Reconstructive Surgery
Proceedings of the National Academy of Sciences
Respiratory Medicine
Science
Surgery

STANDARD ABBREVIATIONS

The following terms are abbreviated in this edition: acquired immunodeficiency syndrome (AIDS), cardiopulmonary resuscitation (CPR), central nervous system (CNS), cerebrospinal fluid (CSF), computed tomography (CT), deoxyribonucleic acid (DNA), electrocardiography (ECG), health maintenance organization (HMO), human immunodeficiency virus (HIV), intensive care unit (ICU), intramuscular (IM), intravenous (IV), magnetic resonance (MR) imaging (MRI), ribonucleic acid (RNA), ultrasound (US), and ultraviolet (UV).

NOTE

The YEAR BOOK OF DERMATOLOGY AND DERMATOLOGIC SURGERY™ is a literature survey service providing abstracts of articles published in the professional literature. Every effort is made to assure the accuracy of the information presented in these pages. Neither the editors nor the publisher of the YEAR BOOK OF DERMATOLOGY AND DERMATOLOGIC SURGERY™ can be responsible for errors in the original materials. The editors' comments are their own opinions. Mention of specific products within this publication does not constitute endorsement.

To facilitate the use of the YEAR BOOK OF DERMATOLOGY AND DERMATOLOGIC SURGERY™ as a reference tool, all illustrations and tables included in this publication are now identified as they appear in the original article. This change is meant to help the reader recognize that any illustration or table appearing in the YEAR BOOK OF DERMATOLOGY AND DERMATOLOGIC SURGERY™ may be only one of many in the original article. For this reason, figure and table numbers will often appear to be out of sequence within the YEAR BOOK OF DERMATOLOGY AND DERMATOLOGIC SURGERY™.

COLOR PLATE I

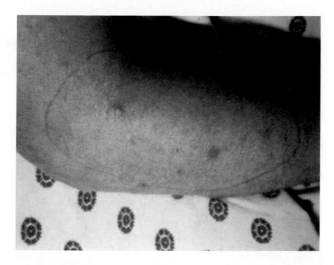

Weisshaar, **Fig 1**

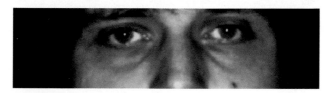

Weisshaar, **Fig 2**

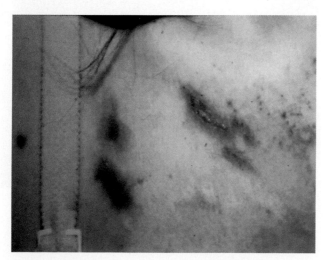

Weisshaar, **Fig 3**

COLOR PLATE II

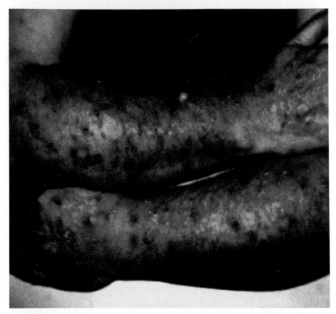

Weisshaar, Fig 4

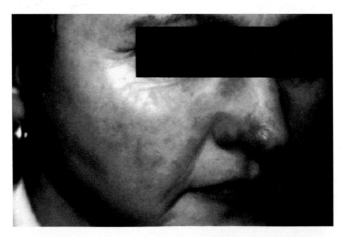

Weisshaar, Fig 5

COLOR PLATE III

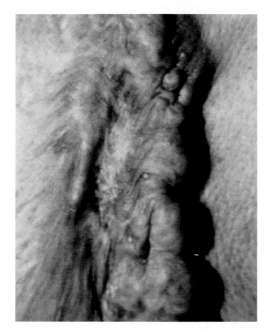

Weisshaar, Fig 6

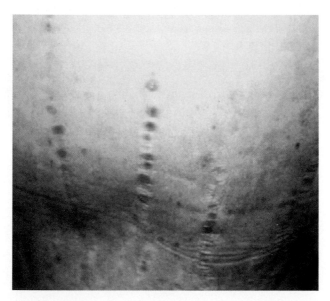

Weisshaar, Fig 7

COLOR PLATE IV

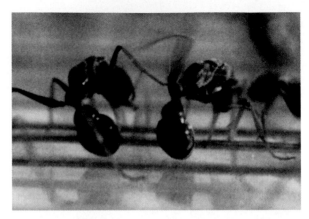

Abstract 1-22, **Fig 1**

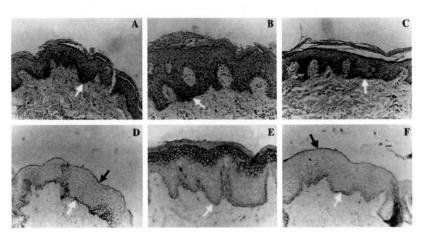

Abstract 1-22, **Fig 2**

(continued)

COLOR PLATE V

Fig 2 (continued)

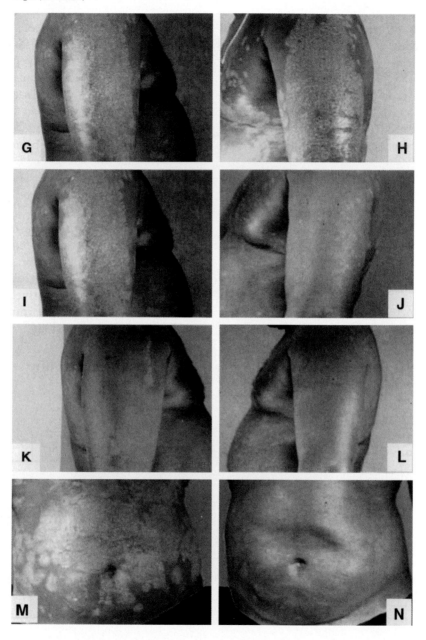

COLOR PLATE VI

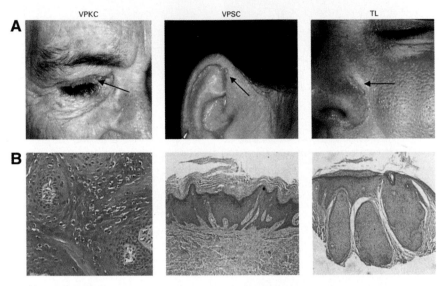

Abstract 5–7, **Fig 1**

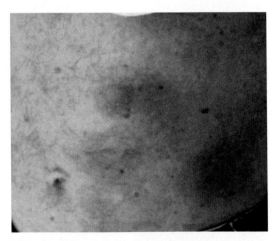

Abstract 6–9, **Fig 1**

COLOR PLATE VII

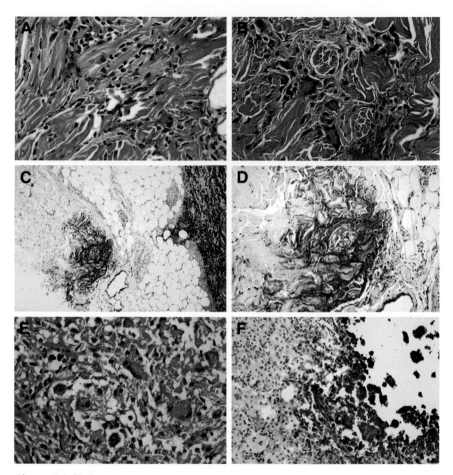

Abstract 6–9, **Fig 2**

COLOR PLATE VIII

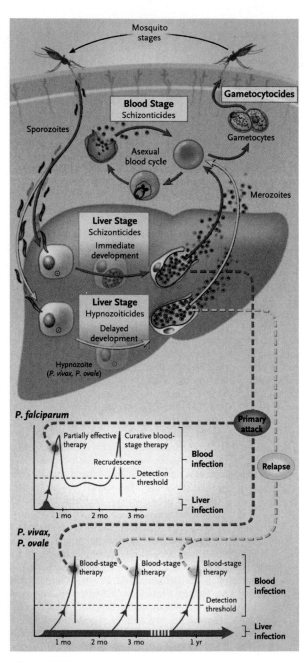

Abstract 7–4, **Fig 1**

COLOR PLATE IX

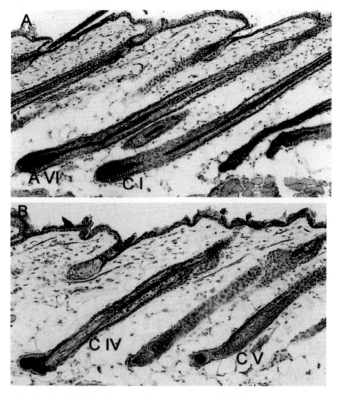

Abstract 7–4, Fig 2

(continued)

COLOR PLATE X

Fig 2 (continued)

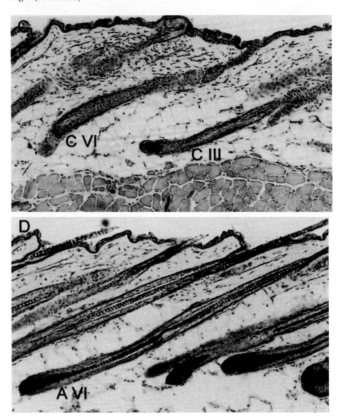

COLOR PLATE XI

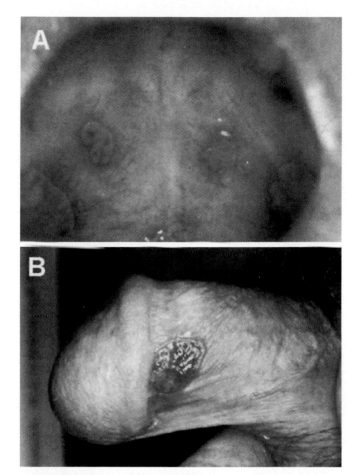

Abstract 10–4, **Fig 2**

(continued)

COLOR PLATE XII

Fig 2 (continued)

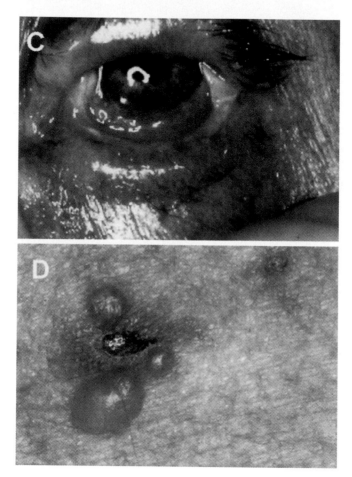

COLOR PLATE XIII

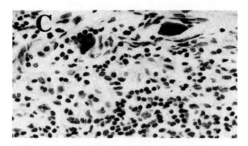

Abstract 16–18, **Fig 1, C**

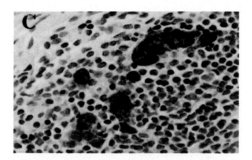

Abstract 16–18, **Fig 2, C**

COLOR PLATE XIV

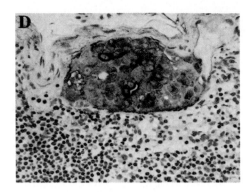

Abstract 16–18, Fig 3, D

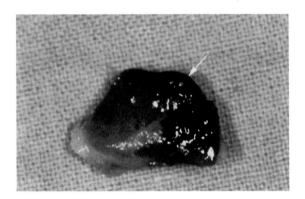

Abstract 17–28, Fig 3

COLOR PLATE XV

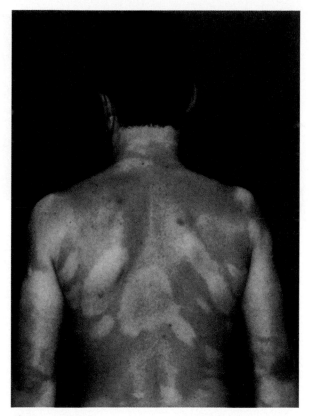

Abstract 18–4, **Fig 6**

COLOR PLATE XVI

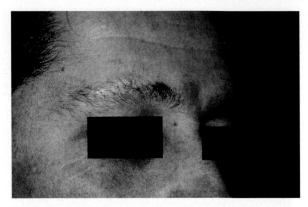

Abstract 18–4, **Fig 7**

Filler Materials

C. William Hanke, MD, MPH
Clinical Professor of Otolaryngology-Head and Neck Surgery, Indiana University School of Medicine, Indianapolis, Indiana; and Medical Director, Laser & Skin Surgery Center of Indiana, Carmel, Indiana

Introduction

Soft tissue augmentation is undergoing a Renaissance period with many new filler materials entering the marketplace. This article will deal only with injectable fillers commonly used by dermatologists and several others that are expected to be approved shortly (Table 1). Cadaveric collagen fillers are not currently in common use by dermatologists and will not be discussed. Injectable liquid silicone, although used off label by a minority of dermatologists, will not be addressed here.[1] Autologous fat transfer, although used effectively by many dermatologists, will not be discussed.[2] Similarly, expanded polytetrafluoroethylene (ePTFE) implants, although used by some dermatologists, will not be covered.[3]

Almost without exception, patients want soft tissue augmentation that is safe, clinically effective, reasonably priced, can be administered painlessly, with minimal down time. Several of the following products fulfill these criteria.

Collagen-Based Dermal Fillers

Zyderm/Zyplast

Product Description. Zyderm I (Zy-I) (Inamed Aesthetics, Santa Barbara, Calif), the first bovine collagen-based injectable filler, was approved by the US Food and Drug Administration (FDA) in 1981. Zyplast (ZP), a more robust filler for deeper contour defects, was approved in 1985. Zy/ZP implants are 95% to 98% type I collagen suspended in phosphate-buffered saline

---

TABLE 1.—Commercially Available Filler Materials

I. Bovine collagen derived fillers
   A. Zyderm/Zyplast (Inamed Aesthetics, Santa Barbara, Calif)
   B. Koken atelocollagen (Koken Co, KTD, Tokyo)
   C. Resoplast (Rofil Medical International BV, Breda, Netherlands)
II. Human collagen derived fillers
   A. CosmoDerm/CosmoPlast (Inamed Aesthetics, Santa Barbara, Calif)
III. Hyaluronic acid–derived fillers
   A. Restylane (Medicis, Scottsdale, Ariz)
     1. Restylane Fine Lines
     2. Perlane
   B. Hylaform (Inamed Aesthetics, Santa Barbara, Calif)
     1. Hylaform Fine Lines
     2. Hylaform Plus
   C. Rofilan (Rofil Medical International, Breda, Netherlands)
   D. Javederm (L.E.A. Derm., Paris, France)
IV. Other new injectable agents
   A. Artecoll (Rofil Medical International, Breda, Netherlands)
   B. Radiance (Bioform, Franksville, Wis)
   C. New-Fill/Sculptra (Dermik Laboratories, Berwyn, Pa)

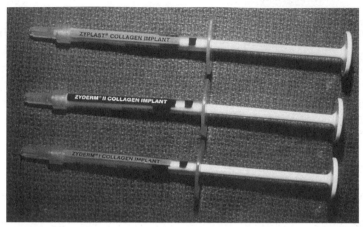

FIGURE 1.—Zyderm I, Zyderm II, and Zyplast are each available in 1 mL syringes. (Used with permission, C. William Hanke, MD, Indianapolis, Indiana.)

containing 0.3 percent lidocaine. The products are prepared from the skin of a closed American herd. Zy-I contains 3.5% bovine collagen by weight. Zy-II, approved in 1983, contains 6.5% bovine collagen. ZP is cross-linked with 0.0075% glutaraldehyde. The cross-linking makes ZP more resistant to proteolytic enzyme digestion. Zy/ZP syringes are preloaded and are stored at 4°C. The low temperature keeps the collagen fibrils in suspension. The fibrils consolidate into a solid gel after injection into the skin (Fig 1).

Indications/Contraindications. A list of indications for Zy/ZP is found in Table 2. ZP should not be used in the glabellar area because of the potential for local necrosis.[4] Treatment is contraindicated in patients who are hypersensitive to bovine collagen or lidocaine, or have had an anaphylactoid reaction. Skin testing is necessary before treatment in order to identify allergic individuals. Skin tests are performed by injecting 0.1 mL of Zy-I into the der-

TABLE 2.—Indications for Zyderm/Zyplast

Indication	Product
Horizontal forehead lines	Zy-I, Zy-II
Glabellar lines	Zy-I, Zy-II
Crow's feet	Zy-I, Zy-II
Nasolabial lines	Zy-I, Zy-II
Fine lip lines	Zy-I, Zy-II
Marionette lines	Zy-I, Zy-II
Soft acne scars	Zy-I, Zy-II
Deep nasolabial folds	ZP
Marionette grooves	ZP
Deep acne scars	ZP
Vermilion-cutaneous border	ZP
Lip mucosa	Zy-I, Zy-II

Abbreviations: Zy-I, Zyderm-I; Zy-II, Zyderm II; ZP, Zyplast.

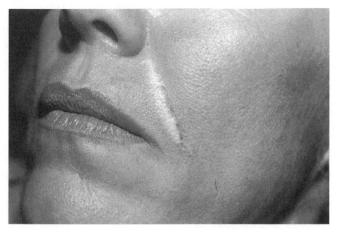

FIGURE 2.—A white blanche in the skin is observed when CosmoDerm or Zyderm has been injected correctly in the papillary dermis. (Used with permission, C. William Hanke, MD, Indianapolis, Indiana.)

mis of the volar forearm. A positive test is manifested by erythema, swelling, induration, or tenderness that lasts more than 6 hours. Of the tested individuals, 3.0% to 3.5% will have a positive skin test and will be excluded from treatment. Skin tests are evaluated at 48 to 72 hours and 4 weeks. Most physicians will perform a second skin test on the opposite forearm 2 to 4 weeks after the first skin test.[5] The second skin test is observed for 2 to 4 weeks before treatment is initiated. If an individual has not received Zy/ZP for 1 year or has been treated elsewhere, a single skin test is usually performed.

Technique/Anesthesia. Most patients do not require topical or local anesthesia. Zy-I is implanted into the papillary dermis with a 30 g or 32 g needle with a serial puncture technique. A white blanche on the surface of the skin is

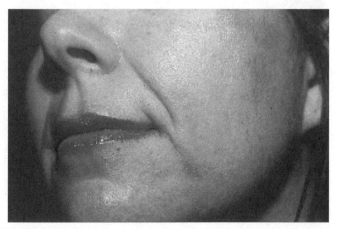

FIGURE 3.—Deep nasolabial folds are present immediately before treatment. (Used with permission, C. William Hanke, MD, Indianapolis, Indiana.)

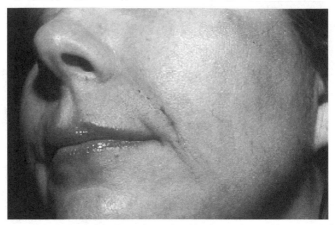

FIGURE 4.—Subtle elevation of the skin without white blanche is indicative of proper mid-dermal placement of CosmoPlast or Zyplast. (Used with permission, C. William Hanke, MD, Indianapolis, Indiana.)

indicative of correct placement (Fig 2). Zy-II has twice the concentration of collagen as Zy-I. Zy-II is injected into the mid-dermis with a 30 g needle. Zy-II is commonly used for soft acne scars and glabellar frown lines. Overcorrection (ie, 100%) is ideal when Zy-I/Zy-II is used.

ZP is a more rigid implant because of its glutaraldehyde cross-linked structure. Therefore, it should not be placed in the superficial dermis. A white blanche should not be observed but rather a subtle elevation of the wrinkle or scar (Figs 3 and 4). Overcorrection should not be done. ZP is ideally placed in the mid-dermis. If ZP is inadvertently placed in the subcutaneous fat, the correction will be lost within a matter of days. Zy-I can be "layered" over ZP during the same treatment session to enhance results.

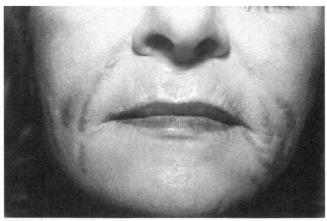

FIGURE 5.—Allergic hypersensitivity granulomas are present 3 months after treatment with Zyplast. (Used with permission, C. William Hanke, MD, Indianapolis, Indiana.)

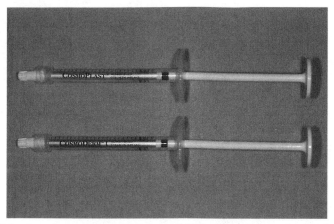

FIGURE 6.—CosmoDerm and CosmoPlast are available in 1 mL syringes similar to Zyderm/Zyplast. (Used with permission, C. William Hanke, MD, Indianapolis, Indiana.)

Results/Duration of Correction. One to 3 treatment sessions 2 to 4 weeks apart are usually necessary for maximum correction of a soft tissue defect. The duration of correction may be 4 to 12 months depending on the area treated.[6-8] In general, correction lasts longer in less mobile defects such as soft acne scars and glabellar frown lines. Correction is lost over time in all areas because of migration of the implant material from the dermis to subcutaneous tissue.[9]

Adverse Reactions. Nonallergic adverse treatment site reactions include infection, bruising, and reactivation of Herpes simplex. These events are uncommon and are self-limited. Another nonallergic adverse reaction is local necrosis due to vascular interruption.[4] This complication is rare, but it usually occurs when ZP has been used in the glabellar area. Therefore, ZP

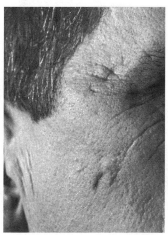

FIGURE 7.—Two depressed acne scars are present on the right cheek. (Used with permission, Inamed Aesthetics, Santa Barbara, Calif.)

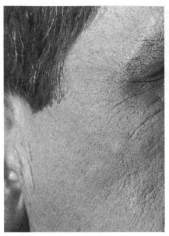

FIGURE 8.—The 2 scars demonstrate correction after treatment with CosmoDerm and CosmoPlast. (Used with permission, Inamed Aesthetics, Santa Barbara, Calif.)

should not be used in the glabellar area. Allergic hypersensitivity reaction to Zy/ZP can occur even when skin testing has been done properly. These patients nearly always have anti-Zyderm antibodies. Most allergic hypersensitivity reactions are characterized by red papules that gradually resolve over 6 months. Rarely, severe allergic hypersensitivity reactions manifested by abscesses can occur[4] (Fig 5). Some of these reactions have required 18 to 24 months to resolve.

CosmoDerm/CosmoPlast

Product Description. CosmoDerm/CosmoPlast (CD/CP) (Inamed Aesthetics, Santa Barbara, Calif) was approved by the FDA in March 2003. It is

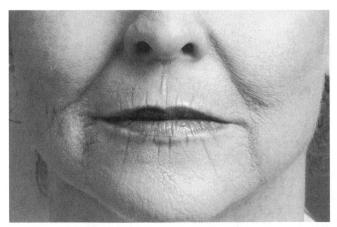

FIGURE 9.—The patient is concerned about vertical rhytids on the lower lips and deep nasolabial folds. (Used with permission, Inamed Aesthetics, Santa Barbara, Calif.)

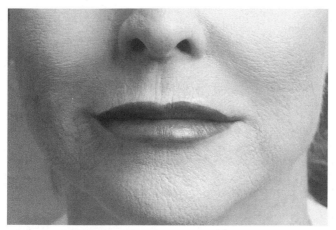

FIGURE 10.—The lip rhytids have been corrected with CosmoDerm and the nasolabial folds corrected with CosmoPlast. (Used with permission, Inamed Aesthetics, Santa Barbara, Calif.)

similar to Zy/ZP except for its human origin. CD/CP is extracted from human fibroblast cultures. The product is supplied as CosmoDerm-I (CD-I), CosmoDerm II (CD-II), and CosmoPlast (CP) in 1 mL syringes (Fig 6) The human collagen is suspended in phosphate-buffered saline containing 0.3% lidocaine. CP is cross-linked with glutaraldehyde.

Indications/Contraindications. Skin testing is not required. Indications are identical to Zy/ZP. CD/CP can be used in patients who are allergic to Zy/ZP.

Technique/Anesthesia. Identical to Zy/ZP. Since CD/CP contains 0.3% lidocaine, additional anesthesia is not usually required. The exception is the lips, where topical or local anesthesia may be necessary. CP is sometimes used to enhance the vermilion-cutaneous junction.

Results/Duration of Correction. Although long-term follow-up is not available, the clinical results are considered to be similar to Zy/ZP (Figs 7-10). The duration of correction is considered similar to Zy/ZP.

Adverse Reactions. Adverse reactions are similar to Zy/ZP, except that allergic hypersensitivity reactions have not been reported.

Hyaluronic Acid–Derived Fillers

Restylane

Production Description. Restylane (Medicis, Scottsdale, Ariz), was the first hyaluronic acid (hyaluronan)–based filler to receive FDA approval (December 2003). It has been available in Europe since 1996. Restylane is produced with the use of bacterial fermentation from streptococcal bacteria. The hyaluronic acid is partially cross-linked with butanediol diglycidyl ether (BDDE) for greater stability over time. Restylane has a higher concentration of hyaluronic acid (20 mg/mL) than Hylaform (6 mg/mL). Restylane is formulated in medium-sized particles for mid-dermal injection. Restylane is supplied in disposable syringes containing 0.7 mL hyaluronic acid gel. A 30 g × ½-inch needle is supplied with each syringe. Restylane Fine Line is a less-viscous (ie, small particle) formulation of Restylane, which can be injected through a 32 g needle. Perlane is a more-viscous (ie, large particle) formulation of Restylane that requires a 27½ g needle for injection. Restylane Fine Line and Perlane are not currently FDA-approved. Restylane is marketed in more than 60 countries.

Indications/Contraindications. Restylane is indicated for mid to deep dermal implantation for the correction of moderate to severe facial wrinkles and folds, such as nasolabial folds. Contraindications include patients with severe allergies manifested by a history of anaphylaxis or history or presence of multiple severe allergies. Restylane contains trace amounts of gram-positive bacterial proteins and is contraindicated for patients with a history of allergies to such material. Restylane is contraindicated for use in breast augmentation and for implantation into bone, tendon, ligament, or muscle. Restylane must not be implanted into blood vessels. Implantation of Restylane into dermal blood vessels may cause occlusion, infarction, or embolic phenomena.

Technique/Anesthesia. Since Restylane is non-animal based, skin testing is not required. Restylane, unlike Zy/ZP or CD/CP, does not contain lidocaine. Therefore, topical and/or local anesthesia is necessary. Lip augmentation with Restylane should be performed with the use of nerve block anesthesia. Restylane should be placed evenly in the mid-dermis using either a linear threading or serial puncture technique. A correction of no more than 100% of the desired effect should be performed. Surface irregularities should be massaged out at the completion of the treatment session.

Results/Duration of Correction. Restylane correction will generally last 6 to 12 months.[10] This is twice as long as Zy/ZP or CD/CP. A recent study by Carruthers[11] demonstrated that pretreatment Botox injections to the glabellar frown lines prolonged the duration of Restylane correction by 14 weeks.

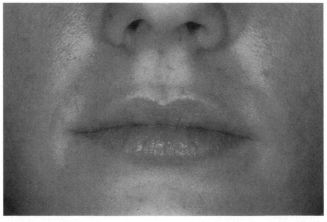

FIGURE 11.—A 25-year-old woman desires augmentation for thin lips. (Used with permission, C. William Hanke, MD, Indianapolis, Indiana.)

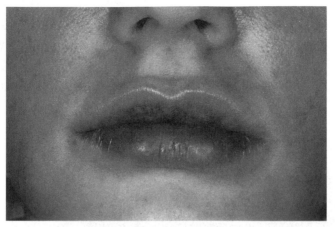

FIGURE 12.—The lips are slightly swollen but not bruised 24 hours after treatment. CosmoDerm 1 mL was utilized for the vermilion-cutaneous junction following infraorbital and mental nerve blocks. Restylane 0.7 mL was given to the vermilion. (Used with permission, C. William Hanke, MD, Indianapolis, Indiana.)

Adverse Reactions. Significant adverse events have not been reported, although long-term safety and effectiveness have not been established beyond 12 months in clinical trials. Bruising and swelling are generally greater with Restylane than collagen. If present, lumpiness usually resolves in a few days. Patients who have had Restylane for lip augmentation will have significant swelling for several days (Figs 11-13).

Hylaform

Product Description. Hylaform gel (Inamed Aesthetics, Santa Barbara, Calif) is extracted from the coxcombs of domestic fowl which contain large amounts of hyaluronic acid.[12] Like Restylane, Hylaform is supplied in different viscosities for different uses. Hylaform is designed for mid-dermal injec-

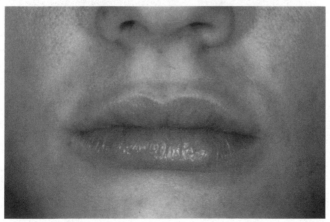

FIGURE 13.—The volume and projection of the lips demonstrate improvement 7 days after treatment. (Used with permission, C. William Hanke, MD, Indianpolis, Indiana.)

tion with a 30 g needle. Hylaform Fine Lines is less viscous than Hylaform and is designed for upper dermal placement with a 32 g needle. Hylaform Plus is more viscous than Hylaform and is designed for deep dermal placement with a 27 g needle.

Indications/Contraindications. Indications are similar to Restylane. Hylaform should not be used in patients who are allergic to avian products.

Technique/Anesthesia. The technique is similar to Restylane. Skin testing is not required.

Results/Duration of Correction. The clinical results should be comparable to Restylane (Figs 14 and 15).

Adverse Reactions. Adverse reactions are similar to Restylane.[13]

Other New Injectable Agents

Artecoll (Artefill)

Product Description. Artecoll (Rofil Medical International B.V., Breda, Netherlands) utilizes 3.5% bovine collagen to suspend smooth-surfaced 30 µg to 42 µg in diameter polymethylmethacrylate (PMMA) beads.[14] The collagen is rapidly degraded after injection, leaving the microscopic beads to act as a nidus for new collagen formation. The beads become encapsulated with new collagen within 2 to 4 months after injection. The beads apparently cannot migrate from the injection site. Artecoll has been used in more than 200,000 patients worldwide in the past 10 years. It was approved for use in Europe in 1996. Clinical trials were completed in the United States in 2001, but FDA approval is still pending as of this date. Once approved, the product will be marketed as Artefill in the United States.

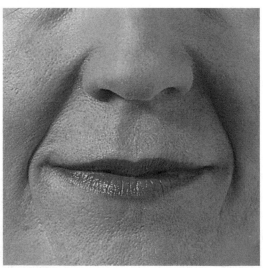

FIGURE 14.—The patient is concerned about deep nasolabial folds. (Used with permission, Inamed Aesthetics, Santa Barbara, Calif.)

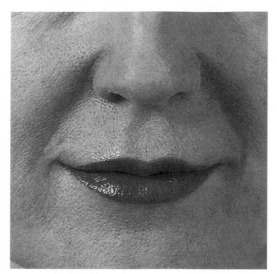

FIGURE 15.—The nasolabial folds are less apparent after treatment with Hylaform. (Used with permission, Inamed Aesthetics, Santa Barbara, Calif.)

Indications/Contraindications. Skin testing is required to screen for bovine collagen hypersensitivity. Common indications and injection volumes are listed in Table 3. The following areas can also be treated: lower lid circles (ie, tear trough), crow's feet in individuals with thick skin, facial wasting, perioral lip rhytids, oral commissures, horizontal chin fold, and distensible acne scars.

Technique/Anesthesia. The Artecoll syringe with attached 26 g needle contains 0.3% lidocaine. However, due to the deep dermal placement of the injection, supplemental topical or local anesthesia is often necessary. Artecoll should not be placed in the papillary dermis. If this occurs inadvertently (observed as a blanching of the skin), the material can be immediately massaged to a deeper level. Only very slight overcorrection should be performed. A linear threading technique is utilized whereby the material is delivered to the deep dermis on withdrawal of the syringe. Repeat injections may be given in 4 to 6 weeks. Treatment sites should be immobilized with tape for 3 days after treatment in order to prevent dislodging of the implant by facial muscle movement.

TABLE 3.—Indications for Artecoll and Injection Volumes

Indication	Volume (mL)
Frontal lines	0.5
Glabellar frown lines	0.5
One nasolabial fold	0.5
One upper or lower lip	0.5
Both oral commissures	0.5
Both marionette lines	0.5
Two neck folds	0.5

Results/Duration of Correction. Clinical improvement with Artecoll occurs gradually after several injections over several months. The improvement that occurs can last 2 years or more. Patient satisfaction has been reported to be 90%.

Adverse Reactions. Swelling of the treatment site will occur for 24 hours. Allergic hypersensitivity reactions can be caused by the bovine collagen carrier. Granulomas can occur, especially when Artecoll has been placed in the upper dermis. Granulomas are usually treated with intralesional steroids or excision.

Radiance

Product Description. Radiance (Bioform, Inc, Franksville, Wis) consists of calcium hydroxylapatite microspheres suspended in a carrier containing carboxymethylcellulose, glycerine, and sterile water. The carrier is degraded, leading to neocollagenesis around the microspheres.

Indications/Contraindications. Radiance has received FDA approval for vocal cord augmentation and radiologic tissue marking. It has been used off label for acne scars, lip augmentation, nasolabial folds, marionette lines, and HIV facial lipoatrophy of cheeks and temples. Radiance should not be placed in the superficial dermis or muscle.

Technique/Anesthesia. Skin testing is not required. Topical and/or local and/or regional nerve blocks are usually utilized. Radiance is injected in several layers into the subdermal plane with a 23 g to 25 g needle with a slow linear threading technique. The treatment site is molded with the fingers immediately after injection. Repeat treatment may be done after several months.

Results/Duration of Correction. Correction is reported to last 3 to 5 years in some patients.

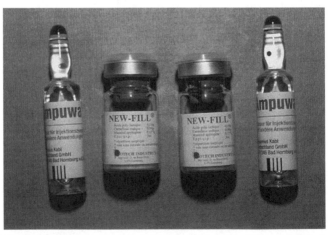

FIGURE 16.—New-Fill (Sculptra) is packaged in vials which contain 150 mg poly-L-lactic acid freeze-dried powder. (Used with permission, C. William Hanke, MD, Indianapolis, Indiana.)

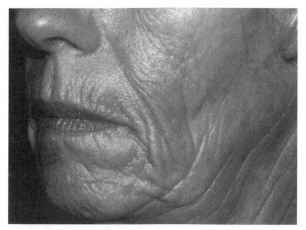

FIGURE 17.—This patient has sun-damaged skin and loss of facial fat as part of the aging process. (Used with permission, Danny Vleggaar, MD, Roussas, France.)

Adverse Reactions. Swelling and sometimes bruising will occur for several days after treatment. If lumpiness is present after 6 to 8 weeks, intralesional injections of triamcinolone 5 mg/mL may be administered. Implants can be removed through small stab incisions made with a No. 11 scalpel blade when necessary.

New-Fill (Sculptra)

Product Description. New-Fill (Dermik Laboratories, Berwyn, Pa) is a poly-L-lactic acid (PLA) filler material that was approved in Europe in 1999 for cosmetic treatment of wrinkles and scars. PLA is a biodegradable inert polymer that has been used in suture materials for many years. Clinical trials

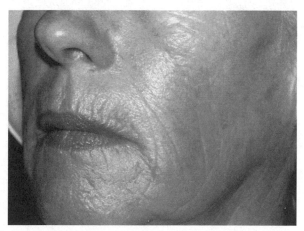

FIGURE 18.—The facial volume is considerably improved after 4 treatment sessions with New-Fill (Sculptra). Two vials of Sculptra were injected during each treatment session. (Used with permission, Danny Vleggaar, MD, Roussas, France.)

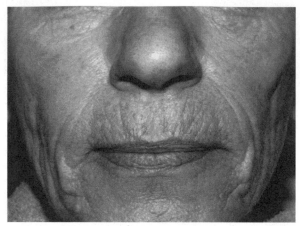

FIGURE 19.—Facial volume loss has caused wrinkles and folds to appear in the lower third of the face. (Used with permission, Danny Vleggaar, MD, Roussas, France.)

are ongoing in the United States. The material will be marketed in the United States as Sculptra.

Indications/Contraindications. Before injection, a 150 mg vial containing PLA freeze-dried powder is reconstituted with 3 mL to 4 mL sterile water (Fig 16). Local anesthesia is necessary. The material is injected at the dermal-subcutaneous junction and in the upper subcutaneous fat with a 26 g needle. Several injections at 4- to 6-week intervals are required to achieve full correction.

Results/Duration of Correction. Correction can last 18 months or more in HIV-lipoatrophy and other soft tissue defects (Figs 17-20).

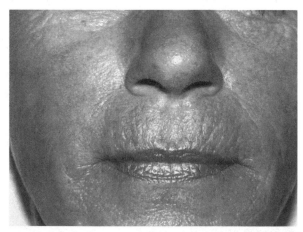

FIGURE 20.—Facial volume has been restored after 4 treatment sessions with New-Fill (Sculptra). Two vials of Sculptra were injected during each treatment session. (Used with permission, Danny Vleggaar, MD, Roussas, France.)

Adverse Reactions. Palpable, nonvisible subcutaneous nodules are occasionally seen.

References

1. Benedetto AV, Lewis AT: Injecting 1000 centistoke liquid silicone with ease and precision. *Dermatol Surg* 29:211-214, 2003.
2. Sattler G, Sommer B: Liporecycling: A technique for facial rejuvenation and body contouring. *Dermatol Surg* 12:1140-1144, 2000.
3. Hanke CW: A new ePTFE soft tissue implant for natural-looking augmentation of lips and wrinkles. *Dermatol Surg* 28:901-908, 2002.
4. Hanke CW, Higley HR, Jolivette DM, et al: Abcess formation and local necrosis after treatment with Zyderm or Zyplast collagen implant. *J Am Acad Dermatol* 25:319-326, 1991.
5. Klein AW: In favor of double testing (editorial). *J Dermatol Surg Oncol* 15:263, 1989.
6. Robinson JK, Hanke CW: Injectable collagen implants: Histopathologic identification and longevity of correction. *J Dermatol Surg Oncol* 11:124, 1985.
7. Klein AW: Implantation techniques for injectable collagen. Two and one-half years of personal clinical experience. *J Am Acad Dermatol* 11:422-432, 1992.
8. Elson ML: Clinical assessment of Zyplast implant: A year of experiences for soft-tissue contour correction. *J Am Acad Dermatol* 18:707-713, 1988.
9. Grosh SK, Hanke CW, DeVore DP, et al: Variables effecting the results of xenogenic collagen implantation in an animal model. *J Am Acad Dermatol* 13:792-798, 1985.
10. Narins RS, Brandt F, Leyden J, et al: A randomized, double-blind, multicenter comparison of the efficacy and tolerability of Restylane versus Zyplast for the correction of nasolabial folds. *Dermatol Surg* 29:588-595, 2003.
11. Carruthers J, Carruthers A: A prospective, randomized, parallel group study analyzing the effect of BTX-A (Botox) and non-animal sourced hyaluronic acid (NASHA, Restylane) alone in severe glabellar rhytides in adult female subjects: Treatment of severe glabellar rhytides with a hyaluronic acid derivative compared with the derivative and BTX-A. *Dermatol Surg* 29:802-809, 2003.
12. Piacquadio D, Jarcho M, Goltz R: Evaluation of hylan b gel as a soft-tissue augmentation implant material. *J Am Acad Dermatol* 36:544-549, 1997.
13. Lowe NJ, Maxwell CA, Lowe P, et al: Hyaluronic acid skin fillers: Adverse reactions and skin testing. *J Am Acad Dermatol* 45:930-933, 2001.
14. Lemperle G, Hazan-Gauthier N, Lemperle M: PMMA microspheres (Artecoll) for skin and soft tissue augmentation, part II: Clinical investigations. *Plast Reconstr Surg* 96:627-634, 1995.

Pruritus in Dermatology: New Advances in Pathophysiology and Therapy

ELKE WEISSHAAR, MD
Department of Social Medicine, Occupational and Environmental Dermatology, University of Heidelberg, Germany

THOMAS L. DIEPGEN, MD
Department of Social Medicine, Occupational and Environmental Dermatology, University of Heidelberg, Germany

ALAN B. FLEISCHER, JR, MD
Department of Dermatology, Wake Forest University School of Medicine, Winston-Salem, North Carolina

Introduction and Classification of Pruritus

Pruritus can be defined as a poor localized, nonadapting, usually unpleasant sensation that provokes a desire to scratch. Pruritus, equivalent to itch, is a frequent sensation in normal and diseased skin and is the most frequently described symptom in dermatology. It can arise from a primary dermatologic etiology but may also be a symptom of underlying systemic disease. Differential diagnoses include metabolic disorders, hematologic disease, malignancy, HIV/AIDS, complication of pharmacologic therapy, and neuropsychiatric disorders. One may consider that there are systemic or central aspects of pruritus in dermatological diseases and of course there are dermatologic factors causing pruritus in systemic diseases.[1] Pruritus can also occur in some patients without visible skin symptoms.[2] One may note that pruritus in systemic diseases can also result from a specific dermatologic disease or infiltrate directly related to the underlying disease (eg, cutaneous infiltrates in Hodgkin's disease). This always needs to be considered in the setting of pruritus in systemic diseases and should be ruled out by the experienced dermatologist and the necessary adequate diagnostic tools (eg, skin biopsy). Pruritus may also occur in dermatologic and systemic diseases not directly related to specific dermatoses or infiltrates. Severe pruritus mostly leads to secondary lesions such as erythema, erosions, excoriations, and crusts. They can be followed by cutaneous infections, which may result in folliculitis, abscess, or erysipelas.

There is no definitive classification of pruritus. It has recently been suggested to classify the following categories[3]:

Pruritoceptive itch: This means itch sensation originating in the skin induced by inflammation, skin damage, dryness and is transmitted by C nerve fibers. Pruritus due to insect bites, urticaria, and scabies, for example, resemble pruritoceptive itch.

Neuropathic itch: This is defined as itch that is caused by a disease of any point along the afferent pathway of the nervous system. Pruritus in postherpetic neuralgia, notalgia paresthetica, brachioradial pruritus (Fig 1; see color plate I), pruritus in multiple sclerosis and brain tumors resemble neuropathic itch.

Neurogenic itch: This is defined as pruritus originating in the CNS centrally without any evidence of neural pathology. Examples are cholestatic

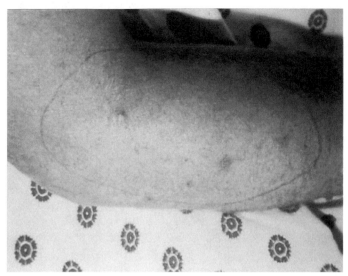

FIGURE 1.—Brachioradial pruritus.

pruritus (Fig 2; see color plate I) that is caused by opioid neuropeptides on μ-opioid receptors, pruritus in neurotic excoriations (Fig 3; see color plate I), and atopic dermatitis.

Psychogenic itch: This describes itch in psychiatric diseases and psychogenic abnormalitis such as delusional state of parasitophobia.

This classification covers clinical relevance and pathomechanisms of pruritus. One should bear in mind that one type of itch can coexist with another one in a patient. It is most likely that, for example, pruritus in atopic dermatitis is pruritoceptive as well as neurogenic.

In summary, when a patient complains of pruritus, there is a rational way to assemble the myriad of etiologies into finite groups, to evaluate the patient in a thoughtful manner, and to then correct the underlying cause and treat the pruritus with currently available therapies.

Epidemiology of Pruritus

There is a high number of dermatoses characterized by pruritus as a main or leading symptom such as atopic dermatitis, urticaria, prurigo nodularis (Fig 4; see color plate II), irritant and allergic contact dermatitis (Fig 5; see color plate II), infectious skin diseases, bullous diseases, mastocytosis, cutaneous T-cell lymphoma, renal itch, hepatic itch, etc. Besides, pruritus occurs

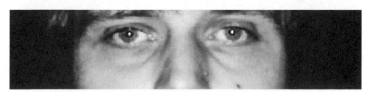

FIGURE 2.—Cholestatic pruritus in a 35-year-old patient with hepatic metastases due to lung cancer.

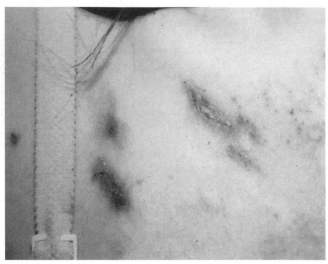

FIGURE 3.—Neurotic excoriations in a young female.

in almost all of the pregnancy-specific dermatological diseases, most frequently in polymorphic eruption of pregnancy (PEP, Fig 6; see color plate III). The overall incidence and prevalence of pruritus remains unknown for several reasons: First, there are no epidemiologic databases for this entity.

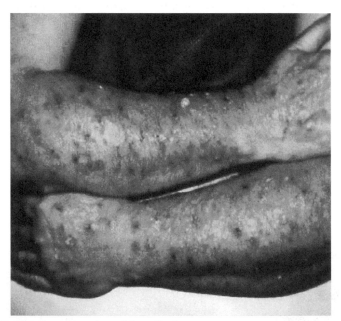

FIGURE 4.—Patient with prurigo nodularis of both arms.

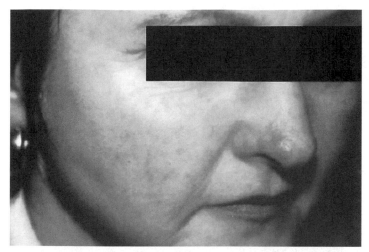

FIGURE 5.—Allergic contact dermatitis caused by a nasal carnival mask.

Second, many studies do not record pruritus as a symptom, especially in nondermatologic fields. Third, most people do not present to a physician for minor pruritic conditions. However, it is reasonable to assume that all humans experience this sensation at some point in their life, even if it is just the itching in insect bites or wound and scar formation. Hereunto, prolonged itching in keloids (Fig 7; see color plate III) needs to be delineated. The latter

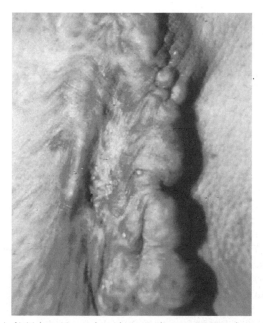

FIGURE 6.—Typical initial pruritic papules within striae distensae in PEP (polymorphic eruption of pregnancy).

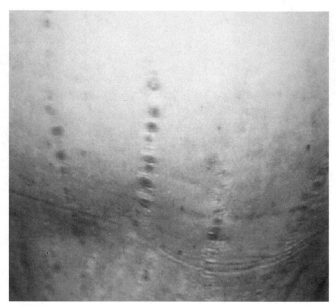

FIGURE 7.—Large keloid causing intense itching.

is most likely a result of a mixture of mechanical and chemical stimuli, nerve regeneration, increased mast cell number, and thus increased production of tumor necrosis factor (TNF)-α.[1]

Epidemiologic data have been lately obtained for single types of pruritus: itching is stated by up to 84% of patients with extensive psoriasis, but this refers to patients living in tropical climate.[4] Whereas in the 1980s, up to 80% of haemodialysis patients suffered from pruritus, the prevalence of renal itch is now decreased in Western countries, which is most likely due to improved dialysis techniques. Prevalence rates varied between 22% in Germany[5] and 66% in Israel[6] in recent studies. There was no relation between renal pruritus and sociodemographic characteristics.[6] Up to 30% of patients with Hodgkin's disease suffer from severe pruritus, and this may precede the diagnosis by many months. As recently described in a case report, paroxysmal itching attacks can be followed by generalized hyperhidrosis.[7] In a retrospective cohort, 48% of patients with polycythemia vera had a history of pruritus.[8] Clinical studies have shown that 16% to 50% of patients presenting with generalized pruritus have a systemic disease. In the most recent study, pruritus of unknown origin was the initial symptom of an underlying systemic disease in just 14% of patients.[9]

Preliminary epidemiologic data could also be obtained about pruritus in herpes zoster: up to 58% of patients reported itch as a symptom experienced in shingles (herpes zoster). Up to 30% of patients with postherpetic neuralgia (PHN) described itch as a symptom. Severe itching as a single symptom is termed postherpetic itch (PHI). Subjects whose shingles affected the head, face, and neck were more likely to experience PHI than other body regions.[10]

Pathophysiology of Pruritus

Generally, no particularly good animal model exists for studies on pruritus, and species differences must be taken into account when models of pruritus are used. Significant progress has been achieved in understanding the pathophysiology of pruritus, especially during the last 7 years. Still, the neural representation of pruritus is not completely known and partly controversial. For many years, pruritus has been considered a subliminal form of pain (intensity theory), explaining the sensation of pruritus as weak activation of noxious stimuli and pain sensations as strong activation of noxious stimuli. However, over the time it was known that pruritic sensations can not be transferred to pain, and microstimulation of fascicles that evoke pain can not produce pruritus. Recent neurophysiological experiments in humans and animals revealed that there is a distinct neuronal pathway for itch, functionally separated from the pain pathway.[11,12] Primary afferent nerve fibers (unmyelinated C fibers) that are mechano-insensitive, have slow conduction velocities, and have excessive terminal branching were discovered in humans encoding histamine-induced itch.[11] Besides, spinal neurons were identified that specifically respond to histamine stimuli.[12] Meanwhile, it could be shown that activity in this specific pathway coincides with itch under pathophysiological conditions in a patient with chronic pruritus.[13] The combination of peripheral and central neurons with a unique response pattern to pruritogenic mediators and anatomically distinct patterns to the thalamus provided the basis for a specific neuronal pathway for itch.[11-15] However, pain and pruritus share common features of being multidimensional, having induction by chemical stimuli, initiating motor response, and presenting negative affective valence. From the clinical point of view, itch sensations can be reduced by painful scratching. This has also been shown experimentally by thermal, chemical, and mechanical stimuli. Also, electrical stimulation, known as cutaneous field stimulation (CFS), has been shown to inhibit itch sensation in patients with localized pruritus.[16,17] The number of epidermal nerve fibers was reduced, which was paralleled by the relief of itch. Patients with generalized pruritus did not have any benefit. It is suggested that CFS acts through endogenous central inhibitory mechanisms that are normally activated by scratching the skin. Interestingly, single and repeated CFS treatments reduce the itch sensation but do not have any adverse effects on contact dermatitis.[18]

Various inflammatory mediators also activate pruritoceptors and concomitant activation of nociceptors decrease itch and increase pain. For example, it is well known that opioids reduce pain but may induce pruritus, and pruritus can strongly be inhibited by noxious stimuli. Thus, the itch sensation is apparently based on both increased activity in the itch pathway and a low level of activity in the pain pathway.[15] In summary, the relative activation of the 2 pathways will finally determine the perceived modality of sensation and may explain different types of pain and pruritus in the clinical setting.

Central Processing

Pruritus can be directly evoked in the skin by chemical mediators, by physical and thermal stimuli. Pruritic stimuli enter into the CNS via unmyelinated C-fibers and possibly A-delta fibers. The axon enters through the dorsal horn for spinal dermatomes or the trigeminal equivalent of the brainstem for head and neck pruritus. After synaptic connection within the ipsilateral gray column of the spinal cord, processing and control of the transmission occurs before crossing the midline. After synaptic transmission with the next neuron, the fiber ascends within the contralateral spinothalamic tract.

Whereas the peripheral pathway of pruritus (unmyelinated C-fibers) is mostly identified but still under investigation, less is known about CNS processing of pruritus and scratching. The "pruritus center" has long been proposed to be at the medulla oblongata.[1] Recent results obtained by positron emission tomography (PET) that measured regional cerebral blood flow (rCBF) as an index of neuronal activity revealed activation of several cortical structures such as anterior cingulate cortex (ACC), supplementary motor area (SMA), premotor (PM) area, and inferior parietal lobule (IPL) substantiating that the posterior sector of the ACC (Brodman 24) is related to sensorial/affectional aspects of the event.[19] The premotoral cortical areas (SMA, PM) may participate in the preparation of an intended action. Another study demonstrated significant activation of the contralateral primary sensory cortex and the ipsilateral and contralateral motor areas (SMA, PM cortex, primary motor cortex).[20] Additional significant activation was found in the prefrontal cortex and the cingulate gyrus. Several cortical areas showed a graded increase in rCBF with the logarithm of the histamine concentration applied by prick testing. Pruritus and pain seem to share common pathways; however, in contrast to pain activation studies, no subcortical activations were detected.[20] In the most recent study using PET, changes in the secondary somatosensory cortex during the itch stimulus (histamine iontophoresis) were not confirmed and, interestingly, the midbrain including periaqueductal gray matter was only activated when a dual stimulus (itch and cold pain) was performed.[21]

The phenomenon of alloknesis (*allos* = different, *knesis* = pruritus) designates a state when a normally nonpruritic stimulus induces pruritus in the skin surrounding a local cutaneous injury (eg, insect bite). It appears clinically as pruritus induced by touching the site (eg, an insect bite that may have occurred several hours before). In many pruritic dermatological diseases such as atopic dermatitis (AD), it is observed when pruritic attacks occur after accidental touch to affected skin lesions and/or the surroundings or are induced by mechanical factors such as clothing. Experimentally, alloknesis can be induced by mechanical stimuli such as stroking a soft brush or a cotton swab along the skin surrounding a histamine stimulus and is considered an important tool in psychophysical studies on pruritus. Alloknesis is explained by the excitation of pruritus-mediating central neurons through interneurons receiving input from low-threshold, fast-conducting mechanoreceptor units that are gated by histamine-induced input from unmyelinated pruritus mediating nerve fibers. Most likely, central and peripheral mechanisms contribute to the phenomenon of alloknesis. In contrast to this well-known A-fibers–mediated alloknesis, new studies provide evidence that central sensitization for itch appears to be elicited by C-nociceptors. It was shown in patients with AD that noxious stimuli primarily evoked itch in lesional skin.[22] It is possible that chronic barrage of pruriceptive input may elicit central sensitization.

Atmoknesis (*atmos = air, knesis* = pruritus) means pruritus provoked by open exposure of the skin after undressing and is common in AD, especially in children, patients with psoriasis, and elderly patients with aquagenic pruritus. Whether air itself really causes pruritus is unclear. It is imaginable that atmoknesis is a consequence of skin temperature changes induced by air draft after undressing or due to mechanical stimuli of clothing while undressing and is thus some type of alloknesis.[1,23]

Mediators of Pruritus

Mediators of pruritus presumably act on nerve fibers or lead to a cascade of mediator release whose final common pathway results in nerve stimulation and the sensation of pruritus. For example, vasoactive inflammatory mediators released during inflammation exert a dual action on nociceptive structures and on blood vessels. Activation of nociceptors leads to a release of neuropeptides, which induce vasodilatation and protein extravasation in the skin that has been termed *neurogenic inflammation*.[24,25] The group of potential chemical mediators is large and steadily increases. It contains amines (eg, histamine, serotonin), proteases (eg, tryptases), neuropeptides (eg, substance P [SP], calcitonin gene-related peptide [CGRP], bradykinin), opioids (morphine, beta-enkephalin, met-enkephalin, leu-enkephalin), eicosanoids, growth factors, and cytokines.[24,25] Endogenous as well as synthetic cannabinoids are known for their analgesic potency.

The cannabinoid receptor antagonist HU210 showed to reduce histamine-induced itch and axon reflex erythema.[26] Very recently, cannabinoid receptors were found to be present on sensory nerve fibers in human skin.[24] The recently confirmed expression of vanilloid receptor subtype 1 (VR1) on cutaneous sensory nerve fibers in humans supports that vanilloid and these receptor types contribute to the induction and modulation of nociceptive cutaneous sensations such as pain and pruritus.[27] Activation of the vanilloid receptors leads to depolarization and release of secretory granules containing neuropetides such as SP and CGRPs. Other members of the vanilloid heat-activated receptor family are identified, but their implication in the pathophysiology is unknown.[27]

Histamine is stored in mast cells and keratinocytes and mediates its effects via H_1 and H_2 receptors located on sensory nerve fibers. H_3 receptors have been shown in some peripheral tissues including abdominal skin; just recently, it could be demonstrated that intradermal injection of H_3 antagonists induces scratching and that chemical mediators other than histamine seem to be involved in the response.[28] Histamine's effects, either from mast cell degranulation or intracutaneous injection, includes the triple response (localized red spot around the injection site, red flush or flare extending around the red spot, and wheal reaction).

Histamine plays a primary role in pruritus of urticaria and mastocytosis. Its mediation in pruritus of other pruritic states and diseases is suspect and best proven by rather poor clinical response to antihistamines in patients with pruritus who do not have urticaria. In atopic dermatitis, one recent microdialysis study demonstrated that mast cell mediators other than histamine cause pruritus in patients with AD.[29] It could be recently shown that afferent neurons activated by histamine (pruritoceptors) were insensitive to mechanical stimulation and had very high electrical and thermal thresholds. Moreover, histamine sensitivity of patients with AD was equal or even reduced when tested in nonlesional skin.[30]

Serotonin (5-hydroxytryptamine) is a potent activator of unmyelinated C-fibers but is less potent in inducing pruritus when compared with histamine.[31] In animal models and humans, it is most likely to act histamine-independently. The potency of serotonin to induce protein extravasation is low, and its differential effect on nociceptors and vasculature is best explained by a weak direct or indirect non-neurogenic effect of this agent on the endothelia, which might be due to lower receptor densitiy or affinity of the vasculature. Whole blood serotonin levels were reported to be elevated in patients receiving hemodialysis while the levels of free plasma serotonin are not.[32] The widespread distribution of 5-HT3 receptors in the peripheral and CNS indicates that they may play a role in various diseases including pruritic diseases. In experimental and controlled clinical trials, antipruritic effects of 5-HT3 receptor antagonists could just be confirmed for chronic liver disease, including cholestatic disease of malignant and non-malignant origin and opioid-induced pruritus[1,33] (also see Therapy section). In summary, serotonin is likely to play a role in some pruritic diseases such as polycythemie vera and hepatic pruritus.

Neuropeptides such as SP and CGRP are the most frequently investigated ones in the skin. Their effects cover a wide range of acute proinflammatory reactions, including vasodilatation and protein extravasation, trophic function, and immunomodulation. SP is a peptide that is synthesized in dorsal root ganglia of nociceptive C-fibers and terminals, is transported peripherally to the nerve endings, and released upon activation. It induces flare reactions by releasing histamine from mast cells by an indirect effect, induces protein extravasation by a direct effect on small skin blood vessels and by a secondary release of histamine from mast cells. As new data demonstrated, SP is also capable of inducing histamine-independent vasodilatation and protein extravasation.[34] SP and CGRP induced marked vasodilatation but did not induce pruritus or pain, even in much higher concentrations above the vasodilatory threshold. These results suggest that vasoactive concentrations of SP and CGRP do not excite nociceptors and that they have no acute sensory function.[34] These results are in contradiction to others who showed that dermal neuropeptides are transmitters of pruritus.[1] Altogether, the role of neuropeptides in protein extravasation, in mast cell activation, and its mediator function of pruritus, is not clear.

Opioids: Morphine induces histamine release from mast cells but does not lead to a triple response. Besides, opioid peptides appear to be involved in the central transmission and regulation of pruritus, but it is still not known in which central or peripheral structure opiate receptors are possibly involved. Recently, the μ-opioid receptor isoform 1A could be localized by immunohistochemistry on nerve fibers of human skin, which may contribute to neurogenic inflammation, pain, and pruritus sensations.[24] In human beings, intrathecal injection of morphine may especially induce intense pruritus without skin lesions. Antihistamines do not prevent or relieve morphine-induced pruritus, which often occurs after 3 to 7 hours, is dose-related, and typically spreads out from the injection site to the trunk, to the face (distribution of the trigeminal nerve), and/or to the whole body. But it can also occur as facial pruritus only. Its incidence is especially high in cesarean delivery. Morphine-induced pruritus usually subsides after the cessation of the treatment. Naloxone is an effective treatment but may have the risk of decreasing the pain threshold. These observations suggest that the μ-opiod receptor system is involved in the processing of pruritus. Less information is known about the role of the κ-opioid receptor. TRK-820, a recently developed κ-opioid receptor agonist, had the ability to suppress antihistamine-sensitive and antihistamine-resistant pruritus in an experimental animal model.[35] In a new study, it is suggested that the central μ-opiod receptors play a role in the processing of itch sensation, and the activation of κ-opioid receptors antagonize the central μ-opiod receptor–mediated itch processing.[36] Pruritus may be induced by an imbalance between μ- and κ-opioid systems in systemic and peripheral pathways.

Elevated serum endorphin levels were found in patients with AD.[1] For renal pruritus, this could not be confirmed, although they had been reported as being accumulated in those patients with hepatic impairement.[1,5] In hepatic/cholestatic pruritus, their role has not been completely clarified yet.[37] One component of the pathopysiology of the syndrome of cholestasis is the increased CNS neurotransmission mediated by endogenous opioid agonists. Animal studies have recently drawn attention to loperamide, a peripherally acting opioid, that was efficacious in models of pruritus and pain.[38]

Cytokines: In various dermatological diseases, pruritus is due to activation of cytokines and lymphokines such as in AD, autoimmune blistering diseases, allergic contact dermatitis, mycological, and viral diseases.[1,23] When patients with AD are treated with cyclosporin A—which inhibits cytokines—pruritus, skin lesions, and peripheral eosinophilia are significantly reduced.[1,23] On the other hand, pruritus and inflammatory skin changes have been reported as side effects of cytokine treatment such as in interleukin-2 (IL-2) treatment in patients with cancer where pruritus and redness, dermal T-lymphocyte infiltrate, and peripheral eosinophilia occur some days after the initiation of the treatment. In patients with AD and control subjects, IL-2 induced a low-intensity intermittent local pruritus that appeared after a few hours' delay and peaked between 6 hours and 48 hours. In another study investigating controls, a weak but significant early pruritogenic effect with no detectable axonic reflex was seen, and in this setting, tumor necrosis factor α (TNF-α) did not induce pruritus. Others showed that peripheral blood mononuclear cells of patients with AD can be stimulated to secrete IL-8 after antigen stimulation, but no measurable quantities of IL-2 and TNF-α were measured.[39] It has been suggested that renal pruritus might be conveyed if not originated by a deranged cytokine pattern with a pronounced pro-inflammatory profile.[5]

In summary, cytokines may play a role in pruritus, but more research regarding the involvement of cytokines in the pathomechanisms of pruritus is needed. Pruritus is most likely due to several mediators functioning together in the sense of an antagonistic effect and/or leading to mast cell depletion and the release of various substances including chymase, tryptase, interleukin-4, and histamine. Each cascade or predominating mediator may differ in each type of pruritus, respectively, according to the underlying disease.

Clinical Aspects and Evaluation of Pruritus

When evaluating the patient, a precise history may provide insight into the disease process. Important characteristics of pruritus that need to be considered are given in Table 1. The onset, duration, and nature of pruritus help to determine the cause. If some general clues are present, the clinician will be able to narrow the diagnosis (Table 2). Questionnaires help to get more information about the patient, the disease process, the characteristics of pruritus, and social factors of the patient. Questionnaires for patients with uremia and other forms of pruritus such as pruritus in psoriasis, urticaria, and AD were found to be reliable and reproducible.[40-44] Concerning the measurement of itch severity and scratching, several modalities have been proposed

---

TABLE 1.—Features to Consider in Patients With Pruritus

Descriptive Features of Pruritus

1. Onset—eg, abrupt, gradual, prior pruritic episodes
2. Time course—eg, continuous, intermittent, cyclical, time of day
3. Nature—eg, prickling, crawling, burning, dysesthesia
4. Duration—eg, minutes, hours, days, weeks, months
5. Severity—eg, interference with activities and habits
6. Location—eg, generalized or localized
7. Relationship to activities —eg, occupation, spare time
8. Provoking factors—eg, water, exercise
9. Patient's personal theory as to etiology of disease

Historical Features of Pruritus

1. Medications and topicals—prescribed, over-the-counter, duration, and onset
2. Allergies—systemic, contact allergies
3. Atopic history—eczema, allergic rhinitis, and asthma
4. Past medical history—thyroid, liver, renal, or other systemic diseases
5. Family history of atopy, skin disease, or similar pruritic conditions
6. Occupation
7. Hobbies
8. Social history—eg, household, food habits, stress
9. Drugs—nicotine, alcohol, intravenous drugs
10. Bathing and cosmetic habits
11. Pets
12. Sexual history
13. Travel history
14. Prior diagnosis made by physician or patient

TABLE 2.—General Clues to Consider in Patients With Pruritus

- Localized pruritus is usually not a consequence of a systemic disease, but generalized pruritus often is.
- Acute onset of pruritus without primary skin lesions over only a few days is less suggestive of an underlying systemic disease than chronic, progressive generalized pruritus.
- Secondary lesions on the upper mid-back suggest that a skin disease is responsible for the symptom, whereas sparing is associated with systemic causes of pruritus. This represents the so-called "butterfly sign" due to the inaccessibility from the patient's hand.
- Most patients with pruritus not related to a primary dermatological disease demonstrate only excoriations or other secondary changes.
- Some severely pruritic dermatoses such as urticaria and mastocytosis rarely lead to scratching and secondary lesions but instead involve pressing and rubbing behavior.
- When multiple family members are affected, scabies or other parasites should be considered.
- Seasonal pruritus often occurs as "winter itch" representing pruritus in the elderly.
- The relationship of pruritus to activities is important and may resemble cholinergic pruritus in association with physical activity. Pruritus provoked by cooling of the skin after emergence from a bath may be a sign of idiopathic aquagenic pruritus or polycythemia rubra vera.
- Nocturnal generalized pruritus in association with chills, sweating, and fever may be a presenting history for Hodgkin's disease. Pruritus may precede the onset of the disease by months to years.
- Whereas psychogenic pruritus rarely interferes with sleep, most pruritic diseases (with or without primary skin lesions) cause nocturnal wakening.
- Pruritus may often occur before, during, and/or after shingles (herpes zoster infection). When reported after the skin infection, it can resemble postherpetic itch (PHI) or can be a symptom of postherpetic neuralgia (PHN).

to aid the clinician and researcher.[1,23] The most commonly used ones are categorical scales, interval scales, and continuous scales like visual analogue scales (VAS).[1,23] Various methods, such as the measurement of nocturnal scratching with an infrared video camera, provide very interesting and impressive data,[45] but most of these methods are not suitable for routine clinical use.[1] In a very recent study, perceptual matching was found to be a reliable method of itch assessment in terms of high reliability and excellent reponsiveness. This method is recommended as an assessment tool for itch intensity in experimental conditions as well as in patients suffering from pruritus.[46] Any drug can cause an adverse reaction in the skin that can be associated with pruritus. Most commonly, pruritic drug reactions are urticarial or morbilliform, but one should remember that adverse drug reactions can also lead to generalized pruritus without any specific skin lesions. Table 3 summarizes the major groups of drugs that may induce pruritus in recognition of their pathomechanism. Just recently, topiramate, a sulfamate-substituted monosaccharide that is intended for use as an antiepileptic drug, has been reported to induce pruritus without any rash or other skin lesions.[47] So far, the pathological mechanism behind it is not clear, especially as there was an improvement of symptoms in some patients when tapering the dose. The patient's history should therefore always include recording of all medications—the prescribed and the over-the-counter ones. The possibility of an underlying neuropathy should be considered in the evaluation of all patients with brachioradial pruritus (BRP).[48] Radiographs should be performed because an association between cervical spine disease and BRP may exist.[49] Besides, further neurologic investigation may be beneficial.

A careful and complete examination of skin, scalp, hair, nails, mucous membranes, and the anogenital area is necessary. Evaluation of primary and

TABLE 3.—Differential Diagnoses of Drug-Induced Pruritus

Pathomechanism	Medication
1. Cholestasis	Valproic acid, chloroform, oral contraceptives, minocycline
2. Hepatotoxicity	Oral contraceptives and other estrogens
	Testosterone and other anabolic steroids
	Phenothiazine, tolbutamide, erythromycin, azathioprine, penicillamine
3. Sebostasis/Xerosis	Beta-blockers, retinoids, tamoxifen, busulfan, clofibrate
4. Phototoxicity	8-methoxypsoralen, doxycyclin
5. Neurologic	Tramadol, codeine, cocaine, morphine, butorphanol, fentanyl
6. Deposition	Hydroxyethyl starch
7. Idiopathic	Chloroquine, clonidine, gold salts, lithium, angiotensin-converting enzyme inhibitors

secondary lesions, morphology, distribution, lichenification, xerosis, and skin signs of systemic diseases must be performed.

The general physical examination of lymph nodes, liver, spleen, etc, may disclose an undiagnosed systemic disease and should be properly performed when the differential diagnosis includes systemic disease and malignancy. There is no general need for laboratory investigation. However, in the setting of generalized pruritus of unknown etiology, further investigation may be pursued (Table 4). A skin biopsy that includes direct immunofluorescence may provide information in presentations where the pruritic skin is otherwise normal in appearance. On occasion, histologic examination of a nonspecific secondary lesion may point to a specific dermatologic disease.

Treatment of Pruritus

In the setting of pruritus, each patient has to be especially seen as unique—there are no therapies that work for all patients. The treatment of pruritus has several categories, all of them emphasizing the cause, which means con-

TABLE 4.—Laboratory Tests When Evaluating Patients With Pruritus

Initial tests:

- Erythrocyte sedimentation rate (ESR)
- Complete blood cell count (CBC) with differential leukocyte count
- Blood urea nitrogen, creatinine
- Liver transaminases, alkaline phosphatase, bilirubin
- Fasting glucose, HbA1C
- Thyroid function test (thyroid stimulating hormone [TSH] and thyroxine levels)
- Parathyroid function (calcium and phosphorus levels)
- Serum iron, ferritin
- Chest x-ray
- Stool for ova, parasites, and occult blood

Then (depending on patient's history, clinical, and previous laboratory findings):

- Serum protein electrophoresis, serum immunoelectrophoresis
- Antinuclear antibody (ANA), extranuclear antibody (ENA)
- Human immunodeficiency virus (HIV)
- Allergy diagnostic investigation: total IgE, specific IgE, histamine, serotonin, prick tests of major atopy antigens and additives, patch tests
- Urine for sediment, 5-hydroxyindolacetic acid (5 HIAA), and mast cell metabolites
- Additional radiographic and sonographic studies

firmation of the exact diagnosis and identification of the underlying etiology.[1,23] In general, provocative factors that enhance pruritus should be avoided and general guidelines should be followed (Table 5). Heat (eg, sauna), hot food, alcoholic drinks, hot drinks, or intake of other hot liquids should be avoided because they may increase itching due to increased blood circulation. Symptomatic treatment includes topical, systematic, and physical treatment modalities such as ultraviolet (UV) phototherapy.[1,23]

Topical Treatment

Topical treatmment encompasses the application of nonspecific emollients on a regular daily basis in order to prevent dryness and xerosis of the skin, which lead to pruritus. A large variety of topical compounds having antipruritic potency are currently available, including glucocorticosteroids, topical immunomodulators, coal tar, cooling agents (menthol, camphor, shake lotions), capsaicin, topical anesthetics, and antihistamines.

Topical anesthetic agents decrease pain and pruritic sensation and may have a great relief on tingling and dysesthesia. The onset of action is usually fast, but the duration is limited. No comparative studies clearly demonstrate one agent being superior.[23] Early preparations such as lignocaine are less effective because they do not penetrate the stratum corneum well. Eutectic mixture of local anesthetics (EMLA [lignocaine/-prilocaine cream]) has shown antipruritic potency in experimentally induced pruritus and may be sufficient in localized pruritic states such as notalgia paresthetica.[1] Effectiveness may be improved by combination of an anesthetic with urea, also known for its antipruritic potency. The therapeutic effect depends on the underlying disease (eg, no therapeutical benefit was seen in AD).[1]

The *topical antihistamine* dimetindene may improve pruritus severity depending on the underlying cause, but no effect was seen in AD.[1] Doxepin has demonstrated modest antipruritic effects in AD and other eczematous dermatoses but has an increased risk of allergic contact dermatitis.[1,23] Promethazine also has antipruritic potency, most likely due to antihistaminergic ac-

---

TABLE 5.—General Guidelines That Are Helpful to Relieve Pruritus in Patients

- Wearing of appropriate clothing (no wool or synthetic fabrics; instead cotton clothing)
- Prevention of excessive bathing; therefore, warm (not cold, not hot) short showers with nondrying detergents such as bath oil. In case of bathing, colloid, tar, oil, or potassium permanganate baths for 10 to 15 minutes
- Avoid factors that aggravate dry skin such as dry climate, excessive exposure to water, alkali, and detergents
- Regular skin hydration on a daily basis with nonspecific emollients that should be selected individually depending on the patient's skin condition and in consideration of the patient's compliance. Rich emollients may be used at night whereas creams are more appropriate for daytime use in order to enable the patient to wear clothing without any restriction
- Teaching adequate methods on how to interrupt the itch-scratch cycle such as application of a cold wash cloth, gentle pressure, etc
- Controlled physical exercise
- Prevention of stress and anxiety
- Prevention of dust and dust mites
- Prevention of heat, hot foods or drinks, hot liquids, large amounts of alcohol
- Relaxation therapy

tivity.[23] Diphenhydramine is widely used in the United States despite no controlled studies to prove its antipruritic potency.[23] Side effects such as drowsiness and xerostomia occur when large portions of the body are covered and young children are treated. Intoxications have been reported with promethazine.[23]

Capsaicin (CAP) is a naturally occurring alkaloid found in many botanical species of the night shade family (solanacea), including the pepper plants. It enhances the release and secondarily inhibits the reaccumulation of neuropeptides such as SP, a very powerful vasodilator releasing histamine from cutaneous mast cells by an indirect effect and inducing plasma extravasation by a direct effect on the small skin blood vessels. It could be shown that hypalgesia produced by CAP results from the degeneration of epidermal nerve fibers (ENF) and discontinuation of CAP was followed by reinervation of the epidermis with a return of all sensations such as tactile, mechanical, heat, and pain sensations except cold. Topical CAP therapy has been successfully reported in various dermatologic disorders such as prurigo nodularis, hemodialysis-related pruritus, notalgia paresthetica, brachioradial pruritus, pruritic psoriasis, aquagenic pruritus, lichen simplex chronicus, hydroxyethyl starch–induced pruritus, and various forms of neuralgia such as postherpetic and diabetic neuralgia.[1,23,50] In some forms of pruritus, such as in patients with AD or those receiving hemodialysis, results have been controversial.[1,51] Available concentrations range from 0.01% to 0.3% and need to be applied 3 to 5 times daily for maximal effect. It has shown to be a safe treatment even on large skin areas. Side effects include stinging, burning, pain, erythema, and irritation, all of which decrease with continued use.[1]

Topical immunomodulators such as tacrolimus reduce pruritus via the modulation and suppression of T-cell invasion and mediators that can provoke pruritus. Controlled trials indicate that topical tacrolimus is a safe and efficient treatment in AD, showing rapid anti-inflammatory and antipruritic effects. Long-term safety appears superior to corticosteroid agents. Burning, pruritus, and erythema are the most commonly reported application-site adverse events. In a very recent study, tacrolimus showed significant improvement of pruritus in hand/foot eczema but did not affect formation of vesicles that are known to be especially itchy. When the topical treatment was discontinued, pruritus reoccurred.[52] SDZ ASM 981 (pimecrolimus) is an ascomycin macrolactam derivative that selectively inhibits proinflammatory cytokines from T-cells and mast cells in vitro. Improvement of pruritus in patients with atopic dermatitis was noted. SDZ ASM 981 is likely to be less effective than tacrolimus in decreasing the pruritus of inflammatory diseases. Side effects are burning and application-site pruritus.

Whereas systemic *aspirin* does not have any antipruritic effect, topical application of an aspirin/dichloromethane solution showed a significant antipruritic potency in patients suffering from localized circumscribed pruritus such as that which occurs in lichen simplex chronicus.[53] A possible mechanism could be a peripheral nociceptive effect of salicylic acid on pruritus. Others did not reconfirm this in detail in a human experimental model.[54]

Crotamiton is an effective scabicide. Some patients anecdotally reported that this agent is highly effective in amelioration of pruritus. A double-blind study did not show a significant antipruritic potency of crotamiton lotion compared with its vehicle.[23]

Topical application of *strontium nitrate* demonstrated significant antipruritic effects in histamine-induced pruritus.[55] The mechanism is unclear but may be due to a direct effect on the C fibers. Further investigations will show if strontium nitrate will also be useful in clinical dermatology.

Zangrado, an extract of the Amazonian ethnomedicine Sangre de Grado, showed antipruritic, anti-inflammatory, and analgesic effects when topically applied in a placebo-controlled study. These actions appear to be mediated by vanilloid receptor antagonism.[56] This substance may offer significant therapeutic potential in the future.

Systemic Treatment

Most drugs with antipruritic potency act centrally by a property or mechanism related to sedation. Placebo responses in pruritus are quite marked and were achieved in 66% of the patients of a study.[23] The application of a systemic drug depends on the underlying disease (eg, antihistamine for urticaria, cyclosporin for severe AD). Systemic drugs with antipruritic potency are antihistamines, glucocorticosteroids, doxepin, cyclosporin, thalidomide, naloxone, naltrexone, nelmefene, TRK-820, and serotonin reuptake inhibitors.[1,23] Thalidomide reduces itch in inflammatory skin disease such as prurigo nodularis, actinic prurigo, eczema, and senile pruritus.[23] It is a powerful central depressant and may thereby have antipruritic properties. The opiate antagonist naltrexone greatly reduced alloknesis whereas the H_1 blocker cetirizine did not.[57] These results indicate a predominantly central effect of naltrexone, compared with a predominantly peripheral effect of cetirizine.[57] Naltrexone was given to patients with pruritus of various etiologies of internal and dermatologic diseases in a clinical trial and achieved antipruritic potency in 35 of 50 patients within 1 week.[58] Experiments in animals suggest that the κ-opioid receptor modulates the perception of itch. TRK-820 is a newly synthesized κ-opioid receptor-selective agonist that showed antipruritic activity in antihistamine-sensitive and antihistamine-resistant pruritus in an animal model.[35] This substance may represent a new entity of drugs to treat pruritus in humans (eg, renal pruritus). Selective serotonin reuptake inhibitors like paroxetine were succesfully applied in polycythemia vera, psychogenic and neurotic excoriations, and pruritus in advanced cancer.[59-61] 5-HT3 receptor antagonists have been reported in the treatment of uremic, hepatic, and opioid-induced pruritus and pruritus in cancer with variable success.[1,33,62] The wide variation in study design restricts the potential for meta-analysis. Another problem is the wide variation in the bioavailability of 5-HT3 receptor antagonists through variable absorption between individuals, route of administration, and dose prescribed. In summary, a role for serotonin receptor antagonists in different types of pruritus such as renal pruritus appears unlikely but not definitely excluded.

Physical Treatment Modalities

UV light (UVA, UVB, UVA/UVB) and psoralen UV A-range (PUVA) therapy have shown most benefit in pruritic diseases such as inflammatory dermatoses, pruritus related to uremia, primary biliary cirrhosis, polycythemia rubra vera, and prurigo nodularis. In a very recent case report, renal pruritus did not respond to narrowband UVB therapy but to classical broadband UVB therapy.[63] Cutaneous field stimulation (CFS) is a new technique stimulating thin afferent fibers including C-fibers. In a recent open-label uncontrolled study, patients with localized itching experienced sufficient relief[17] (see above).

Psychological factors may affect the course of any physical disease process. Pruritus may be precipitated, prolonged, or enhanced by a number of stress-related mediators such as histamine and neuropeptides. One should consider that there are a number of secondary psychosomatic mechanisms through which pruritus may be generated or exacerbated (eg, sweat response, alterations in cutaneous blood flow, and scratching). Studies show that group psychotherapy, behavioral therapy, controlled physical exercise, support groups, and biofeedback help to stop scratching and improve quality of life.[1,23,64]

References

1. Weisshaar E, Kucenic MJ, Fleischer AB: Pruritus: A review. *Acta Derm Venereol (Suppl)* 213:5-32, 2003.
2. Pujol RM, Gallardo F, Llistosella E, et al: Invisible mycosis fungoides: A diagnostic challenge. *J Am Acad Dermatol* 47:S168-S171, 2002.
3. Yosipovitch G, Greaves MW, Schmelz M: Itch. *Lancet* 361:690-694, 2003.
4. Yosipovitch G, Goon A, Wee J, et al: The prevalence and clinical characteristics of pruritus among patients with extensive psoriasis. *Br J Dermatol* 143:969-973, 2000.
5. Mettang T, Pauli-Magnus C, Alscher DA: Uraemic pruritus—New perspectives and insights from recent trials. *Nephrol Dial Transplant* 17:1558-1563, 2002.
6. Zucker I, Yosipovitch G, David M, et al: Prevalence and characterization of uremic pruritus in patients undergoing hemodialysis: Uremic pruritus is still a major problem for patients with end-stage renal disease. *J Am Acad Dermatol* 49:842-846, 2003.
7. Stadie V, Marsch WCH: Itching attacks with generalized hyperhidrosis as initial symptoms of Hodgkin's disease. *JEADV* 17:559-561, 2003.
8. Diehn F, Tefferi A: Pruritus in polycythaemia vera: prevalence, laboratory correlates and management. *Br J Haematol* 115:619-621, 2001.
9. Zirwas MJ, Seraly MP: Pruritus of unknown origin: A retrospective study. *J Am Acad Dermatol* 45:892-896, 2001.
10. Oaklander AL, Bowsher D, Galer B, et al: Herpes zoster itch: Preliminary epidemiologic data. *J Pain* 4:338-343, 2003.
11. Schmelz M, Schmid R, Bickel A, et al: Specific C-receptors for itch in human skin. *J Neurosci* 17:8003-8008, 1997.
12. Andrew D, Craig AD: Spinothalamic lamina I neurons selectively sensitive to histamine: A central neural pathway for itch. *Nat Neurosci* 4:72-77, 2001.
13. Schmelz M, Hilliges M, Schmidt R, et al: Active itch fibers in chronic pruritus. *Neurology* 26:564-566, 2003.

14. Schmelz M, Schmidt R, Weidner C, et al : Chemical response pattern of different classes of C-nociceptive pruritogens and algogens. *J Neurophysiol* 89:2441-2448, 2003.
15. Ikoma A, Rukwied R, Ständer S, et al: Neurophysiology of pruritus. Interaction of itch and pain. *Arch Dermatol* 139: 1475-1478, 2003.
16. Nilsson HJ, Levinsson A, Schouenborg J: Cutaneous filed stimulation (CFS): A new powerful method to combat itch. *Pain* 71:49-55, 1997.
17. Wallengren J, Sundler F: Cutaneous field stimulation in the treatment of severe itch. *Arch Dermatol* 137:1323-1325, 2001.
18. Wallengren J: Cutaneous field stimulation of sensory nerve fibers reduces itch without affecting contact dermatitis. *Allergy* 57: 1195-1199, 2002.
19. Hsieh JC, Hägermark Ö, Ståhle-Bäckdahl M, et al: Urge to scratch represented in the human cerebral cortex during itch. *J Neurophysiol* 72:3004-3008, 1994.
20. Drzezga A, Darsow U, Treede RD, et al: Central activation by histamine-induced itch: analogies to pain processing: a correlation analysis of O-15 H_2O positron emission tomography studies. *Pain* 92:295-305, 2001.
21. Mochizuki H, Tashiro M, Kano M, et al: Imaging of central itch modulation in the human brain using positron emission tomography. *Pain* 105:339-346, 2003.
22. Ikoma A, Fartasch M, Heyer G, et al: Painful stimuli evoke itch in patients with chronic pruritus. Central sensitization for itch. *Neurology* 62:212-217, 2004.
23. Fleischer AB: The clinical management of itching. Parthenon Publishing, New York, London, 2000.
24. Ständer S, Steinhoff M, Schmelz M, et al: Neurophysiology of pruritus. Cutaneous elicitation of itch. *Arch Dermatol* 139:1463-1470, 2003.
25. Steinhoff M, Ständer S, Seeliger S, et al: Modern aspects of cutaneous neurogenic inflammation. *Arch Dermatol* 139:1479-1488, 2003.
26. Dvorak M, Watkinson A, McGlone F, et al: Histamine induced responses are attenuated by cannabinoid receptor agonist in human skin. *Inflam Res* 52:238-245, 2003.
27. Ständer S, Moormann C, Schumacher M, et al: Expression of vanilloid receptor subtype 1 (VR1) in cutaneous sensory nerve fibers, mast cells and epithelial cells of appendage structures. *Exp Dermatol* 13:129-139, 2004.
28. Hossen MA, Sugimoto Y, Kayasuga R, et al: Involvement of histamine H3 receptors in scratching behaviour in mast cell-deficient mice. *Br J Dermatol* 149:17-22, 2003.
29. Rukwied R, Lischetzki G, McGlone F, et al: Mast cell mediators other than histamine induce pruritus in atopic dermatitis patients: A dermal microdialysis study. *Br J Dermatol* 142:1114-1120, 2000.
30. Ikoma A, Rukwied R, Ständer S, et al: Neuronal sensitization for histamine-induced itch in lesional skin of patients with Atopic Dermatitis. *Arch Dermatol* 139:1455-1458, 2003.
31. Weisshaar E, Ziethen B, Gollnick H: Can a serotonin type 3 (5-HT3) receptor antagonist reduce experimentally-induced itch? *Inflam Res* 46:412-416, 1997.
32. Weisshaar E, Dunker N, Domröse U, et al: Plasma serotonin and histamine levels in hemodialysis-related pruritus are not significantly influenced by 5-HT3 receptor blocker and antihistamine therapy. *Clin Nephrol* 59:124-129, 2003.
33. Weisshaar E, Dunker N, Röhl FW, et al: Antipruritic effects of 5-HT3 receptor antagonists in haemodialysis patients. *Exp Dermatol* 13:298-304, 2004.
34. Weidner C, Klede M, Rukwied R, et al: Acute effects of substance P and calcitonin gene-related peptide in human skin—A microdialysis study. *J Invest Dermatol* 115:1015-1020, 2000.
35. Togashi Y, Umeuchi H, Okano K, et al: Antipruritic activity of the opioid receptor agonist, TRK-820. *Eur J Pharmacol* 435:259-264, 2002.
36. Umeuchi H, Togashi Y, Honda T, et al: Involvement of central μ-opioid system in the scratching behavior in mice, and the suppression of it by the activation of κ-opioid system. *Eur J Pharmacol* 477:29-35, 2003.
37. Bergasa NV: Pruritus and fatigue in primary biliary cirrhosis. *Bailliperes Clin Gastroenterol* 14:643-655, 2000.

38. DeHaven-Hudkins DL, Cowan A, Cortes Burgos L, et al: Antipruritic and antihyperalgesic actions of loperamide and analogs. *Life Sci* 71:2787-2796, 2002.

39. Lippert U, Hoer A, Möller A, et al: Role of antigen-induced cytokine release in atopic pruritus. *Int Arch Allergy Immunol* 116:36-39, 1998.

40. Yosipovitch G, Zucker I, Boner G, et al: A questionnaire for the assessment of pruritus: Validation in uremic patients. *Acta Derm Venereol* 81:108-111, 2001.

41. Yosipovitch G, Ansari N, Goon A, et al: Clinical characteristics of pruritus in chronic idiopathic urticaria. *Br J Dermatol* 147:32-36, 2002.

42. Yosipovitch G, Goon AT, Wee J, et al: Itch characteristics in Chinese patients with atopic dermatitis using a new questionnaire for the assessment of pruritus. *Int J Dermatol* 41:212-216, 2002.

43. Darsow U, Mautner VF, Bromm B, et al: The Eppendorf Itch Questionnaire. *Hautarzt* 48:730-733, 1997.

44. Darsow U, Scharein E, Simon D, et al: New aspects of itch pathophysiology: Component analysis of atopic itch using the "Eppendorf Itch Questionnaire." *Int Arch Allergy Immunol* 124:326-331, 2001.

45. Ebata T, Iwasaki S, Kamide R, et al: Use of a wrist activity monitor for the measurement of nocturnal scratching in patients with atopic dermatitis. *Br J Dermatol* 144:305-309, 2001.

46. Stener-Victorin E, Lundeberg T, Kowalski J, et al: Perceptual matching for assessment of itch; reliability and responsiveness analyzed by a rank-invariant statistical method. *J Invest Dermatol* 121:1301-1305, 2003.

47. Ochoa JG: Pruritus, a rare but troublesome adverse reaction of topiramate. *Seizure* 12:516-518, 2003.

48. Cohen AD, Masalha R, Medvedovsky E, et al: Brachioradial pruritus: A symptom of neuropathy. *J Am Acad Dermatol* 48:825-828, 2003.

49. Goodkin R, Wingard E, Bernhard JD: Brachioradial pruritus: cervical spine disease and neurogenic/neurogenic pruritus. *J Am Acad Dermatol* 48:521-524, 2003.

50. Ständer S, Luger T, Metze D: Treatment of prurigo nodularis with topical capsaicin. *J Am Acad Dermatol* 44:471-478, 2001.

51. Weisshaar E, Dunker N, Gollnick H: Topical capsaicin therapy in humans with hemodialysis-related pruritus. *Neurosci Let* 345:192-194, 2003.

52. Thelmo M, Lang W, Brooke E, et al: An open-label pilot study to evaluate the safety and efficacy of topically applied tacrolimus ointment for the treatment of hand and/or foot eczema. *J Dermatol Treat* 14:136-140, 2003.

53. Yosipovitch G, Sugeng MW, Chan YH, et al: The effect of topically applied aspirin on localized circumscribed neurodermatitis. *J Am Acad Derm* 45:910-913, 2001.

54. Thompsen JS: Itch models and effect of topical antipruritic substances. *Forum for Nord Derm Ven* 7(Suppl 5):7-42, 2002.

55. Zhai H, Hannon W, Hahn GS, et al: Strontium nitrate decreased histamine-induced itch magnitude and duration in man. *Dermatology* 200:244-246, 2000.

56. Miller MJS, Vergnolle N, McKnight W, et al: Inhibition of neurogenic inflammation by the Amazonian herbal medicine Sangre de Grado. *J Invest Dermatol* 117:725-730, 2001.

57. Heyer G, Groene D, Martus P: Efficacy of naltrexone on acetylcholine-induced alloknesis in atopic eczema. *Exp Dermatol* 11:448-455, 2002.

58. Metze D, Reimann S, Beissert S, et al: Efficacy and safety of naltrexone, an oral opiate receptor antagonist, in the treatment of pruritus of internal and dermatological disease. *J Am Acad Dermatol* 41:533-539, 1999.

59. Zylic Z, Smith S, Krajnik M: Paroxetine for pruritus in advanced cancer. *J Pain Symptom Manag* 16:121-124, 1998.

60. Biondi M, Arcangeli T, Petrucci RM: Paroxetine in a case of psychogenic pruritus and neurotic excoriations. *Psychother Psychosom* 69:165-166, 2000.

61. Tefferi A, Fonseca R: Selective serotonin reuptake inhibitors are effective in the treatment of polycythemia vera-associated pruritus. *Blood* 99:2627, 2002.

62. Murphy M, Reaich D, Pai P, et al: A randomised, placebo-controlled, double-blind trial of ondansetron in renal itch. *Br J Dermatol* 148:314-317, 2003.

63. Hsu MML, Yang CC: Uraemic pruritus responsive to broadband ultraviolet (UV)B therapy does not readily respond to narrowband UVB therapy. *Br J Dermatol* 149:888-889, 2003.

64. Heyer GR, Hornstein OP: Recent studies of cutaneous nociception in atopic and non-atopic subjects. *J Dermatol* 26:77-86, 1999.

Statistics of Interest to the Dermatologist

MARTIN A. WEINSTOCK, MD, PHD, AND MARGARET M. BOYLE, BS
Brown University Dermatoepidemiology Unit, Providence, Rhode Island

Morbidity and Mortality

Health Care Delivery in the United States

Miscellaneous

TABLE 1.—New Cases of Selected Reportable Infectious Diseases in the United States

	1940	1950	1960	1970	1980	1990	2000	2003*
AIDS	—	—	—	—	—	41,595	40,758	41,832†
Anthrax	76	49	23	2	1	0	1	—
Congenital Rubella	—	—	—	77	50	11	9	—
Congenital Syphilis			—			3865	529	361
Diphtheria	15,536	5796	918	435	3	4	1	1
Gonorrhea	175,841	286,746	258,933	600,072	1,004,029	690,169	358,995	311,922
Hansen's Disease	—	44	54	129	223	198	91	61
Lyme Disease						—	17,730	17,970
Measles	291,162	319,124	441,703	47,351	13,506	27,786	86	42
Plague	1	3	2	13	18	2	6	1
Rocky Mountain Spotted Fever	457	464	204	380	1163	651	495	957
Syphilis (primary and secondary)	—	23,939	16,145	21,982	27,204	50,223	5979	6693
Toxic Shock Syndrome					—	322	135	126
Tuberculosis‡	102,984§	121,742§	55,494	37,137	27,749	25,701	16,377	11,339
US population (millions)	132	151	179	203	227	249	281	291

Note: Dash indicates that data not available.
*For 52 weeks ending December 27, 2003.
†Last update November 30, 2003.
‡Reporting criteria changed in 1975.
§Data include newly reported active and inactive cases.
(Data from Centers for Disease Control and Prevention: Summary of Notifiable Diseases, United States, 2003. *Morb Mortal Wkly Rep* 52[51&52]:1267-1275, 2004; Centers for Disease Control and Prevention: Summary of Notifiable Diseases, United States, 2000. *Morb Mortal Wkly Rep* 49[51&52]:1167-1174, 2001; Centers for Disease Control and Prevention: Annual Summary 1994: Reported morbidity and mortality. *Morb Mortal Wkly Rep* 43[53]:70-71, 1994; Centers for Disease Control and Prevention: Annual Summary 1984: Reported morbidity and mortality. *Morb Mortal Wkly Rep* 33:124-129, 1986.)

TABLE 2.—Estimates of HIV/AIDS, 2003

REGION	Adults and Children Living With HIV/AIDS	Adults and Children Newly Affected With HIV During 2003	Adult Prevalence (%)*	Adult and Child Deaths Due to HIV/AIDS During 2003
Sub-Saharan Africa	25.0-28.2 million	3.0-3.4 million	7.5-8.5	2.2-2.4 million
North Africa and Middle East	470,000-730,000	43,000-67,000	0.2-0.4	35,000-50,000
South and Southeast Asia	4.6-8.2 million	610,000-1.2 million	0.4-0.8	330,000-590,000
East Asia and Pacific	700,000-1.3 million	150,000-270,000	0.1-0.1	32,000-58,000
Latin America	1.3-1.9 million	120,000-180,000	0.5-0.7	49,000-70,000
Caribbean	350,000-590,000	45,000-80,000	1.9-3.1	30,000-50,000
Eastern Europe and Central Asia	1.2-1.8 million	180,000-280,000	0.5-0.9	23,000-37,000
Western Europe	520,000-680,000	30,000-40,000	0.3-0.3	2,600-3,400
North America	790,000-1.2 million	36,000-54,000	0.5-0.7	12,000-18,000
Australia and New Zealand	12,000-18,000	700-1000	0.1-0.1	<100
Total	40 million (34-46 million)	5 million (4.2-5.8 million)	1.10% (0.9-1.3%)	3 million (2.5-3.5 million)

*The proportion of adults (15-49 years of age) living with HIV/AIDS in 2003, using 2003 population numbers.
(Data from AIDS Epidemic Update, Joint United Nations Programme on HIV/AIDS [UNAIDS] World Health Organization [WHO], December, 2003.)

TABLE 3.—AIDS Cases by Age Group and Exposure Category, Through December 2002, and Cumulative Totals Through December 2002, United States

	2002		Cumulative Total*	
	No.	(%)	No.	(%)
Adult/adolescent exposure category				
Men who have sex with men	14,545	(33%)	384,784	(45%)
Injecting drug use	7502	(17%)	209,920	(25%)
Men who have sex with men and inject drugs	1510	(3%)	54,224	(6%)
Hemophilia/coagulation disorder	90	(0%)	5371	(1%)
Heterosexual contact	7953	(16%)	100,071	(12%)
Receipt of blood transfusion, blood components, or tissue†	265	(1%)	9152	(1%)
Other/risk not reported or identified	11,927	(27%)	86,258	(10%)
Adult/adolescent SUBTOTAL	43,792	(100%)	849,780	(100%)
Pediatric (<13 years old) exposure category				
Hemophilia/coagulation disorder	0	(0%)	236	(3%)
Mother with/at risk for HIV infection	139	(88%)	8425	(91%)
Receipt of blood transfusion, blood components, or tissue†	2	(1%)	385	(4%)
Other/risk not reported or identified	17	(11%)	174	(2%)
Pediatric SUBTOTAL	158	(100%)	9220	(100%)
TOTAL	43,950		859,000	

Note: Total includes 2 persons whose sex is unknown.

*Includes persons with a diagnosis of AIDS, reported from the beginning of the epidemic through 2002.

†Forty-six adults/adolescents and 3 children developed AIDS after receiving blood screened negative for HIV antibody. Fourteen additional adults developed AIDS after receiving tissue, organs, or artificial insemination from HIV-infected donors. Four of the 14 received tissue or organs from a donor who was negative for HIV antibody at the time of donation.

(Data from Centers for Disease Control and Prevention: *HIV/AIDS Surveillance Rep* 14:30, 2002.)

TABLE 4.—Selected Causes of Death, United States, 1991 and 2001

	Number of Deaths	
Cause of Death	1991	2001
Malignant melanoma	6451	7542
Infections of the skin	747	1249
Motor vehicle traffic accidents	45,621	42,443
Accident involving animal being ridden	95	116
Accidental drowning and submersion	3967	3281
Lightning	75	44
Homicide and legal intervention	26,513	20,704*
All cancer	514,657	553,788
All causes	2,169,518	2,416,425

*Figures include September 11, 2001, related deaths for which death certificates were filed as of October 24, 2002.

(Data from National Center for Health Statistics, Division of Vital Statistics, personal communication, March 2004.)

TABLE 5.—Annual Change in Cancer Incidence in the United States

	Average Annual Percent Change	
	1992-2000	1973-1990
Liver and intrahepatic bile duct	+3.9	+2.3
Thyroid	+3.4	+0.8
Melanomas of the skin	+2.5	+4.1
Kidney and renal pelvis	+1.3	+2.2
Testis	+1.3	+2.6
Breast (women only)	+0.8	+1.9
Esophagus	+0.3	+0.8
Non-Hodgkin lymphoma	+0.0	+3.6
Lung and bronchus	−0.9	+1.8
Urinary bladder	−0.0	+0.7
Corpus and uterus, NOS	−0.1	−2.1
Pancreas	−0.4	−0.2
Hodgkin lymphoma	−0.4	−0.1
Brain and ONS	−0.5	+1.5
Colon rectum	−0.6	+0.2
Myeloma	−0.7	+1.1
Ovary	−0.8	+0.5
Stomach	−1.3	−1.6
Leukemia	−1.3	+0.1
Oral cavity and pharynx	−2.0	−0.4
Cervix uteri	−2.5	−2.7
Larynx	−2.6	0.0
Prostate	−3.1	+3.6
All sites	−0.7	+1.2

Note: Rates are per 100,000 and age-adjusted to the 2000 US standard million population.

(Data from Ries LAG, Eisner MP, Kosary CL, et al (eds): *Seer Cancer Statistics Review: 1975-2000,* National Cancer Institute, Bethesda, Md, 2003; Surveillance, Epidemiology, and End Results (SEER) Program SEER Stat Database: Incidence— SEER 9 Regs, November 2002 Sub (1973-2000), National Cancer Institute, DCCPS, Surveillance Research Program, Cancer Statistics Branch, released April 2003 based on the November 2002 submission.)

TABLE 6.—Melanoma Incidence and Mortality Rates, United States

Year	Incidence*	Mortality†
1975	7.9	2.1
1976	8.1	2.2
1977	8.9	2.3
1978	8.9	2.3
1979	9.5	2.4
1980	10.5	2.3
1981	11.1	2.4
1982	11.2	2.5
1983	11.1	2.5
1984	11.4	2.5
1985	12.7	2.6
1986	13.3	2.6
1987	13.6	2.6
1988	12.8	2.6
1989	13.7	2.7
1990	13.8	2.8
1991	14.6	2.7
1992	14.7	2.7
1993	14.5	2.7
1994	15.6	2.7
1995	16.3	2.7
1996	17.1	2.8
1997	17.5	2.7
1998	17.7	2.8
1999	17.6	2.6
2000	17.7	2.7

2004 estimate: 55,100 newly diagnosed cases and 7910 deaths

*Surveillance, Epidemiology and End-Results (SEER) Program, (9 registries of the National Cancer Institute).

†National Center for Health Statistics, United States population. Rates per 100,000 per year, and age-adjusted to the 2000 US standard million population. All races.

(Data from American Cancer Society, Inc. Surveillance Research. *Cancer Facts & Figures 2004* 4:2004; Ries LAG, Eisner MP, Kosary CL, et al [eds]: *SEER Cancer Statistics Review: 1975-2000.* National Cancer Institute, Bethesda, Md, 2003.)

TABLE 7.—Melanoma Five-Year Relative Survival

Year	Whites (%)	Blacks (%)
	Year at Diagnosis	
1960-1963	60	—
1970-1973	68	—
1974-1976	80	66
1977-1979	82	51
1980-1982	83	60
1983-1985	85	76
1986-1988	88	65
1989-1996	89	70
1992-1999	90	64
	Stage at Diagnosis (1992-1999)	
Local	97	85
Regional	60	32
Distant	14	—

Notes: Dash indicates insufficient data. Relative survival is the observed survival divided by the survival expected in a demographically similar subgroup of the general population. Survival estimates among blacks are imprecise due to small numbers of cases observed.

(Data from Ries LAG, Eisner MP, Kosary CL, et al [eds]: *SEER Cancer Statistics Review: 1975-2000.* National Cancer Institute, Bethesda, Md, 2003.)

TABLE 8.—Contact Dermatitis in Belgium: Proportion of Positive Patch Tests to Standard Chemicals in 350 Patients With at Least 1 Positive Reaction (Among 618 Patients Tested in 2003)

Chemical	(%)
Nickel sulphate	30.9
Paraphenylenediamine	15.7
Fragrance mix	14.8
Wool alcohols	12.7
Balsam of Peru	11.2
Cobalt chloride	8.2
Colophony	7.9
Potassium dichromate	6.0
Thiuram mix	6.0
Neomycin sulphate	3.6
Formaldehyde	3.3
Benzocaine	2.7
Budesonide	2.7
Cl+ Me-isothiazolinone	2.7
Mercapto mix	2.7
Tixocortol pivalate	2.4
Epoxy resin	2.1
Paraben mix	2.1
Paratertiarybutyl phenol-formaldehyde resin	2.1
Clioquinol	1.5
Mercaptobenzothiazole	1.5
Quaternium-15	1.5
Sesquiterpene lactone mix	0.9
Isopropyl-phenylparaphenylenediamine	0.6
Primin	0.3

(Data from Goossens A, University Hospital, Katholieke Universiteit Leuven, Belgium, personal communication, January 2004.)

TABLE 9.—Non-Federal Dermatologists by Age and Sex, 1993 and 2002

	1993			2002		
Age Group	Men	Women	Total	Men	Women	Total
under 35	691	756	1447	642	853	1495
35-44	1633	933	2566	1246	1288	2534
45-54	1828	333	2161	1751	897	2648
55-64	1133	106	1239	1748	301	2049
65 and over	669	36	665	977	81	1058
TOTAL	5914	2164	8078	6364	3420	9784
Country of Graduation						
United States	7391	(92%)		9025	(92%)	
Canada	116	(1%)		128	(1%)	
Other	571	(7%)		631	(7%)	
TOTAL	8078	(100%)		9784	(100%)	
Board Certification						
Certified	6382	(79%)		8140	(83%)	
Not certified	1696	(21%)		1644	(17%)	
TOTAL	8078	(100%)		9784	(100%)	

(Data from *Physician Characteristics and Distribution in the US, 2004 ed.* Department of Physician Practice and Communication Information, Division of Survey and Data Resources, American Medical Association, 2004; *Physician Masterfile,* Yearend 1993, Chicago, American Medical Association, 1993; and special tabulations.)

TABLE 10.—Number of Dermatologists per Million Population

State	1970		1980		1990		2000		2002	
Alabama	13	(44)	17	(68)	18	(75)	22	(99)	22	(97)
Alaska	3	(1)	0	(0)	9	(5)	11	(7)	14	(9)
Arizona	15	(26)	27	(75)	26	(98)	31	(160)	31	(167)
Arkansas	9	(17)	16	(36)	20	(48)	23	(62)	23	(63)
California	27	(542)	34	(819)	40	(1157)	40	(1353)	40	(1442)
Colorado	17	(38)	21	(61)	26	(91)	27	(116)	26	(122)
Connecticut	21	(65)	28	(87)	41	(136)	48	(162)	48	(166)
Delaware	11	(6)	17	(10)	15	(10)	18	(14)	21	(17)
District of Columbia	49	(37)	58	(37)	60	(37)	72	(63)	103	(59)
Florida	17	(116)	26	(55)	34	(431)	39	(628)	40	(662)
Georgia	13	(58)	21	(116)	24	(162)	30	(249)	31	(264)
Hawaii	23	(18)	26	(25)	30	(34)	33	(40)	34	(42)
Idaho	7	(5)	13	(12)	15	(15)	22	(29)	24	(32)
Illinois	16	(179)	21	(238)	24	(283)	30	(378)	31	(387)
Indiana	10	(54)	13	(73)	19	(104)	23	(140)	23	(143)
Iowa	12	(34)	18	(52)	24	(66)	27	(80)	26	(75)
Kansas	6	(13)	13	(30)	16	(39)	18	(53)	20	(55)
Kentucky	7	(23)	14	(52)	21	(79)	27	(110)	28	(116)
Louisiana	17	(61)	23	(97)	29	(129)	37	(164)	36	(160)
Maine	8	(8)	10	(11)	13	(16)	15	(19)	12	(15)
Maryland	14	(54)	29	(121)	39	(185)	44	(232)	46	(251)
Massachusetts	24	(137)	30	(173)	41	(243)	53	(335)	54	(345)
Michigan	16	(139)	21	(193)	27	(250)	29	(291)	28	(282)
Minnesota	20	(76)	24	(100)	29	(124)	36	(175)	36	(179)
Mississippi	7	(16)	9	(23)	11	(31)	17	(47)	17	(48)
Missouri	15	(70)	19	(94)	23	(120)	29	(160)	30	(168)
Montana	13	(9)	19	(15)	22	(18)	31	(28)	36	(33)
Nebraska	9	(13)	16	(25)	15	(24)	18	(30)	17	(30)
Nevada	12	(6)	19	(15)	20	(21)	25	(49)	21	(46)
New Hampshire	15	(11)	27	(25)	25	(28)	32	(39)	33	(42)
New Jersey	19	(134)	23	(168)	31	(245)	36	(305)	36	(308)
New Mexico	11	(11)	18	(23)	25	(41)	30	(55)	29	(54)
New York	27	(485)	31	(548)	42	(740)	50	(941)	49	(940)
North Carolina	13	(68)	21	(123)	26	(173)	33	(263)	33	(275)
North Dakota	13	(8)	12	(8)	27	(18)	26	(17)	24	(15)
Ohio	16	(166)	18	(196)	25	(265)	29	(327)	30	(339)
Oklahoma	14	(36)	16	(48)	17	(55)	21	(71)	20	(70)
Oregon	22	(47)	27	(71)	34	(95)	34	(118)	33	(115)
Pennsylvania	17	(198)	21	(247)	29	(340)	34	(421)	35	(426)
Puerto Rico	12	(33)	16	(51)	20	(72)	21	(81)	21	(81)
Rhode Island	17	(16)	28	(27)	43	(43)	61	(64)	66	(71)
South Carolina	7	(17)	12	(38)	21	(73)	26	(106)	27	(112)
South Dakota	9	(6)	0	(6)	17	(12)	25	(19)	25	(19)
Tennessee	11	(42)	15	(67)	22	(108)	28	(161)	28	(165)
Texas	15	(173)	20	(284)	23	(400)	26	(536)	25	(553)
Utah	13	(14)	19	(28)	25	(45)	14	(69)	30	(70)
Vermont	9	(4)	12	(6)	27	(15)	30	(18)	32	(20)
Virginia	14	(64)	22	(117)	26	(159)	28	(200)	30	(219)
Washington	14	(47)	22	(91)	29	(133)	28	(192)	33	(198)
West Virginia	8	(14)	13	(25)	13	(24)	15	(28)	15	(27)
Wisconsin	15	(66)	20	(93)	24	(115)	30	(162)	31	(168)
Wyoming	3	(1)	8	(4)	6	(3)	14	(7)	16	(8)
TOTAL	17	(3526)	23	(5207)	29	(7233)	34	(9472)	31	(9770)

Note: Actual number in parenthesis.

(Data from *Physician Characteristics and Distribution in the US*, 2004 ed. Department of Physician Practice and Communication Information, Division of Survey and Data Resources, Chicago, American Medical Association, 2004, and special tabulations.)

TABLE 11.—Dermatology Trainees in the United States

Year Residency to Be Completed	Male Residents	Female Residents	Total
2004	160	183	345
2005	159	216	378
2006	156	231	392
2007	3	5	8

(Data from American Academy of Dermatology, personal communication, February 2004.)

TABLE 12.—Diplomates Certified by The American Board of Dermatology From 1933 to 2003

Decade Totals (Inclusive Dates)	Average Number Certified per Year
1933-1940	69
1941-1950	74
1951-1960	76
1961-1970	112
1971-1980	247
1981-1990	271
1991-2000	295
2001-2003	307
Individual Year Totals	Actual Number Certified
1999	286
2000	283
2001	305
2002	309
2003	307
TOTAL 1933 through 2003	12,228

(Data from The American Board of Dermatology, Inc, personal communication, January 2004.)

TABLE 13.—Physicians Certified in Dermatologic Subspecialties

Physicians Certified for Special Qualification in Dermatopathology, 1974-2003

Year	Dermatologists	Pathologists Average Number Certified	Total
1974-1975	108	44	302
1976-1980	54	49	515
1981-1985	37	34	351
1986-1990	11	14	125
1991-1995	20	20	196
1996-00	14	32	227
		Actual Number Certified	
2001	10	34	44
2002	14	55	69
2003	14	48	62
TOTAL Certified 1974-2003	931	963	1894

Dermatologists Certified for Special Qualification in
Clinical and Laboratory Dermatological Immunology, 1985-2003

Year	Number Certified
1985	52
1987	16
1989	22
1991	15
1993	5
1997	5
2001	6
TOTAL 1985-2003	121

Notes: No special qualification examination for Dermatopathology was administered in 1992, 1994, and 1996. No special qualification examination in Clinical and Laboratory Dermatological Immunology was administered in 1986, 1988, 1990, 1992, 1994, 1995, 1996, 1998, 1999, 2000, 2002, or 2003.
(Data from American Board of Dermatology and American Board of Pathology, personal communication, January 2004.)

TABLE 14.—Visits to Non-Federal Office-Based Physicians in the United States, 2001
(Estimates in Thousands)

Diagnosis	Dermatologist	Type of Physician Other		All Physicians	
Acne vulgaris	5496 (14.5%)	*	*	6405 (0.7%)	
Eczematous dermatitis	3930 (10.4%)	5581	(0.7%)	9511 (1.1%)	
Warts	1837 (4.8%)	2462	(0.3%)	4299 (0.5%)	
Skin cancer	3174 (8.4%)	*1501	(0.2%)	4675 (0.5%)	
Psoriasis	1197 (3.2%)	*	*	1441 (0.2%)	
Fungal infections	746 (2.0%)	*	*	1683 (0.2%)	
Hair disorders	631 (1.7%)	*	*	1388 (0.2%)	
Actinic keratosis	3430 (9.1%)	*	*	4124 (0.5%)	
Benign neoplasm of the skin	2422 (6.4%)	1206	(0.1%)	3629 (0.4%)	
All disorders	37,883 (100%)	842,603	(100%)	880,487 (100%)	

*Figure does not meet standard of reliability or precision.
Note: Percentage of visits for all disorders is in parentheses.
(Data from National Ambulatory Medical Care Survey 2001, National Center for Health Statistics, Centers for Disease Control and Prevention. Personal communication, February 2004.)

TABLE 15.—Health Insurance Coverage of the United States Population, 2002

	Children 1-17 Years (%)	Adults Aged 18-64 Years (%)	Adults Aged 65 Years and Over (%)
Individually purchased insurance	8	6	27
Employer-provided private insurance	60	66	34
Public insurance, any type	27	11	96
Medicaid/State Children's Health Insurance Program	24	7	10
No health insurance	12	20	1

Note: Some individuals have both public and private insurance, so the numbers will not add to 100%.
(Data from the Employee Benefit Research Institute, Washington, DC, personal communication, January 2004.)

TABLE 16.—Nonelderly Population With Selected Sources of Health Insurance, by Family Income, 2002

Yearly Family Income Level	Employment-Based Coverage %	Individually Purchased %	Public %	Uninsured %	Total %
under $5000	12	13	38	40	100
$5000-$9999	12	11	52	29	100
$10,000-$14,999	20	11	40	35	100
$15,000-$19,999	33	8	33	31	100
$20,000-$29,999	47	7	23	28	100
$30,000-$39,999	62	7	16	20	100
$40,000-$49,999	71	6	12	16	100
$50,000 and over	84	5	6	8	100
TOTAL	64	7	16	17	100

Note: Details may not add to totals because individuals may receive coverage from more than one source.
(Data from Fronstin P, "Sources of Coverage and Characteristics of the Uninsured: Analysis of the March 2003 Current Population Survey." *EBRI Issue Brief*, No. 264 [Washington, DC. Employee Benefit Research Institute], December 2003.)

TABLE 17.—Health Maintenance Organization (HMO) Market Penetration in the United States, January 1, 2003

HMO Penetration in Region

Northeast	35%
Mid-Atlantic	32%
South Atlantic	21%
East South Central	14%
West South Central	15%
East North Central	23%
West North Central	26%
Mountain	26%
Pacific	43%

HMO Penetration Top Ten Most Highly Penetrated Metropolitan Statistical Areas

Vallejo-Fairfield-Napa, California	69%
Rochester, New York	65%
Sacramento, Arden, Arcade-Roseville, California	64%
Oakland-Fremont-Hayward, California	64%
Buffalo-Cheektowaga-Tonawanda, New York	62%
Stockton, California	56%
Los Angeles-Long Beach-Glendale, California	54%
Riverside-San Bernardino-Ontario, California	53%
Madison, Wisconsin	53%
San Francisco-San Mateo-Redwood City, California	52%
San Diego-Carlsbad-San Marcos, California	51%
San Jose-Sunnyvale-Santa Clara, California	51%

(Data from The InterStudy Competitive Edge: *Regional Market Analysis 13.2* [January 1, 2003], InterStudy Publications, St Paul, Minnesota, personal communication, February 2004.)

TABLE 18.—National Health Expenditure Amounts: Selected Calendar Years

Spending Category	Billions of Dollars (%)				
	1980	1990	2000	2002*	2003*
Total national health expenditures	246	696	1310	1548	1661
Health services and supplies	234	670	1262	1493	1603
Personal health care	215	609	1138	1331	1424
Hospital care	102	254	417	485	511
Professional services	67	217	425	494	530
Physician and clinical services	47	158	289	334	357
Other professional services	4	18	39	45	48
Dental services	13	32	61	70	74
Other personal health care	3	10	37	46	51
Nursing home and home health	20	65	126	140	146
Home health care	2	13	32	36	38
Nursing home care	18	53	94	104	108
Retail outlet sale of medical products	26	73	171	213	237
Prescription drugs	12	40	122	161	182
Other medical products	14	33	49	52	54
Durable medical equipment	4	11	18	19	20
Other non-durable medical products	10	23	31	33	34
Government administration and net cost of private health insurance	12	40	81	111	124
Government public health activities	7	20	44	51	55
Investment	12	26	48	55	58
Research†	6	13	29	35	37
Construction	7	14	19	29	21

*Projected values
†Research and development expenditures of drug companies and other manufacturers and providers of medical equipment and supplies are excluded from research expenditures but are included in the expenditure class in which the product falls, in that they are covered by the payment received for that product. Numbers may not add to totals because of rounding.
(Data from Centers for Medicare and Medicaid Services, Office of the Actuary, National Health Statistics Group, January 2004.)

TABLE 19.—Spending on Consumer Advertising of Prescription Products, United States

Year	(Dollars in Millions)
2003	3082
2002	2514
2001	2479
2000	2150*
1999	1590
1998	1173
1997	844
1996	595
1995	313
1994	242
1993	165
1992	156
1991	56
1990	48
1989	12

*Estimated.
(Data from TNS MediaIntelligence/CMR, personal communication, March 2004.)

TABLE 20.—Results of the American Academy of Dermatology Skin Cancer Screening Program, 1985-2003

Year	Number Screened	Suspected Diagnosis		
		Basal Cell Carcinoma	Squamous Cell Carcinoma	Malignant Melanoma
1985	32,000	1056	163	97
1986	41,486	3049	398	262
1987	41,649	2798	302	257
1988	67,124	4457	474	435
1989	78,486	6266	761	593
1990	98,060	7959	1069	872
1991	102,485	8110	1193	1062
1992	98,440	8403	1280	1054
1993	97,553	7067	1068	2465*
1994	86,895	6908	1235	1010
1995	88,934	7503	1317	1353
1996	94,363	8713	1656	1399
1997	99,554	8730	1685	1469
1998	89,536	6687	1308	1078
1999	89,916	5790	1136	635
2000	65,854	5074	1053	653
2001	70,562	5192	1102	642
2002	64,492	4733	1009	692
2003	70,692	4481	1032	489
TOTAL	1,478,081	112,976	19,241	16,517

*Number of cases included melanoma, "rule out melanoma," and lentigo maligna.
(Data from American Academy of Dermatology: *2003 Skin Cancer Screening Program Statistical Summary Report*, March 2004.)

TABLE 21.—Leading Dermatology Journals

Journal	Total Citations in 2002	Number of Articles Published in 2002
Acta Dermato-Venereologica	3134	70
AIDS Patient Care	326	64
American Journal of Dermatopathology	1786	94
Annals de Dermatologie et de Venereologie	1179	281
Archives of Dermatology	10,626	183
Archives of Dermatological Research	1991	71
British Journal of Dermatology	11,364	360
Clinics in Dermatology	804	93
Clinical and Experimental Dermatology	1781	150
Contact Dermatitis	3780	121
Current Problems in Dermatology	44	6
Cutis	1411	129
Dermatologic Clinics	1168	65
Dermatologic Surgery	2151	186
Dermatology	3358	184
European Journal of Dermatology	774	180
Experimental Dermatology	809	80
Hautarzt	1060	119
International Journal of Dermatology	2654	225
Journal of the American Academy of Dermatology	12,791	355
Journal of Cosmetic Science	66	61
Journal of Cutaneous Pathology	1564	97
Journal of Dermatological Science	805	80
Journal of Dermatological Treatment	199	29
Journal of the European Academy of Dermatology	491	105
Journal of Investigative Dermatology Symposium Proceedings	211	—
Journal of Investigative Dermatology	15,803	310
Leprosy Review	563	44
Melanoma Research	1218	79
Mycoses	1221	114
Pediatric Dermatology	1265	109
Photodermatology, Photoimmunology, and Photomedicine	710	53

(Data from *Journal Citation Reports on CD-ROM:JCR*, Science ed. Philadelphia, Institute for Scientific Information, 2002.)

CLINICAL DERMATOLOGY

1 Urticarial and Eczematous Disorders

Association Between Novel GM-CSF Gene Polymorphisms and the Frequency and Severity of Atopic Dermatitis
Rafatpanah H, Bennett E, Pravica V, et al (Univ of Manchester, England)
J Allergy Clin Immunol 112:593-598, 2003   1–1

Background.—There is a genetic component to atopic dermatitis (AD). Polymorphisms in factors involved in the maturation and function of the antigen-presenting Langerhans' cell (LC), such as granulocyte-macrophage colony-stimulating factor (GM-CSF), tumor necrosis factor (TNF)-α, and interleukin (IL)-1β, were studied in children with AD.

Study Design.—The study group consisted of 113 children with AD and 114 controls without AD, asthma, or allergic rhinitis. DNA was extracted and amplified by the polymerase chain reaction (PCR) and assessed for well-characterized polymorphisms of the IL-1β and TNF-α genes. Novel polymorphisms of the GM-CSF gene were also detected.

Findings.—A significant difference in the frequency of the novel polymorphisms −677 and −1916 of the GM-CSF gene was detected between children with AD and healthy controls. None of the children with the most severe AD (affecting 27%-100% of their body surface area) had the −677 GM-CSF C/C genotype, but 50% had the A/A genotype. In the control group, 16% had A/A and 16% had C/C. None of the GM-CSF polymorphisms was associated with a significant variation in production of GM-CSF by stimulated peripheral blood mononuclear cells from adult volunteers. There was no significant association between IL-1β and TNF-α alleles or genotype frequencies and AD.

Conclusions.—The findings include 2 novel polymorphisms of the GM-CSF locus that are associated with the propensity for AD in children. This supports the hypothesis that the genetic predisposition to AD is controlled, at least in part, by factors involved in Langerhans' cell maturation.

▶ GM-CSF is an important modulator of Langerhans' cell maturation and behavior, and has been detected at increased levels in the skin of patients with AD. These investigators tested the hypothesis that polymorphisms within the gene encoding GM-CSF are involved in the genetic predisposition to AD. Genotyping of a large population of patients revealed that the GM-CSF −677 A/A genotype was significantly associated with atopic dermatitis, especially in those children with the most severe disease. The significance of this association is not clear, since the authors found no correlation between genotype and cytokine production in stimulated mononuclear cells obtained from healthy adults. This study further underlines the complexity of the pathogenic mechanisms in atopic dermatitis.

G. M. P. Galbraith, MD

Cytokine Milieu of Atopic Dermatitis, as Compared to Psoriasis, Skin Prevents Induction of Innate Immune Response Genes
Nomura I, Goleva E, Howell MD, et al (Natl Jewish Med and Research Ctr, Denver; Univ of Colorado, Denver; McGill Univ, Montreal; et al)
J Immunol 171:3262-3269, 2003   1–2

Introduction.—Atopic dermatitis (AD) and psoriasis differ in their mechanisms for skin inflammation and tendency for skin infection. Such infections are common in AD, but not in psoriasis. The immune response in AD is Th2-mediated, whereas that of psoriasis is Th1-mediated. Thus, high levels of immunoglobulin E (IgE) and eosinophilia are characteristic of AD, whereas local neutrophil infiltration is seen in psoriasis. Skin biopsy specimens from patients with AD and psoriasis were analyzed to better understand the innate immune response in AD.

Methods.—Biopsy specimens were obtained from the lesions of 15 patients with moderate to severe AD, 15 with psoriasis, and 6 healthy individuals. None of the patients had been treated with systemic immunosuppressive drugs, and all were off topical corticosteroids for more than 1 week before biopsy. GeneChip microarray studies, immunohistochemistry, and real-time polymerase chain reaction (PCR) were performed in samples from each group.

Results.—GeneChip microarray analyses examined all known innate immunity genes available in the human U-95Av2 GeneChip Affymetrix probe array. Lower levels of interferon-γ (IFN-γ), interleukin-1β (IL-1β), and tumor necrosis factor α (TNF-α) were seen in AD than in psoriatic skin, but the difference was not statistically significant. Expression of human β defensin 2 (HBD-2), inducible NO synthetase (iNOS), and IL-8, however, was significantly lower in AD skin lesions. There was strong HBD-3 staining in keratinocytes from psoriasis skin lesions, but none in AD skin samples. Decreased expression of this antimicrobial peptide was demonstrated at the messenger RNA level by real-time PCR and at the protein level by immunohistochemistry. Because HBD-2, IL-8, and iNOS are known to be inhibited by Th2 cytokines, the effects of IL-4 and IL-13 on HBD-3 expression were examined in keratinocyte culture in vitro. Both IL-4 and IL-13 inhibited TNF-α and IFN-γ–induced HBD-3 production.

Conclusion.—Levels of the recently identified antimicrobial peptide HBD-3 are extremely low in AD skin and may contribute to patients' increased susceptibility to skin infections, especially *Staphylococcus aureus*. As compared with psoriasis lesions, those of AD contain significantly lower levels of iNOS, IL-8, and HBD-2 transcripts. In AD skin, decreased expression of antimicrobial genes may occur as the result of local upregulation of Th2 cytokines and low levels of TNF-α and IFN-γ despite inflammatory conditions.

▶ AD is characterized by colonization of the skin by *S aureus* and frequent skin infections. These investigators used microarray technology to study the expression of more than 40 genes involved with innate immune function in cells from patients with AD. The control group comprised patients with psoriasis. Although expression of the majority of the genes studied was similar between the patient groups, a number of genes were expressed at a significantly lower level in AD tissues compared with psoriatic cells. The most striking result was a reduction of HBD-2 in AD. HBD-2 is a peptide produced by keratinocytes that possesses antimicrobial activity. This finding prompted the investigators to examine expression of a recently described, more potent antimicrobial peptide, HBD-3, using immunohistology and real-time PCR. The data obtained clearly showed that AD keratinocytes express negligible protein product and severely diminished HBD-3 messenger RNA compared with cells from patients with psoriasis. Interestingly, Th2 cytokines such as IL-4 and IL-13, which are present at high levels in AD lesions, were found to inhibit HBD-3 induction. The authors suggest that inhibition of innate immune mechanisms such as those involving antimicrobial peptides may account for the increased susceptibility to skin infections in patients with AD.

G. M. P. Galbraith, MD

Association Between Antenatal Cytokine Production and the Development of Atopy and Asthma at Age 6 Years
Macaubas C, de Klerk NH, Holt BJ, et al (Univ of Western Australia, Perth)
Lancet 362:1192-1197, 2003   1–3

Introduction.—There is evidence that antenatal factors are important in determining susceptibility to atopy and asthma. Cytokine production is a possible mechanism. It is high throughout gestation and it protects placental integrity by controlling local immunologic homeostasis. Antenatal cytokine concentrations were assessed in a prospective birth cohort that was intensively monitored for atopy and asthma outcomes at age 6 years.

Methods.—Cryopreserved cord blood serum samples from 407 participants were assayed for interleukins 4, 5, 6, 10, 12, and 13; interferon γ; and tumor necrosis factor α. Correlations between family, antenatal and perinatal factors, cord blood cytokine concentrations, and atopy or asthma outcomes were examined via logistic regression analyses. Causal effects of cytokines on outcomes were estimated by propensity scores that were based on family and antenatal and perinatal factors.

Results.—Detectable cord blood concentrations of interleukin 4 and interferon γ were each linked with lower risk of physician-diagnosed asthma (adjusted odds ratios [ORs], 0.60 [95% confidence interval (CI), 0.37-0.99] and 0.60 [0.37-0.97], respectively); current asthma (OR, 0.59 [95% CI, 0.33-1.00] and 0.39 [0.22-0.71], respectively); current wheeze (OR, 0.55 [95% CI, 0.32-0.93] and 0.52 [0.31-0.90], respectively); and some atopic manifestations at 6 years of age. High concentrations of tumor necrosis factor α were linked with a lower risk of atopy but not with asthma risk. These associations were broadly unchanged by propensity score adjustment. Maternal smoking was linked with higher risk of both wheeze at 6 years and lower concentrations of interleukin 4 and interferon γ in cord blood.

Conclusion.—The mechanism underlying attenuated T-helper–1/T-helper–2 cytokine production in high-risk children also seems to influence cytokine production in the fetoplacental unit. The fact that this mechanism is dysregulated by maternal smoking indicates that it is a target for antenatal environmental factors relevant to asthma etiology.

▶ Macaubas et al found an inverse relation between cord blood concentrations of interleukin 4, interferon γ, and tumor necrosis factor α, and risk of asthma, atopy, or both at the age of 6 years. There also was an apparent dysregulation of cytokine production in the fetal placental unit by maternal smoking, an observation that suggests the importance of antenatal environmental factors in predisposing children to atopy and asthma. As discussed by Holberg and Halonen in an accompanying editorial, the findings underscore the importance of the need for additional studies to determine how genetic factors interact with environmental influences to affect the expression of disease.[1] Data from such studies might lead to new diagnostic procedures, treatments, prevention programs, and possibly cures.

B. H. Thiers, MD

Reference

1. Holberg CJ, Halonen M: Cytokines, atopy, and asthma. *Lancet* 362:1166-1167, 2003.

Probiotics and Prevention of Atopic Disease: 4-Year Follow-up of a Randomised Placebo-controlled Trial
Kalliomäki M, Salminen S, Poussa T, et al (Univ of Turku, Finland; STAT-Consulting, Tampere, Finland; Natl Public Health Inst, Turku, Finland)
Lancet 361:1869-1871, 2003   1–4

Background.—In an earlier study, these authors showed that perinatal administration of the probiotic *Lactobacillus rhamnosus* strain GG (ATCC 5310) halved the incidence of atopic eczema in high-risk children during the first 2 years of life. Now they have extended their follow-up to 4 years and have evaluated the persistence of this protective effect.

Methods.—The subjects were 4-year-old children (n = 107) at high risk for atopic eczema who had participated in a prior randomized placebo-controlled study. In that study, 159 mothers were given either 1×10^{10} colony-forming units of *Lactobacillus* GG per day or placebo beginning 4 weeks before expected delivery; the children continued treatment for 6 months after birth. Children were followed at 2 years to compare the incidence of atopic eczema between the active and placebo groups. In the current study, 107 mothers completed a questionnaire about allergic symptoms and medication usage during the 2 years since the previous follow-up, and children were given a physical examination to check for atopic eczema. In addition, 100 children underwent skin prick testing with a panel of common allergens, and 57 nonasthmatic children underwent measurements of exhaled nitric oxide (NO).

Results.—At 4 years, the incidence of atopic eczema was significantly lower in the children who received perinatal *Lactobacillus* GG (14 of 53, or 26.4%) than in the control group (25 of 54, or 46.3%; relative risk, 0.57). The incidence of skin test reactivity was similar in the experimental and control groups (18% and 20%, respectively). The mean exhaled NO concentration was significantly lower in the *Lactobacillus* GG group (10.8 vs 14.5 ppb).

Conclusion.—The efficacy of perinatal *Lactobacillus* GG in preventing atopic eczema in high-risk infants persists at 4 years. The untreated children may have had subclinical respiratory allergic diseases, as reflected by their higher exhaled NO levels, which suggests an even greater benefit from *lactobacillus* use. Perinatal probiotics offers a promising approach to the prevention of allergic diseases.

▶ A heightened risk of allergic diseases has been associated with improved hygienic conditions that reduce early life exposure to microbes. Microbial gut colonization early in life is thought to be crucial for healthy maturation of the naive immune system.[1] A study reviewed in the 2002 YEAR BOOK OF DERMATOLOGY AND DERMATOLOGIC SURGERY showed that perinatal administration of probiotics halved the development of atopic eczema in children at high risk during the first 2 years of life.[2] The current study shows that this preventive effect extends beyond that period. However, because respiratory allergic diseases typically manifest themselves at an older age, further follow-up data would be desirable.

B. H. Thiers, MD

References

1. Kalliomäki M, Isolauri E: Role of intestinal flora in the development of allergy. *Curr Opin Allergy Clin Immunol* 3:15-20, 2003.
2. Kalliomäki M, Salminen S, Arvilommi H, et al: Probiotics in primary prevention of atopic disease: A randomized placebo-controlled trial. *Lancet* 357:1076-1079, 2001. (2002 YEAR BOOK OF DERMATOLOGY AND DERMATOLOGIC SURGERY, pp 72-74.)

Staphylococcal Enterotoxin Induced IL-5 Stimulation as a Cofactor in the Pathogenesis of Atopic Disease: The Hygiene Hypothesis in Reverse?

Heaton T, Mallon D, Venaille T, et al (Inst for Child Health Research, Subiaco, Australia; Fremantle and Princess Margaret Hosps, Perth, Australia)
Allergy 58:252-256, 2003   1–5

Background.—Patients with atopic eczema/dermatitis syndrome (AEDS) have about a 90% incidence of *Staphylococcus aureus* colonization on their skin. Evidence suggests that epidermal staphylococcal infection is a pathogenic factor in atopic dermatitis. The role of staphylococcal enterotoxin B (SEB) in atopic disease was further investigated.

Methods.—The study subjects were 11 healthy nonatopic adults, 11 asymptomatic atopic adults, 17 patients with active AEDS, and 6 patients with active allergic asthma. Peripheral blood mononuclear cells were isolated from the participants and cultured for 24 or 96 hours with house dust mite, SEB and phytohemaglutinin. The supernatants were assayed for cytokine concentrations.

Findings.—SEB selectively stimulated interleukin (IL)-5 production in patients with AEDS but not in asymptomatic atopic or nonatopic persons. Susceptibility was comparable to the IL-5 stimulatory effects of SEB in allergic asthmatic patients.

Conclusion.—Given that IL-5-driven eosinophilia plays a central role in progression from mild atopy to severe disease, the data suggest a plausible mechanism for the AEDS-promoting effects of staphylococcal superantigens. SEB may play a similar role in atopic respiratory illness.

▶ The "hygiene hypothesis" suggests that decreased contact with the immunostimulatory microbial environment in the developed world has resulted in selective weakening of the T-helper 1 (Th1) arm of the immune system, leading to a predominance of Th2-mediated responses. Clinically, manifestations of such an immunologic microenvironment include atopic dermatitis and asthma, chronic inflammatory conditions in which there is a bias toward production of Th2 cytokines such as IL-4 and IL-5 that, in turn, are associated with increased immunoglobulin E production, eosinophilia, and activation of mast cells. Heaton et al argue that additional environmental stimuli, such as toxins released by skin-dwelling bacteria, may play a significant role in the disease process as well.

B. H. Thiers, MD

γ-Linolenic Acid Supplementation for Prophylaxis of Atopic Dermatitis—A Randomized Controlled Trial in Infants at High Familial Risk
van Gool CJAW, Thijs C, Henquet CJM, et al (Maastricht Univ, The Netherlands; Univ Hosp, Masstricht, The Netherlands)
Am J Clin Nutr 77:943-951, 2003   1–6

Background.—Essential fatty acids (EFAs) may be involved in the development of atopic disease. Research has shown that low n-6 long-chain polyene levels in early life appear to be associated with atopic disease later in life. The possible preventive effect of γ-linolenic acid (GLA) supplementation on the development of atopic dermatitis in at-risk infants was investigated.

Methods.—The study included 118 formula-fed infants with a maternal history of atopic disease who were enrolled in a double-blind, randomized, placebo-controlled trial. The babies were fed borage oil supplement containing 100 mg GLA or sunflower oil supplement as a placebo every day until 6 months of age and evaluated at age 1 year.

Findings.—In an intention-to-treat analysis, GLA supplementation was associated with a favorable trend for atopic dermatitis severity compared with that of placebo. However, GLA supplementation had no significant effects on the other atopic outcomes. The increase in GLA levels in plasma phospholipids between baseline and 3 months correlated negatively with atopic dermatitis severity at 1 year. No significant effect on total serum IgE levels was observed.

Conclusions.—Early GLA supplementation in at-risk infants does not appear to prevent the expression of atopy, as reflected by total serum IgE. However, such supplementation tends to reduce the severity of atopic dermatitis later in infancy.

▶ This study was well designed from the standpoint of patient selection, randomization, evaluation of compliance and statistical analysis. Supplementation of infants' diets with γ-linolenic acid through the age of 6 months did not decrease the incidence of atopic dermatitis at 1 year of age. There was a statistically nonsignificant trend for the severity of the dermatitis to be less in the treated group. However, there was apparently no attempt to standardize the skin care regimen or topical corticosteroid application in the infants, and patients appeared to have been evaluated for dermatitis on only 1 occasion, which is not adequate for evaluating a disease which can wax and wane. It is important to confirm whether supplementation of infants' diets with essential fatty acids decreases the severity of the disease, even if only in a subgroup of atopic children. A study of such dietary supplementation in infants with standardization of skin care regimens and frequent evaluation for the presence and severity of dermatitis would be helpful in determining whether supplementation given early in life is beneficial in reducing the severity of atopic dermatitis.

S. Raimer, MD

BCG Vaccination and Risk of Atopy

Krause TG, Hviid A, Koch A, et al (Statens Serum Institut, Copenhagen; Sisimiut Hosp, Greenland; Pharmacia, Copenhagen)
JAMA 289:1012-1015, 2003   1–7

Background.—In Greenland, Bacille Calmette-Guérin (BCG) vaccination (which elicits a strong T_H1-type immune response) was routinely given to all infants shortly after birth in an effort to reduce the incidence of tuberculosis in that country. This practice also was thought to prevent the development of atopy (which is characterized by T_H2-type cytokine expression). However, BCG vaccination was stopped in 1990, which provided the opportunity to compare atopy rates between vaccinated and unvaccinated children.

Methods.—The subjects were 1575 children, 8 to 16 years old, who were surveyed in November 1998 and November 2001. Each child and a parent completed a questionnaire regarding sociodemographic data and each child provided a blood sample. Subjects whose samples showed IgE to any of the 8 most common inhalant allergens were defined as atopic. Vaccination status was determined from a national database.

Results.—About two thirds of the subjects (1065, or 68%) had been vaccinated with BCG. About 15% (235, or 14.95) were atopic. In multivariate analyses, the incidence of atopy was not significantly different in the vaccinated children than in the unvaccinated subjects (16.2% vs 12.2%; odds ratio, 1.03). Furthermore, the age at vaccination was not significantly associated with the risk of atopy.

Conclusion.—The administration of BCG vaccine to infants does not protect them from the subsequent development of atopy.

▶ The ongoing urbanization in Greenland has made it a popular setting to study factors of possible importance in the pathogenesis of atopic disorders.[1] That country is gradually transitioning to a modern society where residents are no longer dependent on traditional activities such as hunting and fishing. Atopy is characterized by overexpression of T_H2-type cytokines, and it has been proposed that childhood exposure to certain infections and vaccinations that induce T_H1-type immune responses might protect against atopic diseases. In the current article, Krause et al demonstrate that the BCG vaccine does not appear to protect against the development of atopy.

B. H. Thiers, MD

Reference

1. Krause TG, Koch A, Friborg J, et al: Frequency of atopy in the Arctic in 1987 and 1998. *Lancet* 360:691-692, 2002. (2003 YEAR BOOK OF DERMATOLOGY AND DERMATOLOGIC SURGERY, pp 101-102.)

Epidemiology and Health Services Research: Comparison of Parent Knowledge, Therapy Utilization and Severity of Atopic Eczema Before and After Explanation and Demonstration of Topical Therapies by a Specialist Dermatology Nurse

Cork MJ, Britton J, Butler L, et al (Sheffield Children's Hosp, England; Royal Hallamshire Hosp, Sheffield, England; General Infirmary Leeds, England; et al)
Br J Dermatol 149:582-589, 2003   1–8

Introduction.—Noncompliance is known to contribute to therapeutic failure when simple oral regimens are involved, but few studies have examined the problem of compliance with complex treatment regimens for atopic eczema. Effective treatment of atopic eczema requires that the patient be knowledgeable about the development of the disease, its provoking factors, and the optimal way to use medicines. Children with atopic eczema were monitored to determine the impact of education by specialist dermatology nurses on therapy utilization and outcome.

Methods.—Fifty-one children were referred because their eczema could not be controlled in the community. At the first visit, the child and parents received an explanation of the nature of atopic eczema and a full skin examination was performed. The use of topical products was demonstrated in detail, and written instructions were given to summarize the explanation and demonstration. Children were seen at 3 weeks, then at 6- and 8-week intervals as control of eczema improved.

Results.—Fewer than 5% of parents had previously received or recalled receiving any explanation of the causes and treatment of eczema, and the disease was poorly controlled in all children. No emollient cream or ointment

---

TABLE 1.—Best Practice Management of Atopic Eczema

1　The key to the successful management of atopic eczema is to spend time to listen and to explain the nature of the disease and how to use topical therapies and dressings.[6,9,10,21,31,32]

2　In addition to explanation, practical demonstrations of how to apply topical products and dressings should be given.[8,10,12,23,33,34]

3　Emollients should be prescribed in adequate amounts and these should be used liberally and frequently, e.g. for emollient cream/ointment a minimum of 500 g per week.[10] Emollient bath oils and soap substitutes should also be used.

4　Topical steroids should be prescribed, considering the age of the patient, site to be treated and extent of the disease. These considerations guide the potency, quantity of steroid and duration of therapy.[35] The fingertip unit is a simple method to demonstrate the correct quantity to apply.[8,12]

5　Patients/parents should be given written instructions and information to reinforce the therapies which have been explained and demonstrated.[10]

6　Deterioration in previously stable eczema may be due to secondary bacterial or viral infection or to the development of contact dermatitis. Prompt diagnosis and treatment are important to prevent exacerbations.[10]

7　Treatments that suit one child may not suit another.[9] Treatments should be individualized to suit each child and their parents.

(Courtesy of Cork MJ, Britton J, Butler L, et al: Comparison of patient knowledge, therapy utilization and severity of atopic eczema before and after explanation and demonstration of topical therapies by a specialty dermatology nurse. *Br J Dermatol* 149:582-589, 2003. By permission of Blackwell Publishing.)

was being used by 24% of children, whereas 25% were being treated inappropriately with potent or very potent topical steroids. After the program of education and demonstration, there was an 89% reduction in the severity of the children's eczema and an 800% increase in the use of emollients.

Conclusion.—Specialty dermatology nurses can play an important role in the treatment of atopic eczema in children. A program of education and demonstration, followed by development of an individualized regimen and monitoring of compliance with topical therapies, offers the best practice management of atopic eczema (Table 1).

▶ Unfortunately, the nonpatient, friendly attitude ensconced in our modern health care system hardly encourages the kind of approach advocated by the authors. Because many patients forget a great deal of what they have been told, I try to provide my patients with as much written material as possible to help reinforce the onsite explanations and instructions they receive while in my office.

B. H. Thiers, MD

Experience With Low-Dose Methotrexate for the Treatment of Eczema in the Elderly
Shaffrali FCG, Colver GB, Messenger AG, et al (Royal Hallamshire Hosp, Sheffield, England; Royal Hosp, Chesterfield, England)
J Am Acad Dermatol 48:417-419, 2003   1–9

Background.—The literature contains little information on the use of methotrexate in patients with eczema. A retrospective study of 5 elderly patients given methotrexate for the treatment of eczema was reported.

Case Reports.—The patients were 3 women and 2 men, aged 67 to 83 years. One patient had vesicular hand dermatitis; 1 had atopic dermatitis; and 3 had unclassified eczema. Routine therapies had been ineffective in all patients. In 1 patient, a 67-year-old woman, recalcitrant vesicular hand dermatitis had been treated for 30 years with potent topical steroids and intermittent courses of oral steroids. In recent years, her dermatitis became more severe and less responsive to steroid treatment. She was unable to tolerate a course of topical psoralen plus ultraviolet A. Thus, oral methotrexate, 5 mg per week, was initiated. Within 3 weeks, dramatic improvement was seen. The patient commented that her skin was the best it had been in many years. Subsequently, she reported increasing fatigue, prompting a dose reduction to 2.5 mg per week. During 18 months of follow-up, no relapses occurred, and no other adverse effects developed.

Conclusions.—Methotrexate treatment was effective in 4 of 5 elderly patients with eczema. In 1 patient, treatment had to be discontinued because of other ongoing medical problems. Thus, methotrexate is an option in managing eczema in elderly persons that is unresponsive to topical therapy.

▶ Eczema and its associated pruritus can be debilitating in the elderly population. The authors report a simple, well-tolerated therapy for this disorder. The effectiveness of unusually low doses of methotrexate in the elderly may reflect the decreased creatinine clearance in these individuals.

B. H. Thiers, MD

The Safety and Efficacy of Tacrolimus Therapy in Patients Younger Than 2 Years With Atopic Dermatitis
Patel RR, Vander Straten MR, Korman NJ (Case Western Reserve Univ, Cleveland, Ohio)
Arch Dermatol 139:1184-1186, 2003   1–10

Background.—Tacrolimus ointment, a recently developed topical immunomodulator, has been approved for the treatment of atopic dermatitis (AD) in patients older than 2 years. Concerns about possible systemic toxicity have limited treatment options for children younger than 2 years. The safety and efficacy of topical tacrolimus was investigated in children with AD younger than 2 years.

Methods.—In a retrospective chart review, 12 children younger than 2 years who were treated for AD with tacrolimus were identified. Data were obtained on AD severity, treatment response, concentration and blood levels of tacrolimus, adverse effects, and laboratory results.

Findings.—All children had symptomatic improvement. No significant adverse effects occurred. Nine children were given 0.03% tacrolimus ointment, and 3 were given 0.1%. Blood levels of tacrolimus were less than 1.5 ng/mL in all children. Tacrolimus levels did not appear to differ between those given 0.03% and those given 0.1% ointment. Platelet counts were increased in 4 children.

Conclusions.—Tacrolimus may be an appropriate treatment for AD in children younger than 2 years. In the current series, there were no measurable tacrolimus blood levels and no adverse effects in the young children treated. Platelet counts were increased in one third of the children treated, possibly indicating the presence of chronic inflammatory disease.

▶ It is somewhat reassuring that in this small retrospective study tacrolimus blood concentrations were below detectable levels in 12 children with moderate to severe AD who had used the drug for at least 1 month. The ointment had not been applied for 24 hours before blood samples were obtained; thus, blood concentrations on days the drug was applied are not known. A larger prospective study of infants with extensive AD with weekly determinations of tacrolimus blood levels would be much more helpful in determining the safety of the drug in this age group.

S. Raimer, MD

Cost-effectiveness Analysis of Tacrolimus Ointment Versus High-Potency Topical Corticosteroids in Adults With Moderate to Severe Atopic Dermatitis

Ellis CN, Drake LA, Prendergast MM, et al (Univ of Michigan, Ann Arbor; Harvard Med School, Boston; Fujisawa Healthcare Inc, Deerfield, Ill; et al)
J Am Acad Dermatol 48:553-563, 2003   1–11

Introduction.—The financial impact of treating patients with atopic dermatitis (AD) is substantial. One recent study that considered medical, hospital, direct, and indirect costs estimated annual costs per patient at more than $4600. A computerized cost-effectiveness analysis combined outcomes and costs to compare high-potency topical corticosteroids (HPTCs) with tacrolimus ointment, a new topical immunomodulator used to treat moderate to severe AD.

Methods.—A Markov model was applied to accurately represent the cyclic nature of AD. The model randomly assigned simulated adult patients to HPTCs (2-week or 4-week cycles of therapy) or to tacrolimus. Patients were considered to be unresponsive or not well controlled with midpotency topical corticosteroids. Treatment efficacy was defined as disease-controlled days (DCDs) on which patients experienced a greater than 75% improvement. Cost analysis focused on prescription drug and physician costs.

Results.—Total costs were $1682 for HPTCs in 2-week cycles, $1317 for HPTCs in 4-week cycles, and $1323 for tacrolimus ointment. Primary drug costs were higher for tacrolimus ($727) than for HPTCs ($304 for 2-week and $366 for 4-week cycles), but secondary treatment costs were higher with HPTCs ($787 for 2-week and $509 for 4-week cycles versus $162 for tacrolimus). Total efficacy in DCDs was 194 with 4-week HPTCs, 190 with tacrolimus ointment, and 185 with 2-week HPTCs. The most costly average cost-effectiveness ratio was for 2-week HPTCs ($9.08/DCD); HPTCs ($6.80) and tacrolimus ointment ($6.97) had similar values.

Discussion.—Tacrolimus ointment was a more cost-effective option for patients with AD when class I/II HPTC use was restricted to 2-week intervals. The considerably higher cost of tacrolimus itself was offset by reduced time and costs associated with secondary therapy, physician costs, and total costs. In addition, total efficacy as measured by DCDs was higher with tacrolimus (but similar to HPTCs in 4-week cycles).

▶ Neither high-potency topical corticosteroids nor topical immunomodulators by themselves represent the ideal long-term treatment for atopic dermatitis. The best approach can be determined only by future studies. Moreover, it is uncertain whether the assumptions used by Ellis et al in their cost-effectiveness analysis represent "real world" assumptions.

B. H. Thiers, MD

Tacrolimus 0·1% Ointment for Seborrhoeic Dermatitis: An Open-Label Pilot Study

Braza TJ, Dicarlo JB, Soon SL, et al (Emory Univ, Atlanta, Ga)

Br J Dermatol 148:1242-1244, 2003   1–12

Background.—Seborrheic dermatitis is a chronic inflammatory dermatosis that affects approximately 2% to 5% of the US population. It is characterized by erythematous, greasy, scaling patches on the sebaceous regions of the head, neck, and trunk. The pathogenesis is controversial. Conventional therapies include antifungal preparations to decrease colonization by lipophilic yeasts, which are thought by some to be involved in the pathogenesis of the disease, and topical corticosteroids to decrease inflammation. However, long-term treatment with topical corticosteroids on the head and neck may result in skin atrophy and telangiectasia. Tacrolimus ointment may be beneficial in the treatment of seborrheic dermatitis because it is a topical noncorticosteroid immunosuppressant without the adverse effects related to long-term topical corticosteroid use. The efficacy and safety of tacrolimus ointment for the treatment of seborrheic dermatitis were assessed.

Methods.—A group of 16 patients (15 men and 1 woman) were enrolled in a 6-week, open-label, uncontrolled trial of daily topical tacrolimus 0.1% ointment. After a 2-week washout period for study subjects using conventional therapy for seborrheic dermatitis, study medication was applied nightly to the affected areas until clinical clearance was observed, and then for 7 days thereafter. The extent and severity of lesions were assessed at baseline and at weeks 2 and 6 by using 4 parameters: clinical assessment of erythema and scaling with a scale from 0 to 3; investigator global assessment; the patient's global assessment with a scale from 0 to 6; and serial photography.

Results.—The study was completed by 13 of 16 patients (81%). Relative to the mean baseline value, the mean lesional erythema scores improved by 66.1% and 70.9% at weeks 2 and 6, respectively. Compared with baseline, the mean scaling scores improved by 63.7% at week 2 and 87.8% at week 6. The mean investigator global assessment scores relative to the mean baseline values improved by 76.6% at week 2 and by 82.7% at week 6. The mean patient global assessment scores improved by 69.4% at week 2 and by 83.5% at week 6, relative to the mean baseline value. There were no serious adverse events, with the exception of transient application site pruritus and burning in 2 patients.

Conclusions.—The findings of this pilot study suggest that topical tacrolimus 0.1% is efficacious in the short-term treatment of seborrheic dermatitis. Further controlled trials are necessary to confirm the efficacy and safety of topical tacrolimus for this condition.

► The results of this uncontrolled trial certainly need to be duplicated under more stringent experimental protocols. Although the use of a nonsteroidal preparation for this chronic facial dermatosis does seem appealing, application of a topical immunosuppressive agent to an area of skin subjected to frequent and intense sun exposure might theoretically increase the risk of cutaneous carcinogenesis. The predisposition to skin cancer of patients receiving systemic treatment with the related immunosuppressive macrolide, cyclosporine, is well documented.

B. H. Thiers, MD

Microbiological Aspects of Diaper Dermatitis

Ferrazzini G, Kaiser RR, Cheng S-KH, et al (Medinova Ltd, Zurich, Switzerland)
Dermatology 206:136-141, 2003   1–13

Background.—In diaper dermatitis, digestive enzymes in stool make affected areas highly susceptible to mechanical abrasion and microbial infection. Evidence suggests superinfection of involved skin with *Candida* species and/or *Staphylococcus aureus* may aggravate the dermatitis. Whether the extent of *Candida* or *S aureus* colonization correlates with the severity of diaper dermatitis was examined.

Methods.—The research subjects were 76 infants 2 months to 2 years of age who had no diseases of the skin or mucosa other than diaper dermatitis. The skin was healthy in 48 patients (control subjects), but 28 infants had mild to moderate diaper dermatitis. Perianal, inguinal, and oral swabs were tested for *Candida* and *S aureus*. In addition, a 5-point scale (0 = not present, 4 = strong symptoms) was used to describe the severity of 4 symptoms of diaper dermatitis (ie, erythema, pustules, maceration, and desquamation); the maximum possible score was 16.

Results. Candida colonization was significantly more common in the infants with diaper dermatitis than in the control subjects at all 3 swab loca-

TABLE 2.—Negative/Positive and Semiquantitative Culture Results for Children With Healthy Skin and for Those With Clinically Manifest Diaper Dermatitis

	S. aureus Colonisation			*Candida* sp Colonisation		
	Perianal	Inguinal	Oral	Perianal	Inguinal	Oral
Collective with healthy skin (n = 48)						
Culture negative	42	43	43	39	43	36
Culture positive	6 (12.5)	5 (10.4)	5 (10.4)	9 (18.8)	5 (10.4)	12 (25.0)
Isolated	3	1	4	6	4	4
Few	0	2	0	2	0	1
Moderate	3	2	1	1	0	4
Many	0	0	0	0	1	3
Collective with diaper dermatitis (n = 28)						
Culture negative	22	24	26	7	14	9
Culture positive	6 (21.4)	4 (14.3)	2 (7.1)	21 (75.0)	14 (50.0)	19 (67.9)
Isolated	3	0	1	7	2	1
Few	0	0	0	4	1	7
Moderate	1	1	0	6	5	7
Many	2	3	1	4	6	4

Note: Figures in parentheses indicate percentages.
(Courtesy of Ferrazzini G, Kaiser RR, Cheng S-KH, et al: Microbiological aspects of diaper dermatitis. *Dermatology* 206:136-141, 2003. Reproduced with permission of S. Karger AG, Basel.)

tions (Table 2). *S aureus* colonization at the 3 swab locations, however, did not differ significantly between the 2 groups. The severity of disease correlated significantly and positively with the extent of *Candida* colonization at all 3 swab locations.

Conclusion.—Both healthy infants and infants with diaper dermatitis have frequent *Candida* and *S aureus* colonization in the perianal, inguinal, and oral areas. However, colonization with *Candida* is significantly greater in infants with diaper dermatitis, and more extensive *Candida* colonization correlates with disease exacerbation. Thus, semiquantitative analysis to determine the extent of *Candida* colonization is preferable to merely identifying the presence or absence of these species and would improve the effectiveness of diaper dermatitis treatment.

▶ The authors suggest that semiquantitative cultures be performed routinely to determine whether antimicrobial therapy should be used to treat diaper dermatitis. Because 75% of children with diaper dermatitis had cultures of the perianal area that grew *Candida*, it would seem more cost-effective to routinely use topical anticandidal therapy, at least for moderate to severe dermatitis, and to do cultures only when clinically indicated.

S. Raimer, MD

Use of an Anti-interleukin-5 Antibody in the Hypereosinophilic Syndrome With Eosinophilic Dermatitis
Plötz S-G, Simon H-U, Darsow U, et al (Technical Univ, Munich, Germany; Univ of Bern, Switzerland; GlaxoSmithKline, Essex, England)
N Engl J Med 349:2334-2339, 2003   1–14

Background.—The hypereosinophilic syndrome consists of a heterogeneous group of disorders in which eosinophil-mediated tissue damage causes hypereosinophilia and organ dysfunction. The effects of mepolizumab, a neutralizing anti-interleukin-5 antibody, in 3 patients are discussed. One case (Patient No. 2) is summarized.

> *Case Report.*—Woman, 62, with eosinophilic dermatitis reported dyspnea, night sweats, low-grade fever, fatigue, weight loss, abdominal pain, and severe, generalized pruritus of 7 months' duration. Examination revealed widespread skin lesions, including pruriginous, urticarial, and eczematous lesions. She also had erythematosus, centrally ulcerated nodules. Numerous eosinophils were found in skin and bone marrow biopsy specimens. Treatment with antihistamines, dapsone, topical corticosteroids, and systemic corticosteroids was attempted with no success, with the proportion of eosinophils in the peripheral blood ranging from 11% to 27%. IV mepolizumab, 750 mg, was then administered. Within 24 hours, the peripheral blood eosinophil count declined markedly. Serum concentrations of eosinophil cationic protein also decreased. Two weeks later, a second infu-

sion of mepolizumab was given, and the patient's clinical condition started to improve. In 3 weeks, the patient was nearly free of pruritus and other symptoms. Her fever, fatigue, and abdominal pain were also markedly diminished. However, the patient's clinical condition started to deteriorate 5 weeks after the second dose, with increases in the peripheral blood eosinophil count. Another dose resulted in immediate improvement. A 750-mg dose was given monthly for another 7 months, and the patient became almost symptom free. No adverse effects occurred. Unfortunately, treatment had to be stopped because mepolizumab became unavailable. The patient's condition again worsened. Currently, corticosteroids and imatinib mesylate are being given, with marginal success.

Conclusions.—Patients with eosinophilic dermatitis and increased interleukin-5 levels in the blood may benefit from treatment with anti-interleukin-5 antibody. Long-term studies of mepolizumab for patients with the hypereosinophilic syndrome are needed.

▶ The hypereosinophilic syndrome is a heterogeneous disorder with a highly variable response to treatments such as systemic corticosteroids, hydroxyurea, interferon-α and imatinib mesylate. Some patients, particularly those who respond to imatinib mesylate, probably have a myeloproliferative disease or a clonal disorder that is largely independent of interleukin-5, a cytokine required for the differentiation, activation, and survival of eosinophils. In contrast, interleukin-5 does seem to have a critical role in other patients with this syndrome, as demonstrated by the striking clinical response reported here to infusions of a humanized anti-interleukin-5 antibody.

B. H. Thiers, MD

IL-18 Binding Protein Protects Against Contact Hypersensitivity

Plitz T, Saint-Mézard P, Satho M, et al (Serono Pharmaceutical Research Inst, Geneva)
J Immunol 171:1164-1171, 2003   1–15

Background.—Contact hypersensitivity (CHS) is a T-cell–mediated inflammation of the skin that manifests as contact dermatitis and is associated with elevated serum levels of interleukin (IL)-18. The activity of IL-18 can be inhibited by its natural binding protein, IL-18BP. The role of IL-18 in CHS was examined in mice sensitized to 2.4-dinitrofluorobenzene (DNFB).

Methods and Results.—Mice were sensitized with the hapten DNFB and then re-exposed 5 days later to elicit CHS. Mice were treated from the time of challenge with human IL-18BP isoform a. This treatment significantly reduced swelling after DNFB challenge. This effect was IS-18BP specific, and could not be elicited with a nonspecific protein. Even after rechallenge, swelling was substantially reduced in IL-18BP treated mice. Interferon (IFN)-γ production was reduced in supernatants from T cells of IL-18BP treated mice. Cell sorting demonstrated that this was due to a reduction in recruitment of αβ T cells to the challenge site.

Conclusions.—The results of this murine study demonstrate that IL-18 contributes to contact hypersensitivity by increasing recruitment of IFN-γ producing αβ T cells to the site. IL-18BP reduces symptoms of contact dermatitis. IL-18BP appears to have therapeutic potential for the treatment of inflammatory skin diseases.

▶ These investigators examined the possible therapeutic effect of a naturally occurring inhibitor of IL-18, IL-18BP, in a murine model of contact hypersensitivity induced by DNFB. IL-18 is produced by human keratinocytes exposed to sensitizers of contact sensitivity; these cells also express IL-18BP in response to IFN-γ. In this study, mice were injected with recombinant human IL-18BP before the primary challenge with DNFB and before re-exposure to the sensitizer in a second group of animals that had previously received the primary challenge without treatment. The data obtained showed that the binding protein protected the animals against both the initial sensitization and the effect of repeated challenge with DNFB, with a significant reduction in the tissue swelling characteristic of contact sensitivity in this model. Furthermore, the levels of IFN-γ produced by cells obtained from the test tissues was dramatically reduced in cells from treated mice compared to those from control animals. This was shown to be due to a significantly reduced infiltrate of T cells in the tissues of animals treated with IL-18BP. This study not only emphasizes the role of IL-18 in contact hypersensitivity, but also suggests that IL-18BP may be of therapeutic benefit in human diseases such as contact dermatitis.

G. M. P. Galbraith, MD

The Detection of Clinically Relevant Contact Allergens Using a Standard Screening Tray of Twenty-Three Allergens
Saripalli YV, Achen F, Belsito DV (Univ of Kansas, Kansas City)
J Am Acad Dermatol 49:65-69, 2003   1–16

Introduction.—Patch testing remains the gold standard for the diagnosis of allergic contact dermatitis. There are, however, more than 3000 known sensitizers, and the commonly used T.R.U.E. test panels include only 23 allergens. Patients evaluated during a 7-year period were retrospectively reviewed to determine the ability of T.R.U.E. test allergens to detect all relevant allergic reactions.

Methods.—Patients underwent patch testing with T.R.U.E. test allergens during the period from 1995 through 2001. All participants completed a North American Contact Dermatitis Group questionnaire that covered occupational, demographic, and medical data, and findings were used to select additional allergens to include in their testing. Those with positive allergic reactions were classified as having reactions only to allergens on the T.R.U.E. test, reactions only to allergens not included on the T.R.U.E. test, or reactions to both T.R.U.E. test allergens and the additional allergens.

TABLE 2.—Fifty Most Common Allergens Detected: 1995-2001

Allergen	Positive Patch Test (N)	Clinically Relevant Patch Text (N)
1. Nickel sulfate	113	90
2. Bacitracin	92	73
3. Neomycin sulfate	88	70
4. Fragrance mix	86	74
5. Quaternium-15	85	78
6. Formaldehyde	80	72
7. Thimerosal	77	15
8. Balsam of Peru	71	61
9. Cobalt chloride	57	36
10. Sodium gold thiosulfate	52	8
11. Thiuram mix	47	40
12. P-phenylenediamine	46	29
13. Ethyleneurea/melamine formaldehyde	43	22
14. MDBG/PE	40	11
15. MCI/MI	38	37
16. 2-bromo-2-nitropropane-1,3-diol	34	12
17. Carba mix	34	28
18. Diazolidinyl urea	33	30
19. Potassium dichromate	30	17
20. DMDM hydantoin	27	25
21. Benzalkonium chloride	25	17
22. Imidazolidinyl urea	25	23
23. Propylene glycol	25	24
24. Colophony	24	15
25. Ethylenediamine dihydrochloride	24	8
26. Glutaraldehyde	24	16
27. Benzocaine	22	6
28. P-tert-butylphenol formaldehyde resin	19	10
29. Cocamidopropyl betaine	17	17
30. Mercaptobenzothiazole	17	12
31. Epoxy resin	16	14
32. Lanolin alcohol	16	12
33. Tixocortol pivalate	16	16
34. Doxepin	15	9
35. Benzophenone-4	14	4
36. Benzoyl peroxide	14	7
37. Disperse blue 106	14	11
38. Melamine formaldehyde	14	11
39. Glyceryl thioglycolate	13	10
40. Urea formaldehyde	13	10
41. Mercapto mix	11	9
42. Tosylamide formaldehyde	11	10
43. Mixed dialkylthioureas	10	8
44. Oleamidopropyl dimethylamine	10	10
45. Black rubber mix	9	6
46. Ethyl acrylate	9	9
47. Grotan BK	9	5
48. Methyl methacrylate	9	8
49. Tetramethylol acetylenediurea	9	6
50. Budesonide	8	8

Allergens in boldface type are those not included among T.R.U.E. test allergens.

Abbreviations: MCI/MI, Methylchloroisothiazolinone/methylisothiazolinone; *MDBG/PE*, methyldibromo glutaronitrile/phenoxyethanol.

(Reprinted by permission of the publisher from Saripalli YV, Achen F, Belsito DV: The detection of clinically relevant contact allergens using a standard screening tray of twenty-three allergens. *J Am Acad Dermatol* 49:65-69, 2003. Copyright 2003 by Elsevier.)

Results.—Six hundred sixteen (68.6%) of 898 patients who were patch tested had at least 1 positive allergic reaction. Only 25.5% of this group would have been fully evaluated with testing limited to the T.R.U.E. panels. No allergens would have been detected by the T.R.U.E panels in 22.4% of patients with allergic contact dermatitis, and 52.1% of patients would have only been partially evaluated. Expanding the panel to include the top 50 allergens detected in this study group (Table 2) would have significantly increased the yield of positive reactions, but even this larger panel would fail to provide a correct and complete diagnosis in more than 50% of patients.

Discussion.—Patch testing for potential allergic contact dermatitis can provide early diagnosis and treatment, with improved quality of life. But the available 23-allergen panels approved by the Food and Drug Administration fail to detect many clinically relevant allergens. Insurance carriers, unfortunately, often limit testing to a very restricted screening series.

▶ This article confirms what all of us know: the Food and Drug Administration–approved T.R.U.E. test panel of 23 allergens simply is not comprehensive enough to diagnose a majority of cases of suspected contact dermatitis. In many regions of the United States, insurers restrict patch testing to no more than 30 allergens; thus, the physician's ability to adequately evaluate a patient is limited even if an expanded number of allergens (chosen according to the patient's environment and history) was available.

B. H. Thiers, MD

Impact of Atopic Skin Diathesis on Occupational Skin Disease Incidence in a Working Population

Dickel H, Bruckner TM, Schmidt A, et al (Univ Hosp of Heidelberg, Germany; Bavarian Health and Safety Executive, Nuremberg, Germany)
J Invest Dermatol 121:37-40, 2003   1–17

Introduction.—The findings of a number of studies indicate that workers with occupational skin disease (OSD) have a high frequency of atopic skin diathesis (ASD) relative to the total population. Within the working population, however, the proportion of OSD attributable to ASD is unknown. This issue was addressed by analyzing data from a population-based register of OSD in northern Bavaria, Germany.

Methods.—All initial reports of OSD reported between 1990 and 1999 were prospectively registered, then assessed for final diagnoses. Of the 5285 cases of OSD reported, 3730 (71%) were confirmed to have occupation as a determining factor or cofactor. Criteria for ASD were a history of flexural involvement, visible flexural eczematous or lichenified dermatitis, and an atopy score of 10 or more.

Results.—An ASD was present in 1366 workers (37%) with confirmed OSD. Assuming the prevalence of ASD in the total population to be 20%, 21.6% of OSD cases within the 24 occupational groups studied may be attributed to individual susceptibility resulting from ASD. Among cases, workers with ASD were found to have OSD diagnosed at a younger age and earlier in working life than workers without ASD. Most cases of OSD (91%) consisted of occupational contact dermatitis of both irritant and allergic types affecting the hands.

Discussion.—A large proportion of OSD may be explained by the attributable risk of ASD. Because ASD makes the development of OSD more likely, workers with ASD would benefit from special advice on skin protection and skin care measures.

▶ The authors show that an underlying ASD predisposes patients to OSD. Because of the high prevalence of atopic tendencies in the general population (approximately 20%), it may be impractical to discourage individuals other than those who are most severely affected from entering occupations that put them at high risk for exacerbation of their skin disease.

B. H. Thiers, MD

Relation Between Vesicular Eruptions on the Hands and Tinea Pedis, Atopic Dermatitis and Nickel Allergy
Bryld LE, Agner T, Menné T (Univ of Copenhagen, Hellerup)
Acta Derm Venereol 83:186-188, 2003   1–18

Background.—Pompholyx is characterized by vesicular eruptions on the palms and sides of the fingers. The cause of this condition has not been determined. Whether tinea pedis, atopic dermatitis, or nickel allergy is a risk factor for the development of such vesicular eruptions was investigated.

Methods.—Three hundred ninety-eight persons participated in the study. Each was queried for a history of previous eczema and atopic dermatitis. Clinical examination and a patch test with nickel were performed. A sample from the fourth interdigital space on the right foot was obtained for tinea pedis testing.

Findings.—Participants with tinea pedis had a 3.58 relative risk for vesicular eruptions. The relative risk was 1.44 for participants with atopic dermatitis and 0.45 for those with nickel allergy.

Conclusions.—These data indicate an association between tinea pedis and vesicular eruptions on the hands. However, in the current series, there was no correlation with atopic dermatitis or nickel allergy.

▶ Although no association was found between pompholyx, atopic dermatitis, and nickel allergy, the authors did illustrate that the so-called dermatophytid is a relatively common occurrence.

B. H. Thiers, MD

Provocative Use Test of Nickel Coins in Nickel-Sensitized Subjects and Controls

Zhai H, Chew A-L, Bashir SJ, et al (Univ of California, San Francisco; Nickel Producers Environmental Research Assoc, Durham, NC; Euromerican Technology Resources Inc, Lafayette, Calif)
Br J Dermatol 149:311-317, 2003   1–19

Background.—The degree to which handling nickel-containing coins can elicit nickel dermatitis has not been established. This question was investigated in nickel-sensitized and control subjects.

Methods.—Ten sensitized and 8 nonsensitized persons participated in the study after history taking, physical examination, and diagnostic patch testing. Each participant handled 10 coins, including nickel-containing and non–nickel-containing coins, at 5-minute intervals, followed by 5 minutes' rest, for 8 hours per day in a crossover design. The total length of coin handling was 12 days, with weekends off. Visual scores and bioengineering measures were obtained at 4 sites on days 1, 5, and 12.

Findings.—No significant differences in visual or bioengineering data were recorded for nickel-sensitized compared with non–nickel-sensitized participants handling nickel-containing coins on days 1, 5, or 12. Scores also did not differ between day 12 and day 1 for nickel-sensitized participants handling nickel-containing coins. There were no differences between the handling of nickel-containing and non–nickel-containing coins by nickel-sensitized participants on days 5 and 12. Scores did not differ between nickel-sensitized participants wearing gloves or not wearing gloves and handling nickel-containing coins on day 12.

Conclusions.—In this study, handling nickel-containing coins daily did not result in allergic contact dermatitis, as determined by visual scoring or bioengineering parameters.

▶ The data suggest that only highly sensitive subjects might be susceptible to clinically evident contact dermatitis as a result of extensive handling of nickel-containing coins.

B. H. Thiers, MD

Factors Associated With the Development of Peanut Allergy in Childhood

Lack G, for the Avon Longitudinal Study of Parents and Children Study Team (Imperial College, London; et al)
N Engl J Med 348:977-985, 2003   1–20

Background.—The prevalence of peanut allergy appears to be increasing. Reports suggest that atopy, a family history of peanut allergy, prenatal maternal consumption of peanuts, or consumption of peanuts or peanut oil by infants may cause sensitization to peanuts, but some of these findings have not been replicated. Previous studies of the causes of peanut allergy have been unable to define this phenomenon on the basis of a double-blind, placebo-controlled food challenge and have not used longitudinal data to identify its antecedents. Data from a longitudinal study in the United Kingdom that was designed to collect information prospectively from early pregnancy and throughout childhood were analyzed.

Methods.—Data for this study were obtained from the Avon Longitudinal Study of Parents and Children, a geographically defined cohort study of 13,971 preschool children. This cohort was reviewed to identify members with a convincing history of peanut allergy and to select a subgroup that reacted to a double-blind peanut challenge. After the collection of prospective data on the entire cohort, detailed information was retrospectively collected by interview from the parents of children with peanut reactions and of children from 2 groups of control subjects. One control group consisted of a random sample from the cohort, and a second control group consisted of a group of children whose mothers had a history of eczema and who themselves had eczema in the first 6 months of life.

Results.—A history of peanut allergy was identified in 49 children, and the allergy was confirmed by peanut challenge in 23 of 36 children tested. No evidence of prenatal sensitization from the maternal diet was noted, and peanut-specific IgE was not detectable in the cord blood. An independent association of peanut allergy was noted with (1) the intake of soy milk or soy formula; (2) a rash over joints and in skin creases; and (3) an oozing, crusted rash. A significant independent association of peanut allergy was noted also with the use of skin preparations containing peanut oil.

Conclusions.—The application of peanut oil to inflamed skin in children may result in sensitization to peanut protein. The association of peanut allergy with soy protein reported in this study could arise from cross-sensitization through common epitopes.

▶ From a cohort of 13,971 preschool children, 49 children were found by interview to have a history of peanut allergy. Thirty-six of them were subjected to a peanut challenge, and 23 were confirmed to have peanut allergy. After comparing diet, skin disease, and treatments used in these children with children who had atopic dermatitis (but not peanut allergy) and to other children who served as control subjects, the authors hypothesized risk factors for the development of peanut allergy that will need to be confirmed by further study.

S. Raimer, MD

Effect of Anti-IgE Therapy in Patients With Peanut Allergy
Leung DYM, for the TNX-901 Peanut Allergy Study Group (Natl Jewish Med and Research Ctr, Denver; et al)
N Engl J Med 348:986-993, 2003   1–21

Background.—Peanut-induced anaphylaxis affects an estimated 1.5 million people annually in the United States, resulting in 50 to 100 deaths each year. Severe reactions can occur at any age, and the previous reaction cannot be used reliably to predict the course of the next. In some individuals, even the first reaction may be severe. The current treatment for peanut allergy is avoidance or rescue with epinephrine. However, only a small proportion of patients with peanut allergy carry epinephrine, and even timely injection may not prevent death. Avoidance is extremely difficult. TNX-901 is a humanized IgG1 monoclonal antibody against IgE that recognizes and masks an epitope in the C_H3 region of IgE responsible for binding to the high-affinity Fcε receptor on mast cells and basophils. The effectiveness of TNX-901 in raising the threshold of sensitivity to peanuts was assessed.

Methods.—The study included 84 patients with a history of immediate hypersensitivity to peanut in a double-blind, randomized, dose-ranging trial. Patients underwent a double-blind, placebo-controlled oral food challenge at screening to confirm hypersensitivity and establish the threshold dose of encapsulated peanut flour. The patients were then randomly assigned in a 3:1 ratio to receive either TNX-901 at 150, 300, or 450 mg, or placebo subcutaneously every 4 weeks for 4 doses. The patients underwent a final food challenge within 2 to 4 weeks after the fourth dose.

Results.—TNX-901 was well tolerated by all patients in every treatment group. From a mean baseline threshold of sensitivity of 178 to 436 mg of peanut flour in the various groups, the mean increases in the oral food-challenge threshold were 710 mg in the placebo group, 913 mg in the group that received 150 mg of TNX-901, 1650 mg in the group that received 300 mg of TNX-901, and 2627 mg in the group that received 450 mg of TNX-901 (Fig 1).

Conclusions.—A 450-mg dose of TNX-901 significantly increased the threshold of sensitivity to peanut on oral food challenge from a level equal to about half a peanut (178 mg) to a level that equaled nearly 9 peanuts (2805

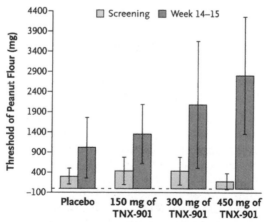

FIGURE 1.—Mean threshold dose of peanut flour eliciting symptoms in patients receiving TNX-901 or placebo. The mean increase in the threshold of sensitivity, as compared with that in the placebo group, reached significance only in the 450-mg group ($P < .001$); however, results of the test for trend with increasing doses were significant ($P < .001$). *I bars* are 95 percent confidence intervals. (Reprinted by permission of *The New England Journal of Medicine* from Sampson HA, for the TNX-901 Peanut Allergy Study Group: Effect of anti-IgE therapy in patients with peanut allergy. *N Engl J Med* 348:986-993, 2003. Copyright 2003, Massachusetts Medical Society. All rights reserved.)

mg). This effect should be sufficient to protect these patients against most instances of unintended peanut ingestion.

▶ The current treatment for peanut allergy is either avoidance or epinephrine injection. Avoidance is difficult, and evidently most individuals allergic to peanuts fail to carry epinephrine on a routine basis. Hyposensitization has been attempted, but the risk:benefit ratio is unfavorable.[1] Leung et al report the successful use of TNX-901, a humanized IgG1 monoclonal antibody against IgE that binds with high affinity to an epitope in the C_H3 domain, in patients proven to have allergy to peanuts by food challenge tests. Monthly injection of the antibody appeared to be safe by all criteria measured. Increased tolerance to peanuts developed in a dose dependent fashion. Treatment with TNX-901 could prove lifesaving to many of the estimated 1.5 million individuals in the United States allergic to peanuts, many of whom are accidentally exposed each year.

S. Raimer, MD

Reference

1. Nelson HS, Lahr J, Rule R, et al: Treatment of anaphylactic sensitivity to peanuts by immunotherapy with injections of aqueous peanut extract. *J Allergy Clin Immunol* 99:744-751, 1997.

Ant Venom Immunotherapy: A Double-blind, Placebo-controlled, Crossover Trial
Brown SGA, Wiese MD, Blackman KE, et al (Royal Hobart Hosp, Tasmania, Australia; Flinders Univ, Bedford Park, South Australia)
Lancet 361:1001-1006, 2003   1–22

Introduction.—Jack jumper ants (Fig 1; see color plate IV), native Australian stinging ants of the aggressive species complex *Myrmecia pilosula*, are implicated in about 90% of allergic reactions to ant venom in southeastern Australia. Treatment has consisted of whole-body extract (WBE), but *M pilosula* WBE was withdrawn in Australia in the early 1990s because of lack of efficacy. Venom immunotherapy (VIT), effective in the treatment of bee and wasp sting allergy, was evaluated in a randomized study.

Methods.—The double-blind, placebo-controlled crossover trial enrolled 68 healthy volunteers who were allergic to *M pilosula* venom. Thirty-three received placebo and 35 received *M pilosula* VIT. Administration of VIT was done in accordance with an outpatient semirush procedure (Table 1). An arbitrary maintenance dose, 100 µg, was chosen on the basis of doses used in bee and wasp VIT. A deliberate sting challenge was conducted in hospital emergency rooms. Systemic allergic reactions were graded on a scale of I to IV.

Results.—The primary analysis included 23 patients receiving VIT and 29 receiving placebo. Twenty-one of those receiving placebo (72%) experienced an objectively defined systemic reaction to sting challenges; 8 of these reactions were grade IV (associated with hypotension). None of the 23 pa-

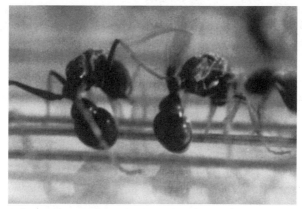

FIGURE 1.—Jack jumper ant, *Myrmecia pilosula*, seen here depositing venom on a glass slide in response to electrical stimulation. This ant is 10 to 12 mm long and jet black except for yellow-orange mandibles and leg tips. It jumps to attack, grasps firmly with its mandibles, and injects venom with an abdominal stinger. (Reprinted with permission from Elsevier Science from Brown SGA, Wiese MD, Blackman KE, et al: Ant venom immunotherapy: A double-blind, placebo-controlled, crossover trial. *Lancet* 361:1001-1006, 2003.)

tients receiving VIT experienced a systemic reaction. The additional 12 patients randomly assigned to VIT had their treatment allocation revealed and were thus excluded from the primary analysis. Only 1 of these 12 patients reacted to the sting challenge, and the reaction was transient urticaria that did not require treatment. After crossover to VIT from placebo, 1 of 26 patients reacted with transient urticaria.

Conclusion.—Venom immunotherapy proved an effective treatment for allergy to jack jumper ant venom. The risk of systemic symptoms was quite high in the placebo group, whereas only transient urticaria occurred in a few

TABLE 1.—Outpatient Semi-Rush Hyposensitization Regimen

	Amount of Venom (µg)		
Visit			
1	0·0001	0·001	0·01
2	0·01	0·1	0·3
3	0·3	1	3
4	3	10	..
5	10	20	..
6	20	30	..
7	30	40	..
8	50	50	..
9	70	30	..
Maintenance	100	..	..

Injections were given at 20- to 60-minute intervals. This regimen was used as a guide only and was adjusted in accordance with patient tolerance. Visits 1 to 10 were 5 to 10 days apart and then gradually extended to monthly maintenance visits. The minimum period of observation after the last injection of each visit was 1 hour.

(Reprinted with permission from Elsevier Science from Brown SGA, Wiese MD, Blackman KE, et al: Ant venom immunotherapy: A double-blind, placebo-controlled, cross-over trial. *Lancet* 361:1001-1006, 2003.)

patients treated with VIT. Ant VIT is recommended for those with skin test venom reactivity and a history of grade III-IV reactions.

▶ Clearly, participants in the study under discussion were, in the authors' words, "highly motivated" and "highly allergic." In southeastern Australia, where *Myrmecia* ant stings occur, about 1% of the population has severe allergy. In this population, VIT may be quite effective in the prevention of life-threatening sting anaphylaxis.

B. H. Thiers, MD

2 Psoriasis and Lichen Planus

The International Psoriasis Genetics Study: Assessing Linkage to 14 Candidate Susceptibility Loci in a Cohort of 942 Affected Sib Pairs
Bowcock AM, for the International Psoriasis Consortium (Washington Univ, St Louis; et al)
Am J Hum Genet 73:430-437, 2003   2–1

Background.—Psoriasis is a common, inflammatory, hyperproliferative skin disorder. Psoriasis appears to have a complex etiology requiring the interaction of unknown environmental factors with genetic predisposition. Evidence for linkage to psoriasis susceptibility has been reported for *PSORS1* located within the major histocompatability complex (MHC). Because *PSORS1* only appears to account for 50% of sibling relative risk, other genes also are likely involved. The International Psoriasis Genetics Consortium was formed to investigate 14 potential psoriasis-susceptibility loci in a cohort of 710 families with psoriasis.

Study Design.—The study group consisted of 942 affected sib pairs (ASPs) from 710 pedigrees. Fifty-three polymorphic microsatellites, spanning the 14 psoriasis candidate gene regions, were selected and genotyping was performed. Risch's maximum LOD score (MLS) was used to determine allele sharing in affected sibs. The association between marker haplotypes and psoriasis was evaluated with the multilocus transmission/disequilibrium test.

Findings.—MLS analysis of ASPs revealed an allele sharing of 60% for 6p21, confirming the presence of a susceptibility locus within the MHC. The strongest evidence of linkage outside of the MHC was for chromosomes 10q and 16q22-q23. Strong linkage disequilibrium was detected between the MHC and psoriasis. Two psoriasis-associated MHC haplotypes were identified. Analysis limited to families carrying those haplotypes significantly increased the chromosome 16q LOD score.

Conclusions.—This large international study provides unequivocal support for the role of the MHC in psoriasis. Other loci, such as those at 16q and 10q, also appear to have a role in disease susceptibility.

A Putative RUNX1 Binding Site Variant Between *SLC9A3R1* and *NAT9* Is Associated With Susceptibility to Psoriasis

Helms C, Cao L, Krueger JG, et al (Washington Univ, St Louis; Rockefeller Univ, New York; Univ of Washington, Seattle; et al)

Nature Genet 35:349-356, 2003   2–2

Introduction.—Psoriasis is a common, inflammatory, chronic skin disorder. Psoriasis susceptibility has previously been associated with HLA class I alleles. This report describes 2 genetic regions on chromosome 17q25 strongly associated with psoriasis.

Methods.—The study group consisted of 572 patients with psoriasis from 242 European families. Single nucleotide polymorphisms (SNPs) were used for semiautomated genotyping of regions of interest. Association analysis was performed by the TDT-AE method.

Results.—SNPs associated with psoriasis were near *SLC9A3R1* and *NAT9*, a member of the N-acetyltransferase family of proteins. SLC9A3R1 is a PDZ domain-containing phosphoprotein that associates with members of the ezrin-radixin-moesin family. SLC9A3R1 expression is highest in the uppermost Malphigian layer of psoriatic and normal skin. The other associated locus is near *RAPTOR*. A psoriasis-associated SNP in the 6-Mb region between SLC9A3R1 and RAPTOR leads to loss of a RUNX1 binding site associated with autoimmune disease.

Conclusions.—These results support the existence of 2 regions on chromosome 17q25 associated with susceptibility to psoriasis in a European population. This region has also been linked to susceptibility to other autoimmune diseases.

▶ The first of these articles (Abstract 2–1) describes a heroic, international, multi-investigator study of 942 sibling pairs affected by psoriasis designed to clarify the genetic contributions to the pathogenesis of the disease. More than 50 candidate microsatellites were analyzed in this population. Linkage analysis confirmed the finding of a major psoriasis susceptibility locus within the MHC on chromosome 6, with evidence for other loci on chromosomes 10q and 16q. Association analysis also revealed strong linkage disequilibrium between psoriasis and MHC alleles. The authors suggest the need for a more detailed analysis of putative loci on chromosomes 10 and 16.

The second study of 572 psoriasis patients and their family members (Abstract 2–2) yielded persuasive evidence for several disease association gene loci located on chromosome 17, including single nucleotide polymorphisms found close to the *SLC9A3R1* gene within 17q25, which has been implicated in both epithelial cell and T lymphocyte function. Interestingly, linkage between 17q25 with childhood atopic dermatitis has also recently been reported.

These 2 reports highlight the extreme genetic complexity of psoriasis and will no doubt further stimulate the search of the human genome for additional disease susceptibility loci.

G. M. P. Galbraith, MD

High Frequency of Detection of Human Papillomaviruses Associated With Epidermodysplasia Verruciformis in Children With Psoriasis

Mahé E, Bodemer C, Descamps V, et al (Institut Pasteur, Paris; Groupe Hospitalier Necker-Enfants Malades, Paris; Groupe Hospitalier Bichat-Claude Bernard, Paris; et al)

Br J Dermatol 149:819-825, 2003   2–3

Background.—The mechanism and the antigen(s) responsible for the T-cell activation seen in psoriasis has not been identified. Some evidence suggests human papillomaviruses (HPVs) associated with epidermodysplasia verruciformis (EV) (particularly HPV5) may be involved in the pathogenesis of psoriasis. Up to 90% of scrapings from skin lesions in patients with psoriasis contain DNA sequences of EV-HPVs, and up to one third of patients with psoriasis have antibodies against HPV5; in contrast, only 5% of patients with atopic dermatitis (AD) have HPV5 antibodies. Whether EV-HPV infection is involved in early psoriasis and, thus, might play a pathogenetic role was investigated.

Methods.—The research subjects were 26 children 1.5 to 13 years of age with psoriasis, 15 children 0.6-14.9 years of age with atopic dermatitis, 28 adults with psoriasis, and 28 age- and sex-matched adults with no history of HPV infection, psoriasis, cutaneous carcinoma, diseases with epidermal repair, or immunosuppression. Scrapings of involved skin (or normal skin in the control subjects) were analyzed by nested polymerase chain reaction to detect EV-HPV DNA sequences and HPV5 and HPV36 variants.

Results.—The children with psoriasis were similar to adults with psoriasis in terms of the prevalence of EV-HPVs (38.5% vs 35.7%, respectively), HPV5 (46.2% vs 46.4%), and HPV36 (15.4% vs 25.0%). Corresponding prevalences were significantly lower in children with atopic dermatitis (6.7% for EV-HPV, 6.7% for HPV5, and 6.7% for HPV36) and in adult control subjects (7.1% for EV-HPV, 10.1% for HPV5, and 7.1% for HPV36). In all, EV-HPVs were detected in 65.4% of children with psoriasis and in 71.4% of adults with psoriasis but in only 20.0% of children with atopic dermatitis and 21.4% of adult control subjects. The prevalence of EV-HPVs did not correlate significantly with clinical findings. Of note, HPV5 was detected in an 18-month-old girl with psoriasis and in a boy whose psoriasis had developed only 1 week earlier. Systemic treatment within the past 3 months (particularly with cyclosporine) was associated with a significantly higher prevalence of EV-HPVs and HPV5.

Conclusion.—The high prevalence of several EV-HPVs in children with psoriasis further supports a link between EV-HPV infection and the development of psoriasis. The association between cyclosporine treatment and an increased incidence of EV-HPV infection has also been reported in renal transplant recipients and in an adult with psoriasis. Exactly how EV-HPVs are involved in the pathogenesis of psoriasis remains unclear, but it may be that growth-promoting properties of some EV-HPVs (eg, E6, E7) induce keratinocyte proliferation or that capsid proteins or nonstructural viral proteins in EV-HPVs increase antigen recognition by autoreactive T cells.

▶ The authors note an increase in prevalence and an apparent increase in susceptibility to HPV infection in children with psoriasis in comparison with children with atopic dermatitis. It is not known whether HPV infection plays a role in the pathogenesis of psoriasis.

S. Raimer, MD

Streptococcal Throat Infections and Exacerbation of Chronic Plaque Psoriasis: A Prospective Study

Gudjonsson JE, Thorarinsson AM, Sigurgeirsson B, et al (Landspitali Univ Hosp, Hringbraut, Reykjavik, Iceland)
Br J Dermatol 149:530-534, 2003   2–4

Introduction.—Guttate psoriasis is characterized by the sudden onset of diffuse red and scaling papules and is known to be associated with streptococcal throat infections. In a previous study, about 30% of patients with chronic psoriasis noted worsening of the disease when they experienced a sore throat. Patients with chronic plaque psoriasis were studied prospectively to determine whether they had an increased frequency of throat infections with M protein-positive streptococci and whether such infections could exacerbate psoriasis.

Methods.—The study group included 208 patients and 116 unrelated age-matched household controls. None of the patients with chronic plaque psoriasis was on systemic treatment when recruited. Participants were asked to report when they experienced a sore throat and/or a worsening of their skin condition. Throat swabs were taken at these times. Patients and controls were monitored for 1 year.

Results.—Sore throat was reported significantly more often by patients with psoriasis (61 of 208) than by controls (3 of 116). Patients were also more likely than controls to have β-hemolytic streptococci of Lancefield groups A, C, and G (M protein-positive streptococci) cultured (19 of 208 vs 1 of 116, respectively). An increase in the Psoriasis Area and Severity Index was observed in 10 of 14 patients who were examined 4 days or later after onset of throat infection with M protein-positive streptococci. Episodes of streptococcal sore throat were less frequent in patients who had undergone tonsillectomy (4.5%) than in those who had not (11.3%).

Conclusion.—Patients with psoriasis were significantly more likely than individuals without psoriasis to experience sore throat and to have β-hemolytic streptococci isolated. Because the streptococcal throat infections were associated with exacerbations of chronic plaque psoriasis, patients might benefit from early treatment of these infections and from tonsillectomy.

▶ Gudjonsson et al provide data to confirm the association between strepto-coccal throat infection and psoriasis. Still to be determined is the effect of appropriate therapy in limiting the associated flare of the skin disease. Clinical trials would be necessary to assess the possible benefit of tonsillectomy in patients with psoriasis.

B. H. Thiers, MD

Allelic Variants of Drug Metabolizing Enzymes as Risk Factors in Psoriasis
Richter-Hintz D, Their R, Steinwachs S, et al (Universität Düsseldorf, Germany; Institut für Arbeitsphysiologie Dortmund, Germany; Institut für Umwelt-medizinische Forschung, Düsseldorf, Germany; et al)
J Invest Dermatol 120:765-770, 2003   2–5

Introduction.—Psoriasis has a genetic basis, but environmental factors play a role in the onset and severity of the disease. Drugs such as antimalarials and β-blockers may provoke psoriasis, and xenobiotics may also be involved in the T cell response and the development of psoriasis. To test the hypothesis that the genetic setup of xenobiotic metabolizing enzymes (XMEs) is linked to psoriasis, allelic variants of a wide range of XMEs in patients with psoriasis were analyzed.

Methods.—Study participants were 327 patients with psoriasis and 235 healthy controls. Blood samples were obtained for isolation of genomic DNA. Alleles tested included 4 phase I and 3 phase II enzymes. Patients with psoriasis and controls were compared for allele frequencies.

Results.—Compared with the patient group, significantly more healthy controls were carriers of variant alleles of *CYP1A1* (alleles *2A and *2C), a finding that suggests a protective role for these alleles. The patient and control groups did not differ significantly in proportions from the other phase I alleles: *1B1 *1* and *1B1 *3*, *2C19 *1A* and *2C19 *2A*, and *2E1 *1A* and *2E1 *5B*. Of the variant alleles coding for phase II enzymes, only *GSTM1* was correlated with a risk of contracting psoriasis. Certain combinations of several phase I and phase II enzyme alleles appeared to have synergistic risk/ protective effects. Heterozygosity for *CYP2C19* alleles *1A and 2A was associated with an increased risk of "late onset" (after age 40) psoriasis, but this genotype was protective for psoriatic arthritis.

Discussion.—Psoriasis has many autoimmune features, and T cells are known to be essential. A role for genetic factors, including XMEs, is suggested by the varied effects of different chemical/environmental triggers. In this first large-scale study on these enzymes, the findings support the view that different activities of XMEs can contribute to the onset and progression of psoriasis.

Cutaneous Expression of Cytochrome P450 CYP2S1: Individuality in Regulation by Therapeutic Agents for Psoriasis and Other Skin Diseases

Smith G, Wolf CR, Deeni YY, et al (Ninewells Hosp and Med School, Dundee, Scotland)

Lancet 361:1336-1343, 2003
                                                                      2–6

Introduction.—Most patients with psoriasis are able to tolerate drug therapy, but some experience adverse events or are resistant to treatment. An important determinant of systemic drug handling is individuality in hepatic expression of drug-metabolizing enzymes. A similar variation in cutaneous gene expression might contribute to individuality in responses to topical therapies used to treat psoriasis. The recently identified cytochrome P450 CYP2S1 was studied for its functional role in the metabolism of topical drugs.

Methods.—Quantitative real-time RT-PCR was used to demonstrate the expression of P450 CYP2S1 in the skin of 27 healthy volunteers and 29 patients with chronic plaque psoriasis. Three patients were scheduled to start PUVA with oral 8-methoxypsoralen and 26 were scheduled to start UVB phototherapy. Biopsy samples were obtained from participants, and triplicate measurements of skin mRNA expression were made from each sample to calculate a mean value.

Results.—In the 26 patients undergoing UVB radiation, CYP2S1 was induced with a geometric mean expression 1.78 times higher in nonlesional irradiated skin than in nonlesional control skin. The dose of UV radiation did not appear to correlate with induction of CYP2S1 in irradiated skin. Similarly, cutaneous expression of CYP2S1 was induced by PUVA, coal tar, and *all-trans* retinoic acid, with expression significantly higher in lesional psoriatic skin than in nonlesional skin (overall geometric mean expression 3.38 times higher in psoriatic skin). *All-trans* retinoic acid was found to be metabolized by CYP2S1, which has higher cutaneous expression than CYP26, a P450 enzyme recently identified as a substrate-inducible and highly specific cutaneous retinoic-acid–metabolizing enzyme.

Conclusion.—The findings suggest that CYP2S1 has a functional role in the metabolism of topical drugs and in mediating the response to photo-chemotherapy in psoriasis. Differences in expression of CYP2S1 might explain the variability in clinical response or risk of toxicity from topical agents or photochemotherapy.

▶ Studies such as those carried out by Richter-Hintz et al (Abstract 2–5) and Smith et al (Abstract 2–6) may explain why certain drugs exacerbate skin diseases in only a select group of patients. They also could help define which patients are more likely to respond favorably to different therapeutic modalities and which patients are more likely to suffer from drug-related toxicities.

B. H. Thiers, MD

Quantitative Real-Time Reverse Transcription–Polymerase Chain Reaction Analysis of Drug Metabolizing and Cytoprotective Genes in Psoriasis and Regulation by Ultraviolet Radiation
Smith G, Dawe RS, Clark C, et al (Univ of Dundee, Scotland)
J Invest Dermatol 121:390-398, 2003   2–7

Introduction.—The response to ultraviolet radiation in the treatment of psoriasis and other common skin diseases is unpredictable and varies by individual. It is essential to identify phenotypic markers that correlate with individual treatment outcomes. As the largest organ of the body, the skin should be a rich source of drug metabolizing and cytoprotective genes.

Methods.—Quantitative real-time reverse transcription–polymerase chain reaction was used to assess interindividual differences in the cutaneous expression of a variety of drug metabolizing and cytoprotective genes, including cytochrome P450s, glutathione S-transferases, and drug transporters. The regulation of gene expression by ultraviolet radiation and in lesional psoriatic skin was also examined.

Findings.—Significant induction of cyclo-oxygenase 2 (mean, 3.63-fold; range, 0.14-22.6; $P < .0001$) by ultraviolet radiation was verified. More modest (approximately 2-fold) inductions of glutathione peroxidase and novel inductions of glutathione S-transferase P1 and the drug transporter multidrug resistance–associated protein-1 were observed. Glutathione S-transferase P1 (3.74-fold; 1.3-33.1; $P < .0001$) and multidrug resistance–associated protein-1 (4.06-fold; 1.3-24.8; $P < .0001$) were significantly higher in psoriatic plaques, as was heme oxygenase-1 (10.19-fold; 2.9-49.7; $P < .0001$), indicating a differential adaptive response to oxidant exposure in lesional psoriatic skin.

Conclusion.—Marked interindividual differences were observed in constitutive gene expression and inducibility, suggesting that these genes may be linked to individuality in response to ultraviolet radiation.

▶ It is commonly observed in dermatology, and indeed in all of medicine, that patients with apparently similar diseases respond differently to identical therapies. Smith et al measured various liver and skin enzymes that metabolize drugs commonly used in the treatment of psoriasis and found that some of these enzymes are particularly active and inducible in psoriatic plaques. There was considerable interindividual variation. The authors speculate that such differences may help determine therapeutic responsiveness.

B. H. Thiers, MD

Narrowband (312-nm) UV-B Suppresses Interferon γ and Interleukin (IL) 12 and Increases IL-4 Transcripts: Differential Regulation of Cytokines at the Single-Cell Level
Walters IB, Ozawa M, Cardinale I, et al (Rockefeller Univ, New York)
Arch Dermatol 139:155-161, 2003   2–8

Introduction.—Narrowband (312-nm) ultraviolet-B (UV-B) delivered from TL-01 fluorescent bulbs is reportedly more effective than broadband UV-B delivered from other fluorescent sources in the treatment of inflammatory cutaneous disorders. Although 312-nm UV-B induces T-cell apoptosis in psoriatic lesions, as many as 90% of the original T cells remain in the dermis of fully resolved lesions after therapy. Biopsy specimens from patients given narrowband (312-nm) UV-B were examined to determine whether this treatment alters production of effector and regulatory cytokines by viable T cells remaining in the psoriatic lesions.

Methods.—The patients, 4 men and 6 women with moderate to severe plaque psoriasis, received narrowband UV-B daily as inpatients or 3 times a week as outpatients. After starting at 50% of a minimum erythema dose, increases of 10% to 15% per treatment were employed unless marked erythema developed. Sessions continued until maximal benefit was seen. Numbers of cytokine-producing cells from epidermal and peripheral T cells were quantified with the use of flow cytometry. Quantitative reverse transcription-polymerase chain reaction measured total mRNA in psoriatic skin biopsy material.

Results.—Treatment of psoriatic lesions with UV-B eliminated production of interleukin (IL)-12 messenger RNA and decreased production of interferon (IFN)-γ messenger RNA by more than 60%. After 1 to 2 weeks of treatment, the frequency of viable T cells producing IFN-γ decreased by 40% to 65%, but mRNA for IL-4 increased during UV-B treatment, and after 1 week of the therapy the number of IL-4–producing cells increased by 228%. The findings of in vitro experiments demonstrated that, on the single-cell level, survival and cytokine production by type 1 T cells were differentially regulated by UV-B.

Conclusion.—Therapeutic UV-B has a direct effect on modulating the type 1 polarized response in tissue. Both IL-2 and IFN-γ, and tumor necrosis factor (TNF)-α to a lesser extent, show the greatest decreases. A major effect of UV-B irradiation in psoriatic lesions is normalization of the proinflammatory versus regulatory cytokine imbalance.

▶ The increased levels of IL-4 in UVB-treated patients correlates nicely with the therapeutic efficacy of this cytokine when administered to a small group of psoriasis patients in a recently published study.[1]

B. H. Thiers, MD

Reference

1. Ghoreschi K, Thomas P, Breit S, et al: Interleukin-4 therapy of psoriasis induces Th2 responses and improves human autoimmune disease. *Nature Med* 9:40-46, 2003.

Narrowband UV-B (TL-01) Phototherapy vs Oral 8-Methoxypsoralen Psoralen–UV-A for the Treatment of Chronic Plaque Psoriasis
Markham T, Rogers S, Collins P (City of Dublin Skin and Cancer Hosp)
Arch Dermatol 139:325-328, 2003   2–9

Introduction.—Oral 8-methoxypsoralen photochemotherapy (8-MOP psoralen-UV-A [PUVA]) is an effective treatment for psoriasis, it but carries a risk of skin cancer. At the study institution, narrowband UV-B (TL-01) phototherapy has replaced PUVA as first-line treatment for patients with chronic plaque psoriasis (CPP). Advantages of TL-01 include fewer adverse effects and its suitability for pediatric use and in pregnancy. The efficacy of TL-01 was compared with that of PUVA in an open, randomized, controlled study of 54 patients with CPP.

Methods.—The patients were 30 men and 24 women, 29 randomly assigned to TL-01 and 25 to PUVA. All had at least 8% psoriasis extent on the trunk and limbs. The 2 treatment groups were well matched for age, sex, skin type, extent of disease, and Psoriasis Area and Severity Index (PASI) score. Patients were treated until completely clear, receiving a whole-body threshold erythemogenic dose of either 3-times weekly TL-01 or twice-weekly oral 8-MOP PUVA. A blinded observer assessed outcome once weekly during the study and monthly after clearance for 12 months. Relapse was defined as 50% of the original psoriasis extent.

Results.—Forty-five patients completed the study, 25 in the TL-01 group and 23 in the PUVA group; 3 patients, 1 in the TL-01 group and 2 in the PUVA group, were withdrawn because of flaring. Patients who received PUVA required significantly fewer treatments to clear, but the 2 groups did not differ significantly in number of days to clear or number of days in remission. The 2 regimens were equally erythemogenic, but grade 2 erythema occurred only in the PUVA group. Pruritus and polymorphic light eruption were reported equally in the 2 groups; only patients treated with PUVA experienced nausea.

Conclusion.—Three-times weekly treatment with TL-01 was as effective as twice-weekly PUVA in patients with CPP. In addition, TL-01 has a lower long-term risk factor profile, is more popular with patients because they do not need to take tablets or wear protective eyewear, and can be used during pregnancy and by children.

▶ Markham et al determined that narrowband UVB therapy used 3 times weekly was as effective as twice-weekly PUVA for the treatment of chronic plaque psoriasis. Other studies have suggested PUVA to be a more effective, although probably more hazardous, therapy. Even if somewhat less effective,

most of this reviewer's patients have elected narrowband UVB over PUVA because of its convenience and reduced toxicity.

B. H. Thiers, MD

Infliximab Monotherapy Provides Rapid and Sustained Benefit for Plaque-Type Psoriasis
Gottlieb AB, Chaudhari U, Mulcahy LD, et al (Univ of Medicine and Dentistry of New Jersey-The Robert Wood Johnson Med School, New Brunswick; Centocor Incorporated, Malvern, Pa)
J Am Acad Dermatol 48:829-835, 2003   2–10

Introduction.—Infliximab, a chimeric monoclonal antibody currently approved for the treatment of rheumatoid arthritis and Crohn's disease, offers
the promise of a clinical benefit in psoriasis. Initial results of a double-blind
trial indicated that a large proportion of patients treated with infliximab
achieved at least a 75% reduction in the Psoriasis Area and Severity Index
(PASI). The durability of the response to infliximab monotherapy was evaluated in an open-label extension of the trial.

Methods.—Thirty-three adult patients with moderate to severe plaque
psoriasis were included in the study. In the double-blind 10-week period, 11
patients were randomly assigned to placebo, 11 patients were randomly assigned to 5 mg/kg infliximab, and 11 patients were randomly assigned to 10
mg/kg infliximab. The open-label period randomly assigned 15 patients to 5
mg/kg and 14 patients to 10 mg/kg infliximab, and follow-up continued
through week 26.

Results.—One patient from each double-blind treatment group discontinued the study within the first 10 weeks; 25 patients treated with infliximab
completed the 26-week trial. Among patients who received the 5 mg/kg dose
of infliximab, 40% maintained at least a 50% PASI improvement, and 33%
maintained at least a 75% improvement from baseline. For those receiving
infusions of 10 mg/kg infliximab, 73% maintained at least 50% improvement, and 67% maintained at least a 75% improvement from baseline. Nine
patients who initially responded to infliximab, then relapsed and were re-
treated with 1 or 2 infusions, had improved PASI scores with retreatment;
however, gains were less than those achieved with the full 3-dose induction
regimen. No infusion reactions occurred in the 3-dose regimen, but 3 patients had generally mild reactions at the time of retreatment.

Conclusion.—A 3-dose induction regimen of infliximab produced rapid
and effective results in patients with moderate to severe psoriasis. Improvement was maintained during 26 weeks of follow-up, and patients who received the 10 mg/kg dose were likely to maintain their initial response for
longer periods than were those given the 5 mg/kg dose.

▶ The efficacy of infliximab in the treatment of psoriasis is well known, and
the article by Gottlieb et al documents the sustainability of the response.
Whether patients with a response to treatment should continue to be treated

with intermittent infusions of infliximab or transitioned to less aggressive therapies should be a subject of future studies. The apparent superiority of higher doses in maintaining the initial response and the observation of infusion reactions in the re-treated patients should be correlated with the possible development of anti-infliximab antibodies.

B. H. Thiers, MD

Case Reports of Heart Failure After Therapy With a Tumor Necrosis Factor Antagonist
Kwon HJ, Coté TR, Cuffe MS, et al (US Food and Drug Administration, Rockville, Md; Duke Clinical Research Inst, Durham, NC)
Ann Intern Med 138:807-811, 2003   2–11

Background.—Etanercept and infliximab are tumor necrosis factor (TNF) antagonists. Etanercept has been approved for the treatment of rheumatoid, juvenile rheumatoid, and psoriatic arthritis, whereas infliximab is approved for the treatment of Crohn's disease and, in conjunction with methotrexate, rheumatoid arthritis. Congestive heart failure is frequently accompanied by elevated TNF-α levels; however, controlled trials in patients with heart failure have shown no benefits from TNF antagonists and, in the case of infliximab, have suggested worse outcomes. In this study, adverse event reports of heart failure after TNF antagonist therapy for arthritis or Crohn's disease were described.

Methods.—Data were obtained from the US Food and Drug Administration's MedWatch program. The study group included 47 patients who had new or worsening heart failure develop, as determined by clinical and laboratory reports, while receiving TNF antagonist therapy.

Results.—According to the MedWatch program, 38 of 47 patients developed new-onset heart failure and 9 patients experienced exacerbation of heart failure after TNF antagonist therapy. Of the 38 patients with new-onset heart failure, 19 (50%) had no identifiable risk factors. Ten patients younger than 50 years had new-onset heart failure develop after TNF antagonist therapy. After termination of TNF antagonist therapy and initiation of heart failure therapy in these 10 patients, 3 patients had complete resolution of heart failure, 6 patients improved, and 1 patient died.

Conclusions.—The cases presented in this report, along with recent data from clinical trials, suggest that TNF antagonists may induce new-onset heart failure or exacerbate existing heart disease in a subset of patients.

▶ Previous studies have demonstrated increased serum levels of TNF in patients with advanced heart failure and have suggested that TNF levels may correlate with its severity. Although early clinical studies indicated that blocking TNF in heart failure patients could yield promising results, later studies were terminated either because of lack of improvement in clinical symptomatology or mortality or, in 1 trial, excessive mortality in patients receiving the TNF-blocking drug, infliximab.[1] Kwon et al suggest that TNF antagonists may *in-*

duce heart failure in a subset of patients, although the exact mechanism underlying this phenomenon is unknown. The bottom line is that the adverse effects of many new drugs are not revealed in premarketing clinical trials designed to gain US Food and Drug Administration approval. In these trials, patients are generally healthy except for the particular disease under study. The true side effects of some drugs may not become evident until patients in the general population, with all their associated co-morbidities, are exposed to them. The current article is reminiscent of experience with itraconazole, which was found to have clinically significant cardiac suppressant effects well after it was initially approved for marketing.[2]

B. H. Thiers, MD

References

1. Dear healthcare professional (Letter). Malvern, Pa; Centocor, October 23, 2001.
2. Ahmad SR, Singer SJ, Leissa BG: Congestive heart failure associated with itraconazole. *Lancet* 357:1766-1767, 2001.

Bilateral Anterior Toxic Optic Neuropathy and the Use of Infliximab
ten Tusscher MPM, Jacobs PJC, Busch MJWM, et al (Laurentius Hosp, Roermond, The Netherlands; Maxima Med Ctr, Eindhoven, The Netherlands; The Netherlands Pharmacovigilance Centre Lareb, s-Hertogenbosch; et al)
BMJ 326:579, 2003   2–12

Introduction.—Infliximab, used to treat various conditions including rheumatoid arthritis and Crohn's disease, was introduced in The Netherlands in the autumn of 1999. In the 3 patients reported here, bilateral optic neuropathy was diagnosed after they received their third dose of infliximab for rheumatoid arthritis.

Case Reports.—Woman, 62, and 2 men, both 54, experienced visual problems at periods ranging from 14 to 40 days after receiving the third infusion of infliximab. Additional drugs taken by 1 or more patients included prednisone, diclofenac, fluoxetine, and diazepam. Findings after treatment with infliximab consisted of severe disc swelling, dilation of the capillaries of the optic nerve, and vascular leakage in the optic nerve heads. All patients were given steroids to exclude temporal arteritis, but none improved.

Discussion.—Defects in the central and cecocentral visual fields in these patients indicate that they had the toxic form of anterior optic neuropathy. The appearance of symptoms after the third dose of infliximab suggests a cumulative effect or that the drug's effects increased with time. None of the other drugs that the patients used have been linked with optic neuropathy. An alternative explanation is that rheumatoid arthritis might be a risk factor for optic neuropathy. Optic neuritis has occurred in rare cases of rheumatoid arthritis, but the clinical picture in these 3 patients was quite different.

▶ An article by Mohan et al discussed the association of TNF-α inhibitors with symptoms of demyelinating disease.[1] However, the clinical picture of demyelinating optic neuritis differs considerably from the clinical picture in the patients reported by ten Tusscher et al.

B. H. Thiers, MD

Reference

1. Mohan N, Edwards ET, Cupps TR, et al: Demyelination occurring during anti-tumor necrosis factor alpha therapy for inflammatory arthritides. *Arthritis Rheum* 44:2862-2869, 2001.

Influence of Immunogenicity on the Long-term Efficacy of Infliximab in Crohn's Disease
Baert F, Noman M, Vermeire S, et al (Univ Hosp Gasthuisberg, Leuven, Belgium; Leuven Univ, Belgium)
N Engl J Med 348:601-608, 2003   2–13

Background.—Infliximab is a chimeric monoclonal immunoglobulin G1 antibody against tumor necrosis factor that has been approved for the treatment of Crohn's disease in patients who do not respond adequately to conventional therapy and for the management of enterocutaneous fistulas. In 50% to 81% of patients with refractory luminal disease, a single IV infusion of infliximab induced a response at 4 weeks, with remission induced in 25% to 48% of patients. This response can be maintained with repeated infusions. However, infliximab therapy can lead to the formation of antibodies against infliximab. The clinical significance of these antibodies was evaluated in patients with Crohn's disease.

Methods.—The study group consisted of 125 consecutive patients with refractory or luminal or fistulizing Crohn's disease who began infliximab therapy between December 1998 and July 2000. The main outcome measures were the concentrations of infliximab and antibodies against infliximab; clinical data; infusion reactions and other side effects; and the use of concomitant medications before and 4, 8, and 12 weeks after each infusion.

Results.—The patients received a mean of 3.9 infusions (range, 1-17 infusions) over a mean of 10 months. Antibodies against infliximab developed in 61% of patients. Concentrations of infliximab antibodies of 8.0 µg or greater before an infusion were predictive of a shorter duration of response (35 days vs 71 days for patients with concentrations of less than 8.0 µg) and a higher risk of infusion reactions. Patients who had a history of infusion reactions had significantly lower infliximab concentrations at 4 weeks compared with patients who had never had an infusion reaction (median, 1.2 vs 14.1 µg/mL). Patients who had an infusion reaction had a shorter duration of clinical response (38.5 days) compared with 65 days for patients who never had an infusion reaction. Concomitant treatment with immunosuppressive agents was found to be predictive of low titers of antibodies against infliximab and high concentrations of infliximab at 4 weeks after infusion.

Conclusions.—Patients who had antibodies develop against infliximab therapy have a greater risk of infusion reactions and a reduced duration of response to infliximab treatment. The concomitant use of immunosuppressive therapy reduces the magnitude of the immunogenic response.

▶ The authors demonstrate a correlation between the development of antibodies against infliximab, an increased risk of infusion reactions, and a reduced duration of response to treatment. They suggest that concomitant immunosuppressive therapy reduces the magnitude of the immunogenic response. Traditionally, rheumatologists have favored methotrexate therapy to provide protection against such immunogenicity. Whether methotrexate is more effective than azathioprine or mercaptopurine in this regard is uncertain. Studies of infliximab in the treatment of psoriasis have generally been structured without concomitant administration of immunosuppressive agents. How this affects the efficacy and safety of long-term infliximab therapy in the psoriasis population remains to be seen. The more recent introduction of humanized and human antibodies against TNF-α may help overcome the immunogenicity problem and lead to treatments with an increased benefit/risk ratio.

B. H. Thiers, MD

An International, Randomized, Double-blind, Placebo-controlled Phase 3 Trial of Intramuscular Alefacept in Patients With Chronic Plaque Psoriasis
Lebwohl M, for the Alefacept Clinical Study Group (Mount Sinai School of Medicine, New York; et al)
Arch Dermatol 139:719-727, 2003   2–14

Background.—Psoriasis appears to be an autoimmune disease involving skin-directed T cells. Most T cells in psoriatic plaques are memory T cells, such as $CD4^+CD45RO^+$ and $CD8^+CD45RO^+$ cells. Alefacept selectively targets and binds $CD45RO^+$ T cells, and thus may be effective against psoriasis. The efficacy and tolerability of IM alefacept in the treatment of moderate to severe psoriasis were examined in a phase 3 trial.

Methods.—A total of 507 adults with chronic plaque psoriasis (333 men and 174 women; mean age, 45.2 years) were studied. Most patients (85%) had moderate to severe disease; the median Psoriasis Area and Severity Index (PASI) was 14.2. Patients were randomly assigned in a 1:1:1 ratio to receive either placebo, 10 mg alefacept, or 15 mg alefacept. Study drugs were injected IM once a week for 12 weeks, and patients were monitored for 12 weeks after the last dose. The percentage changes in PASI from baseline to weeks 12 and 24 were compared between the 3 groups.

Results.—All 3 groups had a decrease in mean PASI from baseline to week 12. However, the mean percentage change in PASI at 12 weeks was significantly greater in the 2 active drug groups than in the controls. All 3 groups reached their maximum percentage change in PASI at 6 weeks; at that time, the mean reductions in PASI in the 15-mg alefacept, 10-mg alefacept, and placebo groups were 46%, 41%, and 25%, respectively. Improvement with alefacept persisted during 12 weeks of follow-up, as PASI scores remained stable until about week 20, then increased slightly. The proportion of patients who achieved at least a 50% reduction in PASI from baseline throughout the study was significantly higher in the alefacept groups (57% with 15 mg, 53% with 10 mg) than in the controls (35%). Alefacept's benefits were apparent in patients with moderate and severe disease, regardless of whether they had received prior systemic therapy or phototherapy. IM alefacept was well tolerated, and none of the patients had rebound disease or opportunistic infection during the study.

Conclusion.—Weekly IM injections of 10 or 15 mg of alefacept over 12 weeks were effective for these patients with moderate to severe psoriasis. Symptoms improved in a dose-dependent manner, and the remission was durable. IM administration appears to be an effective, safe, and convenient alternative to IV dosing for patients with chronic plaque psoriasis.

▶ The percentage of patients responding with at least a 75% reduction in the PASI score was 33% in patients receiving 15 mg of IM alefacept and 28% in those receiving the 10-mg dose weekly during the 12-week trial. These results are consistent with those reported in previous studies of alefacept. Krueger et al[1] noted that after a 12-week course of IV alefacept, the remittive nature of the drug permitted a 12-week rest period before embarking on a second 12-week course, which appeared to enhance the therapeutic effect. Although the safety profile in this 12-week study was good, the safety of long-term, albeit intermittent, alefacept therapy, with its associated minor but definite T-cell depletion, needs further investigation.

B. H. Thiers, MD

Reference

1. Krueger GG, Papp KA, Stough DB, et al: A randomized, double-blind, placebo-controlled phase III study evaluating efficacy and safety of two courses of alefacept in patients with chronic plaque psoriasis. *J Am Acad Dermatol* 47:821-833, 2002.

Treatment of Psoriasis With Alefacept: Correlation of Clinical Improvement With Reductions of Memory T-Cell Counts
Gordon KB, for the Alefacept Clinical Study Group (Loyola Univ, Maywood, Ill; et al)
Arch Dermatol 139:1563-1570, 2003   2–15

Introduction.—Scientific and clinical evidence exists to support a pivotal role for T cells in the pathogenesis of psoriasis. Alefacept targets CD4$^+$ and CD8$^+$ T cells that belong to the memory subsets and express high levels of CD2 on their surface. It has been postulated that decreasing the level of circulating memory T cells might correlate with clinical efficacy and the prolonged responses observed with alefacept. The association between the pharmacodynamic and antipsoriatic effects of IV alefacept was studied in a large phase 3, randomized, double-blind, placebo-controlled investigation involving patients with chronic plaque psoriasis.

Methods.—The study included 553 patients from 51 centers who were randomly selected (1:1:1) to treatment with either alefacept, 7.5 mg, in 2 courses; alefacept, 7.5 mg, in the first course and placebo in the second course; or placebo in the first course and alefacept, 7.5 mg, in the second course. For each course, alefacept or placebo was administered via IV bolus once weekly for 12 weeks, followed by 12 weeks of observation. The primary outcome measures were circulating lymphocyte levels and the score in the Psoriasis Area Severity Index.

Results.—One or 2 course of alefacept decreased CD4$^+$ and CD8$^+$ memory T-cells counts, while sparing the naive population. At 12 weeks after the last dose of alefacept in courses 1 and 2, 88% and 83% of patients, respectively, had CD4$^+$ cell counts higher than the lower limit of normal. In course 1, alefacept-treated patients with the largest reductions in memory T-cell counts experienced the greatest decreases in disease activity ($P < .001$). The duration of clinical benefit appeared to be longer for patients who had the greatest decreases in CD4$^+$ and CD8$^+$ memory T-cell counts.

Conclusion.—The decrease in levels of circulating memory T-cells with alefacept treatment correlates with improvement in psoriasis and suggests an association between the length of response to alefacept and alterations in the memory T-cell population.

▶ A reduction in circulating T-cells has been a concern in patients treated with alefacept. Gordon et al suggest that this reduction is likely secondary to apoptosis of circulating memory T-cells, which are thought to play a key role in the pathogenesis of the disease. Interestingly, there appeared to be a correlation between the reduction in disease activity, the duration of the response, and the magnitude of the drop in CD4$^+$ and CD8$^+$ memory T-cell counts. The sparing of the native T-cell population is reassuring; nevertheless, as suggested by the authors, long-term, multiple-course studies are needed to completely assess the safety of alefacept in clinical practice.

B. H. Thiers, MD

CD4$^+$ T-Cell–Directed Antibody Responses Are Maintained in Patients With Psoriasis Receiving Alefacept: Results of a Randomized Study

Gottlieb AB, Casale TB, Frankel E, et al (Univ of Medicine and Dentistry of New Jersey, New Brunswick; Creighton Univ, Omaha, Neb; Clinical Partners LLC, Johnston, RI; et al)

J Am Acad Dermatol 49:816-825, 2003   2–16

Background.—Memory-effector (CD45RO$^+$) T cells are a source of the pathogenic mediators of psoriasis. Alefacept is a human LFA-3/IgG$_1$ fusion protein that selectively decreases memory-effector T cells. The effects of alefacept on immune function, T-cell–dependent humoral responses to a neoantigen and recall antigen were reported.

Methods.—Forty-six patients with chronic plaque psoriasis were enrolled in the study at 8 centers. Equal numbers of patients were assigned randomly to a control group or to alefacept, 7.5 mg, intravenously every week for 12 weeks. The active treatment group received neoantigen (ϕX174) immunizations at 6, 12, 20, and 26 weeks, as well as a recall antigen (tetanus toxoid) at 21 weeks. The control group received ϕX174 at weeks 6 and 12 and tetanus toxoid at week 10.

Findings.—The 2 groups had similar mean anti-ϕX174 titers. The percentage of responders did not differ between groups, being 86% in the alefacept group and 82% in the control group. Also comparable, at 89% and 91%, respectively, were the percentages of patients with antitetanus toxoid titer increases 2 times baseline or higher.

Conclusions.—Alefacept given for 12 weeks does not appear to hinder primary or secondary antibody responses to a neoantigen or memory responses to a recall antigen. Maintenance of a significant aspect of immune function to fight infection and respond to vaccinations is associated with the selective immunomodulatory effect of alefacept against a potentially pathogenic T-cell subset.

▶ The authors studied the effect of alefacept on specific T-cell–dependent humoral responses to a neoantigen (ϕX174) and a recall antigen (tetanus toxoid). The patients were studied before and after a 12-week course of IV alefacept. Although the results showed no impairment of primary effector antibody responses after a single 12-week course of the drug, at least 2 questions remain unanswered. First, psoriasis is a chronic disease requiring continuous or perhaps, in the case of alefacept, intermittent therapy. Thus, it would be important to study the immune system after multiple courses of the drug. Second, different immunization schedules were used in the control group and in the alefacept group, suggesting that the 2 groups may not be strictly comparable. Interestingly, CTLA4Ig (see Abstract 9–17) and efalizumab have been shown to suppress T cell-dependent humoral responses to ϕX174.[1,2]

B. H. Thiers, MD

References

1. Abrams JR, Lebwohl MG, Guzzo CA, et al: CTLA4Ig-mediated blockade of T-cell costimulation in patients with psoriasis vulgaris. *J Clin Invest* 103:1243-1252, 1999.
2. Gottlieb A, Krueger JG, Bright R, et al: Effects of administration of a single dose of a humanized monoclonal antibody to CD11a on the immunobiology and clinical activity of psoriasis. *J Am Acad Dermatol* 42:428-435, 2000.

A Novel Targeted T-Cell Modulator, Efalizumab, for Plaque Psoriasis

Lebwohl M, for the Efalizumab Study Group (Mount Sinai School of Medicine, New York; et al)
N Engl J Med 349:2004-2013, 2003   2–17

Introduction.—Phase 1 and 2 studies have demonstrated the biologic and clinical activity of efalizumab in patients with psoriasis. Efalizumab, a humanized monoclonal antibody, binds to the α subunit (CD11a) of leukocyte-function-associated antigen type 1 (LFA-1) and inhibits the activation of T cells. A phase 3 trial was conducted to assess the efficacy and safety of efalizumab in patients with moderate to severe plaque psoriasis.

Methods.—Patients eligible for the study were aged 18 to 70, had a psoriasis area-and-severity index of at least 12.0 at screening, and were candidates for systemic therapy. A total of 597 patients participated in the double-blind, parallel-group, multicenter trial that involved 3 consecutive phases. In the first phase, randomization was to 1 or 2 mg of subcutaneous efalizumab per kilogram of body weight per week or to an equivalent volume of matching placebo. Those with a response 50% or greater received an additional 12 weeks of efalizumab (2 mg/kg weekly or every other week) or placebo. Patients with less than 50% improvement received an increased dose of efalizumab (4 mg/kg per week) or placebo. Follow-up continued for 12 weeks after the 24-week treatment period.

Results.—Significantly more patients who received efalizumab versus placebo showed an improvement of 75% or greater in the psoriasis area-and-severity index (22%, 28%, and 5%, respectively, for 1 mg efalizumab, 2 mg efalizumab, and placebo). Differences between the active and placebo groups were apparent as early as week 4. Only 30% of those who continued on efalizumab to week 24 maintained at least half of their improvement 12 weeks after discontinuation of the drug. Adverse events related to the therapy were generally mild to moderate.

Conclusion.—Patients with moderate to severe plaque psoriasis showed significant improvement when treated with efalizumab. The benefits of this agent were rapid and sustained. The adverse events that occurred primarily after the first or second dose of efalizumab did not preclude further treatment.

Etanercept as Monotherapy in Patients With Psoriasis

Leonardi GL, for the Etanercept Psoriasis Study Group (Saint Louis Univ; et al)
N Engl J Med 349:2014-2022, 2003   2–18

Introduction.—The knowledge that T cells and inflammatory cytokines contribute to the pathogenesis of psoriasis had led to the development of new biologic treatment strategies. Etanercept, a recombinant human tumor necrosis factor receptor antagonist, has improved psoriatic skin lesions in patients with psoriatic arthritis. The safety and efficacy of etanercept as a treatment for plaque psoriasis was evaluated in a randomized study.

Methods.—Patients eligible for the study had active but clinically stable plaque psoriasis and had received or were candidates for phototherapy or systemic psoriasis therapy. The 24-week double-blind study included 652 patients, 166 assigned to placebo, 160 to low-dose etanercept (25 mg once weekly), 162 to medium-dose etanercept (25 mg twice weekly), and 164 to high-dose etanercept (50 mg twice weekly). Patients in the placebo group were switched to the medium etanercept dose after 12 weeks. Efficacy was defined as an improvement of at least 75% from baseline in the psoriasis area-and-severity index.

Results.—Patients included in the study were predominantly male (67%) and white (87%). The mean affected body-surface area was 28.7% and the mean duration of psoriasis was 18.7 years. Treatment efficacy, as defined above, was noted after 12 weeks in 4% of patients in the placebo group, 14% in the low-dose etanercept group, 34% in the medium-dose etanercept group, and 49% in the high-dose etanercept group. All dosages of etanercept were significantly more efficacious than placebo. After 24 weeks, at least a 75% improvement in the psoriasis area-and-severity index was reported for 25%, 44%, and 59% of patients in the low-, medium-, and high-dose groups, respectively. Etanercept was generally well tolerated.

Conclusion.—Patients with psoriasis showed significant improvement in the psoriasis area-and-severity index after 12 weeks of treatment with etanercept, and greater benefits were seen after 24 weeks. These responses were paralleled by improved scores on the Physician's Static Global Assessment and the Patient's Global Assessment.

Efalizumab for Patients With Moderate to Severe Plaque Psoriasis: A Randomized Controlled Trial
Gordon KB, for the Efalizumab Study Group (Loyola Univ, Maywood, Ill; et al)
JAMA 290:3073-3080, 2003   2–19

Introduction.—Efalizumab, a humanized monoclonal immunoglobulin G1 antibody that targets T-cell interactions central to the pathophysiology of psoriasis, was examined in a phase III trial for its impact on health-related quality of life measures in patients with moderate to severe plaque psoriasis.

Methods.—The multicenter, parallel-group trial enrolled and randomized 556 patients. Eligible participants were aged 18 to 75 years, had a minimum Psoriasis Area and Severity Index (PASI) score of 12.0 at screening, and were candidates for systemic therapy. Patients received 12 weekly doses of either subcutaneous efalizumab (1 mg/kg) or placebo equivalent. After 12 weeks, all were enrolled in a separate long-term open-label extension study. Emollients could be continued during the study, but phototherapy and systemic therapy were excluded. The primary efficacy outcome was the proportion of patients with at least 75% improvement in PASI at week 12 relative to baseline (PASI-75). Secondary efficacy measures were several global physician assessments and patient-reported outcome scales.

Results.—Compared with placebo-treated patients, those who received efalizumab had significantly greater improvement on all study end points. The percentage of patients achieving PASI-75 was 27% with efalizumab versus 4% with placebo. Mean percentages of improvement on the overall Dermatology Life Quality Index were 47% with efalizumab and 14% with placebo. Outcome after treatment with efalizumab was also significantly better relative to placebo when the Itching Visual Analog Scale and the Psoriasis Symptom Assessment frequency and severity subscales were considered (38%, 48%, and 47% versus -0.2%, 18%, and 17%, respectively). The first 2 injections of efalizumab caused mild to moderate flulike symptoms in some patients, but no clinically significant laboratory abnormalities occurred during the treatment. Few patients in either the efalizumab (3%) or placebo (1%) groups withdrew from the study because of adverse events.

Conclusion.—Efalizumab therapy yielded significant benefits in both primary and secondary end points when administered to patients with moderate to severe plaque psoriasis. With its favorable safety profile, efalizumab may provide a valuable treatment option.

A Randomized Trial of Etanercept as Monotherapy for Psoriasis
Gottlieb AB, Matheson RT, Lowe N, et al (Robert Wood Johnson Med School, New Brunswick, NJ; Oregon Med Research Ctr, Portland; Southern California Dermatology, Santa Monica; et al)
Arch Dermatol 139:1627-1632, 2003   2–20

Background.—Research has established the role of the proinflammatory cytokine, tumor necrosis factor (TNF), in psoriasis. A double-blind, placebo-controlled, multicenter study of the efficacy of TNF blockade in patients with psoriasis was reported.

Methods.—The study included 112 adults with plaque psoriasis involving at least 10% body surface area who were assigned randomly to etanercept, 25 mg, or placebo, subcutaneously twice a week for 24 weeks. Other treatments for psoriasis were restricted. Efficacy was assessed by the Psoriasis Area and Severity Index (PASI).

Findings.—At 12 weeks, 30% of etanercept recipients and 2% of placebo recipients had a 75% improvement in the PASI. At 24 weeks, these percentages for the recipients were 56% and 5%, respectively. By this time, psoriasis was clear or minimal, according to a global evaluation, in more than half the etanercept recipients. A PASI response of less than 50%, defined as treatment failure, was observed in 23% of patients at 24 weeks. The occurrence of adverse events was similar in the 2 groups.

Conclusions.—Etanercept treatment is an effective treatment for psoriasis. Its safety profile is also favorable.

Immunologic Targets in Psoriasis

Kupper TS (Brigham and Women's Hosp, Boston)
N Engl J Med 349:1987-1990, 2003   2–21

Introduction.—Two new biologic drugs, etanercept and efalizumab, are available for use in psoriasis. Etanercept targets the pleiotropic inflammatory cytokine tumor necrosis factor α (TNF-α); efaluzimab is a humanized monoclonal antibody against CD11a that blocks leukocyte-function–associated antigen 1 (LFA-1) interactions with intercellular adhesion molecules 1 and 2 (ICAM-1 and ICAM-2).

Process.—The elegant system of immunosurveillance in the skin, a powerful means of protection against environmental pathogens, is subverted in psoriasis. In this disorder, the immune system appears to perceive putative psoriatic autoantigens as foreign. Skin-homing memory T cells flood into the skin in response to TNF-α–mediated danger signals, and those that are reactive to psoriatic autoantigens are activated. Both processes involve LFA-1. Cytokines are produced by the T cells activated in the skin, and those involved in psoriasis produce type 1 cytokines, including interferon-γ and TNF-α. In patients with psoriasis, the inflammatory response is amplified and a hyperproliferative response of the epidermis occurs. This process is reversible only by blocking activation of T cells within the lesions.

Discussion.—Blocking either LFA-1 or TNF-α has therapeutic effects in psoriasis, but the new biologic agents that achieve this end interfere with important immunologic processes. The activity of these agents may vary from person to person, perhaps because of polymorphisms in genes that control expression of the relevant molecules.

▶ Recent publications outlined above (Abstracts 2–17 to 2–21) have helped define reasonable expectations for results of therapy with the new biologic agents. On average, approximately one third of patients with moderate to severe psoriasis will achieve 75% improvement in the psoriasis area and severity index (PASI) after a 12-week course of alefacept, efalizumab, or etanercept (in the case of the latter, using standard doses currently approved to treat rheumatoid and psoriatic arthritis). Whether this degree of improvement is worth the rather substantial cost of these injectable drugs is an issue that physicians, patients, and indeed our entire health care system will have to decide. Hopefully, more cost-effective drugs will be available in the not too distant future.

B. H. Thiers, MD

Methotrexate Versus Cyclosporine in Moderate-to-Severe Chronic Plaque Psoriasis

Heydendael VMR, Spuls PI, Opmeer BC, et al (Univ of Amsterdam)
N Engl J Med 349:658-665, 2003   2–22

Background.—Chronic plaque psoriasis is characterized by sharply demarcated, erythematous scaly lesions and has an estimated worldwide prevalence of 0.1% to 3%. A variety of therapies are available for the treatment of psoriasis, including topical ointments, phototherapy, systemic drugs such as acitretin, and the systemic immunosuppressant drugs methotrexate and cyclosporine. Guidelines for the treatment of psoriasis state that UVB radiation should be tried first and, if ineffective, should be followed in sequence by psoralen with UVA radiation (PUVA), methotrexate, acitretin, and cyclosporine. Methotrexate and cyclosporine were compared in a randomized controlled trial in terms of effectiveness, side effects, and quality of life for patients with moderate to severe plaque psoriasis.

Methods.—Eighty-eight patients with moderate to severe psoriasis were randomly assigned to 16 weeks of treatment with either methotrexate (44 patients, initial dose 15 mg/wk) or cyclosporine (44 patients, initial dose 3 mg/kg/d). The patients were monitored for an additional 36 weeks. The primary outcome measure was the difference between groups in the psoriasis area and severity index (PASI) after 16 weeks of treatment, after adjustment for baseline values.

Results.—The final analysis included 42 patients in the cyclosporine group and 43 patients in the methotrexate group. After 16 weeks of treatment, the mean (± standard error) score for the PASI declined from 13.4 ± 3.6 at baseline to 5.0 ± 0.7 in the methotrexate group and from 14.0 ± 6.6 to 3.8 ± 0.5 in the cyclosporine group. After adjustment for baseline values, the mean absolute difference in values after the 16-week treatment period was 1.3 ($P = .09$). The 2 groups were similar in terms of the physician's global assessment of the extent of psoriasis, the time to and rate of remission, and the quality of life.

Conclusion.—There was no significant difference in efficacy between methotrexate and cyclosporine for the treatment of moderate to severe psoriasis.

▶ The percentage of patients achieving PASI 75, or 75% improvement in the PASI score, was 60% in the methotrexate group and 71% in the cyclosporine group, demonstrating that both drugs are highly effective agents for the control of moderate to severe chronic plaque-type psoriasis and certainly should be considered part of our therapeutic armamentarium, even in this "new era" of biological therapies. The significant incidence of reversible elevations of liver enzyme levels (12 of 44 patients in the methotrexate group) is inconsistent with this reviewer's experience. I rarely have observed liver enzyme abnormalities in my own patients. Perhaps stricter exclusion criteria and more diligent patient selection might have avoided this problem in the patients presented here.

B. H. Thiers, MD

Ultraviolet-B Irradiation Decreases IFN-γ and Increases IL-4 Expression in Psoriatic Lesional Skin In Situ and in Cultured Dermal T Cells Derived From These Lesions
Piskin G, Koomen CW, Picavet D, et al (Academic Med Ctr, Amsterdam)
Exp Dermatol 12:172-180, 2003   2–23

Introduction.—Several lines of evidence suggest that T cells are important in the pathogenesis of psoriasis. Ultraviolet B (UVB) irradiation, used to treat extensive or persistent psoriasis, decreases the number of lesional T cells. In normal skin, changes in the dermal environment caused by UVB lead to a decrease in the number of interferon (IFN)-γ expressing type 1 T cells together with an increase in the number of interleukin (IL)-4 expressing type 2 T cells. Patients with moderate to severe plaque-type psoriasis were studied to determine whether UVB irradiation causes a similar shift in type 1 and type 2 responses in psoriatic skin.

Methods.—Patients were 4 men and 1 woman with an average age of 53.6 years. The minimal erythema dose (MED) was determined for each patient. Biopsy specimens were obtained from lesional skin before, 2 days after, and 14 days after a single exposure to 4 MED UVB. Biopsy sections were immunostained (CD3, IFN-γ, and IL-4) or RNA was extracted and analyzed for expressions of IFN-γ and IL-4 by polymerase chain reaction. Primary cultures of T cells from dermal cell suspensions were stained intracellularly for IFN-γ and IL-4 expression. Flow cytometry was used to analyze CD4+ and CD8+ T subsets.

Results.—In all patients, locally irradiated skin lesions healed clinically 14 days after 4 MED UVB. Epidermal T-cell numbers determined by CD3 staining decreased progressively after UVB irradiation; changes in dermal T cells were not statistically significant. A decrease in IFN-γ, highly expressed in untreated psoriatic lesions, was observed in all patients after UVB irradiation. Expression of IL-4 was variable before and increased by different amounts after irradiation. Both CD4+ and CD8+ dermal T cells produced less IFN-γ and more IL-4 after UVB exposure.

Conclusion.—A single UVB irradiation of psoriatic lesional skin with 4 MED resulted in decreased IFN-γ and increased IL-4 expression in situ and in primary cultures of dermal T cells derived from in vivo UVB-exposed skin. A cytokine shift from type 1 to type 2 in lesions might contribute to the therapeutic effects of UVB in psoriasis.

▶ Psoriasis is considered by many investigators to be a T$_H$1-dominant disease in which proinflammatory cytokines participate in the pathogenesis of the skin lesions characteristic of the disease. Conversely, anti-inflammatory T$_H$2 cytokines have been studied for their possible therapeutic benefit in psoriasis. Piskin et al found changes in cytokine expression after UVB irradiation that support this hypothesis. Indeed, improvements in psoriasis after UVB phototherapy may be mediated, at least in part, by a shift from a T$_H$1-dominant profile to one in which T$_H$2 cytokines, such as IL-4, are more heavily expressed. These findings support a possible role for IL-4 administration in the treatment of psoriasis, as reported in the 2003 YEAR BOOK OF DERMATOLOGY AND DERMATOLOGIC SURGERY.[1]

B. H. Thiers, MD

Reference

1. Ghoreschi K, Thomas P, Breit S et al: Interleukin-4 therapy of psoriasis induces Th2 responses and improves human autoimmune disease. *Nat Med* 9:40-46, 2003. (2003 YEAR BOOK OF DERMATOLOGY AND DERMATOLOGIC SURGERY, pp 145-146.)

Altered Cutaneous Immune Parameters in Transgenic Mice Overexpressing Viral IL-10 in the Epidermis

Ding W, Beissert S, Deng L, et al (Cornell Univ, New York; Univ of Muenster, Germany; State Univ of New York, Stony Brook; et al)
J Clin Invest 111:1923-1931, 2003   2–24

Introduction.—The pleiotropic cytokine interleukin-10 (IL-10) negatively regulates a variety of immune responses and may be a mediator of suppression of cell-mediated immunity induced by exposure to UVB radiation. Evidence that IL-10 can suppress the efferent phase of delayed-type hypersensitivity and contact hypersensitivity responses suggests that the cytokine plays an important role in the regulation of type IV immune reactions. Transgenic mice that overexpress viral IL-10 (vIL-10) in the epidermis were engineered to investigate the effects of IL-10 on the cutaneous immune system. The protein product of vIL-10 shares many biologic properties with both murine and human IL-10.

Findings.—The vIL-10 transgenic mice were found to have a reduced number of I-A$^+$ epidermal and dermal cells, and fewer I-A$^+$ hapten-bearing cells in regional lymph nodes after hapten painting of the skin. Levels of expression of the costimulatory molecules CD80 and CD86 by I-A$^+$ epidermal cells were also reduced. Upon challenge, vIL-10 transgenic mice exhibited a smaller delayed-type hypersensitivity response to allogeneic cells, but contact hypersensitivity to an epicutaneously applied hapten was normal. Both fresh epidermal cells and splenocytes from the vIL-10 transgenic mice had a decreased ability to stimulate allogeneic T-cell proliferation. Chronic exposure of vIL-10 mice and WT control mice to UVB radiation produced significantly fewer tumors in the vIL-10 mice, suggesting that vIL-10 may inhibit the formation of skin tumors in response to UVB radiation. In addition, these transgenic mice had increased splenic natural killer cell activity against YAC-1 targets.

Conclusion.—Experiments in a transgenic system confirm that IL-10 inhibits a number of cutaneous immune functions. Together with previously published data, these findings support the concept that contact hypersensitivity and delayed-type hypersensitivity are regulated differently, and confirm the function of IL-10 in inhibiting delayed-type hypersensitivity responses.

▶ Numerous previous studies have demonstrated the immunosuppressive properties of the Th2 cytokine, IL-10. High levels of IL-10 seem to predispose to tuberculosis,[1,2] and high levels of IL-10 in melanoma patients are associated with metastasis and a poor prognosis.[3,4] The elegant work by Ding et al confirms that IL-10 inhibits the delayed-type hypersensitivity response. The authors suggest that expression of IL-10 by certain viruses helps to protect them against attack by the host immune system. They further suggest the possibility that IL-10 may be therapeutically useful in the treatment of cutaneous immune-mediated diseases. Unfortunately, published studies of the usefulness of this cytokine for the treatment of psoriasis have yielded disappointing results.[5] The decreased incidence of skin tumors in the vIL-10 mice was an unexpected finding and requires further investigation.

B. H. Thiers, MD

References

1. Turner J, Gonzalez-Juarrero M, Ellis DL, et al: In vivo IL-10 production reactivates chronic pulmonary tuberculosis in C57BL/6 mice. *J Immunol* 169:6343-6351, 2002.
2. Awomoyi AA, Marchant A, Howson JM, et al: Interleukin-10, polymorphism in SLC11A1 (formerly NRAMP1), and susceptibility to tuberculosis. *J Infect Dis* 186:1808-1814, 2002.
3. Nemunaitis J, Fong T, Shabe P, et al: Comparison of serum interleukin-10 (IL-10) levels between normal volunteers and patients with advanced melanoma. *Cancer Invest* 19:239-247, 2001.
4. Muller G, Muller A, Tuting T, et al: Interleukin-10-treated dendritic cells modulate immune responses of naive and sensitized T cells in vivo. *J Invest Dermatol* 119:836-841, 2002.
5. Kimball AB, Kawamura T, Tejura K, et al: Clinical and immunologic assessment of patients with psoriasis in a randomized, double-blind, placebo-controlled trial using recombinant human interleukin 10. *Arch Dermatol* 138:1341-1346, 2002.

Keratinocyte Unresponsiveness Towards Interleukin-10: Lack of Specific Binding Due to Deficient IL-10 Receptor 1 Expression

Seifert M, Gruenberg BH, Sabat R, et al (Humboldt Univ Berlin; Schering AG, Berlin)
Exp Dermatol 12:137-144, 2003   2–25

Introduction.—Previous research indicates that human keratinocytes (KC) express the interleukin-10 (IL-10) receptor, and that the abnormal behavior of KC in several dermatoses suggests a therapeutic role for IL-10. Administration of IL-10 has yielded inconsistent results in psoriasis, and it is not known whether the mode of action of IL-10 involves direct targeting of KC. An experimental study further investigated the direct effects of IL-10 on KC and the reason for potential IL-10 unresponsiveness using KC such as the cell line HaCaT as well as primary foreskin KC.

Methods and Results.—Human epidermal cell suspensions were provided by normal donors (aged 3 to 40 years) undergoing foreskin surgery. The human KC cell line HaCaT was initially derived from an adult donor. Peripheral blood mononuclear cells were isolated from citrated venous blood of healthy volunteers. Real-time reverse transcription polymerase chain reaction was used to demonstrate that IL-10 was not able to induce its typical early gene product suppressor of cytokine signaling (SOCS) 3, or modulate the interferon (IFN)-γ–induced expression of SOCS 1 and 3. Flow cytometric analyses demonstrated binding of biotin-labelled IL-10 to HaCaT cells, but blocking experiments suggested that nonspecific binding had occurred. In addition, Scatchard plot analyses excluded specific binding to primary KC and HaCaT cells. Performance of real-time mRNA analyses and Western blot experiments linked the absence of any specific binding to the absence of clear IL-10R1 (alpha chain) expression; the IL-10R2 (beta chain), however, was strongly expressed.

Conclusion.—KC do not bind specifically to IL-10, a major anti-inflammatory, immunosuppressive cytokine, and KC do not respond to IL-10 by the induction of early gene products such as SOCS 1 and 3. The cause of this is lack of IL-10R1 expression, which is necessary for IL-10 binding and signalling. Because IL-10 does not primarily target KC, the effects on KC noted during IL-10 therapy appear to be indirectly mediated.

▶ A previous article reviewed in the 2003 YEAR BOOK OF DERMATOLOGY AND DERMATOLOGIC SURGERY demonstrated only a marginal effect of IL-10 administration to patients with psoriasis despite changes in circulating cytokine levels.[1] This disappointingly modest benefit may reflect the lack of certain specific receptors for IL-10 on KC.

B. H. Thiers, MD

Reference

1. Kimball AB, Kawamura T, Tejura K et al: Clinical and immunological assessment of patients with psoriasis in a randomized, double-blind, placebo-controlled trial using recombinant human interleukin 10. *Arch Dermatol* 138:1341-1346, 2002. (2003 YEAR BOOK OF DERMATOLOGY AND DERMATOLOGIC SURGERY, pp 144-145.)

Resolution of Psoriasis Upon Blockade of IL-15 Biological Activity in a Xenograft Mouse Model

Villadsen LS, Schuurman J, Beurskens F, et al (Gentofte Univ Hosp, Copenhagen, Denmark; Genmab BV, Utrecht, The Netherlands; Marselisborg Univ Hosp, Aarhus, Denmark; et al)
J Clin Invest 112:1571-1580, 2003   2–26

Introduction.—Psoriasis is a chronic, inflammatory skin disease that is characterized by epidermal hyperplasia, dermal angiogenesis, infiltration of activated T cells, and increased cytokine levels. Interleukin (IL)-15 is a proinflammatory cytokine whose expression is upregulated in inflammatory conditions such as psoriasis. It triggers inflammatory cell recruitment, angiogenesis, and production of other inflammatory cytokines, including interferon gamma (IFN-γ), tumor necrosis factor alpha (TNF-α), and IL-17, which are likewise upregulated in psoriatic lesions. The generation of human antibodies directed against human IL-15 in a murine model is described.

Methods.—The antibodies were acquired through transgenic mice containing an unrearranged human antibody repertoire in which endogenous murine antibody expression had been knocked out. Human IL-15-specific monoclonal antibodies (mAbs) were prepared and selected based on in vitro features. Keratome biopsy specimens from patients with moderate-to-severe plaque psoriasis were transplanted onto the back of 12 C.B-17 SCID mice. The animals were randomly stratified into 3 groups 3 weeks after transplantation for either treatment with intraperitoneal injection of phosphate-buffered saline (PBS) (vehicle); or mAb 146B7 at a dose of 20 mg/kg on day 1 and 10 mg/kg on days 5 and 15; or cyclosporine A (CsA) at a dose of 10 mg/kg every second day for 15 days. The mice were killed 1 week after final injection, and a 4-mm punch biopsy specimen was obtained from each xenograft.

Results.—One of the IL-15-specific antibodies that was generated, 146B7, did not compete with IL-15 for binding to its receptor; however, it potently interfered with the assembly of the IL-15 receptor α, β, γ complex. The 146B7 antibody effectively blocked IL-15-induced T cell proliferation and monocyte TNF-α release in vitro. Light microscopy revealed that mice treated with PBS retained a characteristic psoriatic skin phenotype; treatment with mAb 146B7 resulted in near resolution of psoriasis; and treatment with CsA also resulted in attenuation of psoriasis, but not to the extent seen with mAb 146B7 treatment.

Conclusion.—In a human xenograft model, antibody 146B7 decreased the severity of psoriasis, as determined by epidermal thickness, grade of parakeratosis, and numbers of inflammatory cells and cycling keratinocytes. The findings suggest a prominent role for IL-15 in the pathogenesis of psoriasis.

▶ Clearly, the era of biological therapy for psoriasis is in its infancy. IL-15 induces T-cell proliferation and release of monocyte TNF-α in vitro. The experimental data reported by Villadsen et al suggest that blockade of IL-15 activity may be a viable therapeutic strategy for psoriasis.

B. H. Thiers, MD

Transgenic Delivery of VEGF to Mouse Skin Leads to an Inflammatory Condition Resembling Human Psoriasis
Xia Y-P, Li B, Hylton D, et al (Regeneron Pharmaceuticals, Tarrytown, NY; Harvard Med School,Charlestown, Mass)
Blood 102:161-168, 2003   2–27

Introduction.—Vascular endothelial growth factor (VEGF) is a potent mediator of angiogenesis, a fact that has prompted recent efforts to therapeutically exploit this characteristic in conditions involving pathologically reduced blood flow, including ischemic heart disease and nonhealing skin ulcers. The surprising observation that the transgenic delivery of VEGF to the skin results in a profound inflammatory skin condition with many of the cellular and molecular characteristics of psoriasis was discussed, and the impact of excess VEGF expression in mouse skin was assessed.

Findings.—A keratin-14 (K14)—based expression vector and a mouse cDNA encoding VEGF$_{164}$ were used to generate K14-VEGF transgenic mice on the *FVB* genetic background, with mice homozygous for this transgene used in each experiment. An initial histologic screen of the ear skin from young K14-VEGF transgenic mice, 3 months old, showed a mild and potentially prepsoriatic phenotype. In contrast to the mild changes observed under basal conditions, the creation of an excisional wound in the dorsal ear skin of 3-month-old K14-VEGF transgenic mice produced dramatic invaginations of the epidermis on the ventral side of the ear opposing the wound. The invaginations were similar to the prominent rete ridge structures seen in early human psoriasis. As the mice aged, they spontaneously began to develop dramatic lesions that resembled full-fledged psoriasis, including pronounced epidermal rete ridges and marked cutaneous inflammation in animals older than 5 months. Immunocytochemical investigation revealed hyperplastic and inflamed cutaneous blood vessels. Epidermal analysis of the psoriasiform lesions showed hyperkeratosis and parakeratosis, findings similar to those observed in human psoriasis. Neutrophil-filled lesions that resembled the epidermal microabscesses found in advanced human psoriasis were identified in the epidermis of 6-month-old K14-VEGF transgenic mice. Treatment with VEGF Trap (25 mg/kg every 3 days for 12 days), a potent VEGF inhibitor, resulted in pronounced visual improvement in the lesions on gross inspection in 4 of 6 mice so treated. The other 2 mice showed moderate improvement.

Conclusion.—Vascular changes may be among the earliest markers of the human psoriatic state. It may be that VEGF has a causative role in the vascular changes observed in psoriasis and in epidermal and inflammatory alterations. Prolonged VEGF overexpression had powerful proinflammatory capabilities in vivo, leading to a skin prototype resembling human psoriasis. It is likely that VEGF is a key factor in the link between inflammation and angiogenesis.

▶ As the old saying goes, "What goes around comes around." The suggestion by Dr Irwin Braverman (Yale University School of Medicine) that abnormal angiogenesis could be a key factor in the pathogenesis of psoriasis goes back more than 2 decades and antedates theories related to cyclic nucleotides, prostaglandins, polyamines, immune disregulation, etc. In the current article, Xia et al make the surprising observation that the transgenic delivery of VEGF to the skin results in a profound inflammatory skin disorder with many of the characteristic cellular and molecular features of psoriasis. Such changes could be effectively reversed by the addition of a potent VEGF antagonist. These findings support the importance of vascular factors in the etiology of psoriasis and open new avenues for future research into innovative treatments for this condition.

B. H. Thiers, MD

Efficacy of Acitretin and Commercial Tanning Bed Therapy for Psoriasis
Carlin CS, Callis KP, Krueger GG (Univ of Utah, Salt Lake City)
Arch Dermatol 139:436-442, 2003   2–28

Introduction.—Some patients use commercial tanning beds to treat their psoriasis, and several reports indicate that a majority of users experience clinical improvement in the Psoriasis Area and Severity Index (PASI) score. Forty-three patients with moderate to severe chronic plaque-type psoriasis were studied to determine whether commercial tanning bed irradiation enhances the therapeutic response to retinoids.

Methods.—Twenty-six patients were studied retrospectively, and 17 were enrolled in a prospective study. All lived in rural areas of Utah without easy access to PUVA and UV-B phototherapy. Twenty-five patients in the retrospective review received acitretin and 1 received isotretinoin. In the prospective study, patients were prescribed acitretin (25 mg/d) and received 4 to 5 tanning sessions per week for a maximum of 12 weeks. Tanning beds had a mean UV-B output of 4.7%. Patients were assessed at study entry and every 2 weeks for 12 weeks with use of the PASI score and the National Psoriasis Foundation (NPF) psoriasis score.

Results.—Nineteen patients in the retrospective review (83%) had clearance or near clearance, 2 (9%) experienced moderate improvement, and 2 (9%) showed no improvement. Both patient satisfaction and compliance with treatment were high (mean, 71.7% and 76.9%, respectively). In the prospective trial, the PASI and NPF scores decreased an average of 78.6% and 79.0%, respectively, from baseline. Nearly all adverse effects in both studies were mild and resolved with completion of therapy. Cheilitis was reported by 17 patients in the retrospective review and by 5 in the prospective trial. The other common side effects were dry skin and a mild tanning burn.

Conclusion.—The combination of acitretin and commercial tanning bed therapy proved an effective and useful alternative for patients whose access to physician-directed phototherapy is limited. Tanning bed salons should be evaluated, however, for safety precautions, good equipment, and the presence of well-trained technicians.

▶ The use of a commercial tanning bed as part of psoriasis therapy is not ideal. As noted by the authors, tanning salons differ considerably in the nature of their equipment, the intensity and age of their lamps, and the skill of the operator. Safety is also an issue, especially with coexistent intake of acitretin, a drug that has photosensitizing properties. Nevertheless, both UVL and acitretin are independently effective in the treatment of psoriasis and work even better in combination. For many patients, office-based phototherapy is simply not feasible. For such patients, re-TBUV may be an option if they are carefully monitored. Interestingly, PASI 75 was reached by 59% of patients at 12 weeks in the prospective trial, a figure significantly higher than that reported with the new biologic therapies.

B. H. Thiers, MD

Climatotherapy at the Dead Sea is a Remittive Therapy for Psoriasis: Combined Effects on Epidermal and Immunologic Activation

Hodak E, Gottlieb AB, Segal I, et al (Tel Aviv Univ, Israel; Univ of Medicine and Dentistry of New Jersey, New Brunswick)

J Am Acad Dermatol 49:451-457, 2003   2–29

Introduction.—Climatotherapy at the Dead Sea (CDS) has been used successfully for over 25 years in the treatment of moderate to severe psoriasis. It appears to confer long disease remission. There is a lack of trials evaluating the in vivo effect of CDS at both the molecular and cellular levels. The response to CDS of activated immunologic cells and keratinocytes in psoriatic lesions was examined.

Methods.—Twenty-seven patients with chronic, stable, plaque-type psoriasis treated with CDS for 28 consecutive days were assessed with the use of the Psoriasis Area and Severity Index score, along with quantitative histologic measures.

Results.—After 4 weeks of therapy, the overall Psoriasis Area and Severity Index score dropped by 81.5%. Complete clearance was observed in 48% of patients and moderate to marked improvement in 41%. The average duration of remission was 3.3 months. Histologically, there was an overall decrease in malpighian layer thickness by 63.4%. Keratinocyte hyperplasia, determined by Ki-67 cell cycle antigen expression, was reduced by 78%; residual cell proliferation was restricted primarily to the basal layer.

These changes were accompanied by normalization of keratin 16 expression in 90% of the cohort. T lymphocytes were nearly totally eliminated from the epidermis (depletion of over 90% of CD3+ and CD25+ cells), with only a low number remaining in the dermis (depletion of 69.4% of CD3+ cells and 77.4% of CD25 cells). This decrease in activated T cells was accompanied by a substantial decrease in HLA-DR expression by epidermal keratinocytes.

Conclusion.—CDS seems to be an effective remittive therapy for moderate to severe plaque-type psoriasis. The immunopathologic basis for the clinical efficacy of CDS has been described.

▶ The authors comment that CDS may be the most cost-effective modality for treating psoriasis, with an annual cost calculated at approximately $2300.[1]

B. H. Thiers, MD

Reference

1. Shani J, Harari M. Hristakieva E, et al: Dead Sea climatotherapy versus other modalities of treatment for psoriasis: Comparative cost effectiveness. *Int J Dermatol* 38:252-262, 1999.

308-nm Excimer Laser for the Treatment of Psoriasis: Induration-Based Dosimetry

Taneja A, Trehan M, Taylor CR (Harvard Med School, Boston)
Arch Dermatol 139:759-764, 2003   2–30

Background.—Interest in the the use of the 308-nm excimer laser for the treatment of psoriasis has been growing, because of its ability to selectively target and rapidly debulk lesions that have not responded to conventional treatment. Determining the optimal laser protocol may be difficult, however, as psoriatic lesions differ in erythema, induration, and scaling. The efficacy and safety of a dosimetry schedule based on the thickness of each plaque were examined.

Methods.—Fourteen patients (9 men and 5 women, Fitzpatrick skin types I-III) with plaque psoriasis whose lesions had not responded to at least 2 months of topical therapy, phototherapy, or systemic therapy were studied. Facial or genital lesions were excluded from treatment. One lesion on each patient was selected as a control, and a total of 44 plaques (25 on the knees and elbows, 10 on other parts of the extremities, and 9 on the trunk) were treated with the 308-nm excimer laser. The modified Psoriasis Area and Severity Index (PASI) score for each lesion was determined, and the initial laser dose was based on the induration score: induration score of 1, 0.4 J/cm²; score of 2, 0.6 J/cm²; and score of 3, 0.9 J/cm². Subsequent doses were given twice a week, and dosages were increased by up to 50% depending on the change in induration. Once the induration score was reduced to 0, four final consolidation doses were delivered.

Results.—At baseline, 7 lesions had an induration score of 1, 32 had a score of 2, and 5 had a score of 3. Plaques were treated a mean of 10 times (range, 4-14 treatments), and the mean cumulative dose was 8.8 J/cm² (range, 2.2-22.8 J/cm²). Treatments were quick, generally taking less than 1 minute for a 10-cm² lesion. The modified PASI score improved steadily and significantly in the treated plaques, with mean scores of 6.2 at baseline and 2.6, 1.2, and 1.0 after treatments 5, 10, and 13, respectively. Modified PASI scores increased somewhat after the end of therapy, from a mean of 1.0 to 2.0 after 3 months, and 3.1 after 6 months. The only adverse event was a mild sunburn-like reaction, which occurred in 2 patients after the first treatment; this reaction resolved spontaneously after they skipped a treatment.

Conclusion.—This subblistering dosage schedule based on induration allows the dermatologist to tailor each plaque's treatment plan for maximal effect. These stubborn psoriatic lesions cleared quickly and safely, and the relapse rate is similar to that of other therapies. The 308-nm excimer laser can be recommended as an adjunct to other conventional treatments (perhaps especially in combination with topical therapy) and as the primary method in patients with only a few lesions.

▶ This reviewer would argue that intralesional steroid injections for isolated recalcitrant plaques of psoriasis are quicker, cheaper, and more effective than the approach reported in this article, in which patients received a mean of 10 laser treatments.

B. H. Thiers, MD

The Time Course of Topical PUVA Erythema Following 15- and 5-Minute Methoxsalen Immersion
Man I, Kwok YK, Dawe RS, et al (Univ of Dundee, Scotland)
Arch Dermatol 139:331-334, 2003   2–31

Introduction.—Bath psoralen UV-A irradiation (PUVA) therapy is a widely used and effective alternative to oral PUVA treatments. Limited data are available on the time course and dose-response characteristics of PUVA erythema in skin photosensitized by bath methoxsalen, but recent reports suggest that a 5-minute soak before UV-A exposure may be as therapeutically effective as 10- or 15-minute soaks.

Methods.—Twenty-two healthy adult volunteers were enrolled in a study to determine the characteristics of PUVA erythema after 15- and 5-minute immersion in methoxsalen solution. No participant was receiving photoactive medication or had UV-A exposure in the 3 months before recruitment. One forearm was immersed in 1.2% methoxsalen solution for 15 minutes or for 5 minutes; then UV-A was delivered by means of a broad-spectrum UV-A fluorescent lamp. Erythema was assessed at 24-hour intervals for 7 days.

Results.—In the 15-minute immersion group, erythema was seen in 95% of participants at the first assessment time. PUVA erythema exhibited a broad peak, with the lowest median minimal phototoxic dose (MPD) at 96, 120, and 144 hours after UV-A irradiation. Peak erythema was experienced by 73% of the participants at 120 hours. An increase in the erythema index of 0.025 (equivalent to the MPD) was significantly lower when determined at 120 hours versus 72 hours after UV-A irradiation. The median maximum slope of the dose-response curves occurred at 144 hours (317 versus 165 at 72 hours, a significant difference). Erythema was observed at 24 hours in 11 volunteers (85%) in the 5-minute immersion group, and PUVA erythema exhibited a broad peak from 72 hours. Time trends were similar in 5- and 15-minute immersion groups, but erythemal intensity was significantly lower at all evaluation times with the 5-minute immersion.

Conclusion.—Erythema induced by PUVA therapy is assumed to occur 48 to 72 hours after UV-A irradiation, but recent evidence suggests that maximum PUVA erythema occurs beyond 72 hours. Peak erythema in this study occurred at 120 hours. Thus, the minimum phototoxic dose reading at 72 hours underestimates the phototoxic effect of topical methoxsalen PUVA.

▶ The authors show that the currently accepted MPD assessment time of 72 hours underestimates the phototoxic potential of topical PUVA. Potentially, this could result in cumulative erythema and an increased risk of burning during PUVA when treatments are administered twice weekly before maximum erythema is reached.

B. H. Thiers, MD

Topical Calcitriol Is Degraded by Ultraviolet Light
Lebwohl M, Quijije J, Gilliard J, et al (Mount Sinai School of Medicine, New York; Galderma Inc, Nice, France; SGS Lab Simon, Wavre, Belgium)
J Invest Dermatol 121:594-595, 2003   2–32

Background.—Calcitriol ointment, an approved psoriasis treatment in many countries worldwide, may be prescribed in conjunction with photo-therapy. The effects of various ultraviolet modalities on the stability of this agent were investigated; the effects of the ointment on the transmission of different forms of ultraviolet light were also determined.

Methods.—Calcitriol ointment, 3 µg/g, was irradiated with 10 J/cm² UV-A, 100 mJ/cm² broadband UV-B, and 3 J/cm² narrowband UV-B. The stability of the ointment under these conditions was compared with samples exposed to fluorescent light and ambient sunlight. UV-A and UV-B transmissions were assessed through thin and thick layers of calcitriol ointment, 3 µg/g, as well as vehicle.

Findings.—More then 90% of calcitriol ointment was degraded with exposure to UV-A, broadband UV-B, and narrowband UV-B. UV-A transmission was decreased through calcitriol ointment by 17% to 31% and by its vehicle by 17% to 41%. UV-B transmission was reduced by 50% to 83% through calcitriol ointment and by 67% to 87% through its vehicle.

Conclusions.—Calcitriol ointment used in conjunction with photo-therapy should be applied after rather than before UV exposure. Calcipotri-ene, the only vitamin D analog approved in the United States, has been successfully combined with UV-B and psoralen plus UV-A.

▶ A previous study[1] has documented degradation of calcipotriene by UV light. The current study shows that another vitamin D analog, calcitriol, may be subject to the same fate. This product is not yet in human testing in the United States. The authors bring up the possibility that degradation products of calcitriol might be active against psoriasis and suggest that clinical testing be done to refute or support that possibility.

B. H. Thiers, MD

Reference

1. Lebwohl M, Hecker D, Martinez J, et al: Interactions between calcipotriene and ultraviolet light. *J Am Acad Dermatol* 37:93-95, 1997.

Topical PTH (1-34) Is a Novel, Safe and Effective Treatment for Psoriasis: A Randomized Self-controlled Trial and an Open Trial

Holick MF, Chimeh FN, Ray S (Boston Univ)
Br J Dermatol 149:370-376, 2003   2–33

Introduction.—Expression of parathyroid hormone (PTH) related peptide (PTHrP) occurs in a wide variety of tissues, including skin. Psoriatic skin, however, shows no expression of PTHrP. The safety and efficacy of PTH in a liposomal cream formulation that enhances its percutaneous absorption were assessed for the treatment of plaque psoriasis.

Methods.—The study included 15 adult patients with chronic plaque psoriasis who were selected randomly in a double-blinded manner to be treated with 0.1 g of either Novasome A cream alone or Novasome A cream that contained 20 µg of human PTH (1-34). The preparations were topically applied, twice a day for 2 months, to a 25-cm² psoriatic lesion. At the end of the clinical trial, patients were invited to enroll in an open large area study. Ten patients then applied PTH once daily to their psoriatic lesions. Lesion sever-

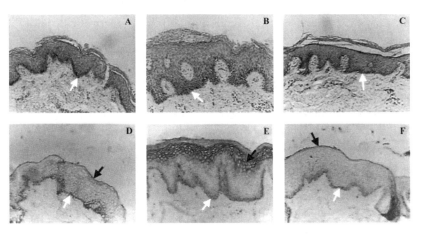

FIGURE 2.—Effect of topical PTH (1-34) and placebo Novasome A cream on the histology of skin biopsies and clinical improvement. A 53-year-old African-American male, who had had plaque psoriasis for > 10 years, had a 25-cm² lesion on the right lower abdomen treated with placebo Novasome A cream and a comparable 25-cm² psoriatic area on the left lower abdomen treated with 20 µg of PTH (1-34) Novasome A cream twice daily for 8 weeks. Skin biopsies were taken from (**A**) an unaffected area, (**B**) a placebo-treated lesion and (**C**) a PTH (1-34) treated area (hematoxylin and eosin; original magnification × 20). The placebo-treated lesion had focal parakeratosis, intracorneal neutrophilic infiltration, keratinocytic hyperplasia, epidermal hypogranulosis, dermal papillary edema, and lymphocytic perivascular cuffing, all of which are compatible with psoriasis and were not present in the unaffected skin biopsy (**A**) or PTH (1-34)-treated skin (**C**). The biopsies were immunohistochemically stained for transglutaminase K: (**D**) unaffected area, (**E**) placebo-treated lesion and (**F**) PTH (1-34)-treated lesion. The *white arrows* designate the pigmented melanocytes and the *black arrows* designate the staining for transglutaminase K. The right arm (**G**) and the left arm (**H**) are shown at the baseline visit. The control-treated lesions on the upper right arm (**I**) are compared with the PTH (1-34)-treated lesions on the left arm (**J**) after 2 months of treatment. The right arm and all the other psoriatic lesions were then treated with PTH (1-34) (**K,L**). Severe psoriatic lesions of the abdomen are shown at the baseline visit of the open trial phase (**M**) and after 2 months of treatment with PTH (1-34) (**N**). *Abbreviation: PTH,* Parathyroid hormone. (Courtesy of Holick MF, Chimeh FN, Ray S: Topical PTH (1-34) is a novel, safe and effective treatment for psoriasis: A randomized self-controlled trial and an open trial. *Br J Dermatol* 149:370-376, 2003. Published by permission of Blackwell Publishing.)

FIGURE 2 (cont.)

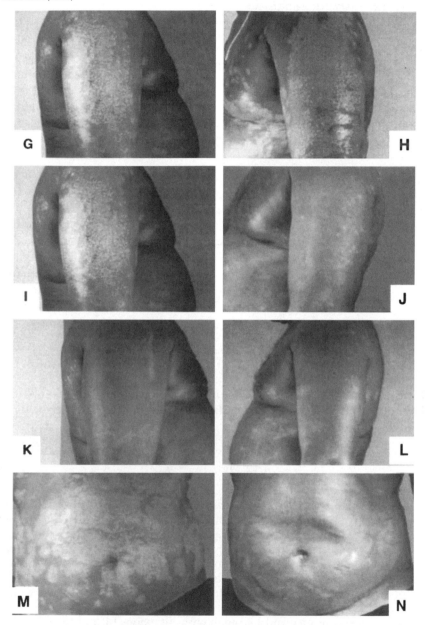

ity was evaluated during follow-up, and patients had blood and urine collected and punch biopsies of skin taken for analysis.

Results.—The lesions that received the cream containing PTH showed
marked improvement in scaling, erythema, and induration. Complete clear-

ing of psoriatic lesions occurred in 65% of those treated with PTH, and 85% showed at least partial improvement. Significantly less improvement, similar to that obtained with a hydrating placebo ointment or cream, was seen in Novasome A placebo-treated lesions (Fig 2); see color plates IV and V). The 10 patients who applied PTH on all their lesions showed an overall improvement of 42.6% in the Psoriasis Area and Severity Index score. No side effects were associated with PTH, and no patient experienced hypercalcemia or hypercalciuria.

Conclusion.—Patients with chronic plaque psoriasis who had failed to respond to at least 1 standard therapy showed marked improvement when PTH was applied to their lesions. Topical PTH offers promise as a safe and effective new therapy.

▶ PTHrP is produced by human skin and appears to be a potent inhibitor of epidermal growth. The data presented by Holick et al suggest some potential for this compound as a topical treatment for psoriasis. Interestingly, data presented more than a decade ago demonstrated no expression of PTHrP in psoriatic skin but restoration of its expression after treatment with topical vitamin D analogues.[1]

B. H. Thiers, MD

Reference

1. Juhlin L, Hagforsen E, Juhlin C: Parathyroid hormone related protein is localized in the granular layer of normal skin and in the dermal infiltrates of mycosis fungoides but is absent in psoriatic lesions. *Acta Derm Venereol* 72:81-83, 1992.

Lichen Planus Associated With Hepatitis C Virus: No Viral Transcripts Are Found in the Lichen Planus, and Effective Therapy for Hepatitis C Virus Does Not Clear Lichen Planus

Harden D, Skelton H, Smith KJ (Natl Naval Med Ctr, Bethesda, Md; Quest Diagnostics, Tucker, Ga)

J Am Acad Dermatol 49:847-852, 2003   2–34

Background.—Acute hepatitis C virus (HCV) infection is often relatively mild, but chronic liver disease develops over time in 70% to 80% of affected patients. Half of these patients may remain asymptomatic for up to 40 years. Lichen planus–like eruptions (LP) are among a number of associated cutaneous manifestations, affecting up to 15% of patients with HCV. Whether viral transcripts are present in the skin of patients with HCV and LP was investigated. Whether systemic virologic response to interferon alfa and ribavirin is associated with LP response was also studied.

Methods.—Four men and 1 woman with cutaneous LP and chronic HCV were included in the study (Fig 2). One patient had oral LP. Biopsy specimens were analyzed by immunohistochemical stains for lymphoid markers and reverse-transcriptase polymerase chain reaction (RT-PCR) for HCV, in ad-

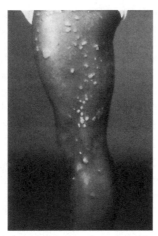

FIGURE 2.—Lichen planus–like lesions on leg of patient who is positive for hepatitis C virus with active liver disease. (Reprinted by permission of the publisher from Harden D, Skelton H, Smith KJ: Lichen planus associated with hepatitis C virus: No viral transcripts are found in the lichen planus, and effective therapy for hepatitis C virus does not clear lichen planus. *J Am Acad Dermatol* 49:847-852, 2003. Copyright 2003 by Elsevier.)

dition to pathologic examination. Treatment for all patients consisted of interferon alfa and ribavirin.

Findings.—Biopsy specimens from 4 of 5 patients showed scattered eosinophils. The predominant component of the lymphoid infiltrate was CD3$^+$ T cells and scattered KP-1$^+$ mononuclear cells, with no CD20$^+$ B cells. About one fourth of the T cells did not mark with CD4. All patients were seropositive for HCV RNA at the time of biopsy. However, HCV RNA could not be detected by RT-PCR in any of the biopsy specimens. Lichen planus–like eruptions responded to treatment inconsistently.

Conclusions.—RT-PCR revealed no HCV in these LP lesions. Therefore, LP may be related to the pattern of immune dysregulation induced by HCV, most likely in a patient susceptible to autoimmune disease. Treatment with interferon alfa and ribavirin may effectively clear the virus, but viral response was unassociated with LP clearing.

▶ The absence of HCV RNA in LP suggests that the virus causes the skin disease by some indirect mechanism.

B. H. Thiers, MD

Treatment of Severe Lichen Planus With Mycophenolate Mofetil
Frieling U, Bonsmann G, Schwarz T, et al (Univ of Münster, Germany)
J Am Acad Dermatol 49:1063-1066, 2003   2–35

Introduction.—Mycophenolate mofetil (MMF), an immunosuppressive agent that specifically and reversibly inhibits the proliferation of activated T cells, has been successfully used in the treatment of autoimmune and inflammatory skin disorders and graft-versus-host disease (GVHD). Both GVHD and lichen planus (LP) are characterized by activated T cells, which have a central role in lesion formation. The successful use of MMF in the management of 2 patients with extensive, disseminated LP was described.

> *Case Reports 1 and 2.*—Woman, 34, and adolescent boy, 17, both had a 2- to 3-month history of extensive, generalized LP, including nonpainful Wickham's striae of the buccal mucosa. The disease worsened with treatment with systemic (20 mg/d over 2 weeks) and potent topical corticosteroids (class II and III over 5 weeks) in the woman and with potent topical corticosteroids (class III) in the adolescent boy. Both patients had extreme pruritus. A review of systems and laboratory analyses, including hepatitis serologies, were unremarkable. After exclusion of potential underlying disease that would contraindicate immunosuppressive therapy (eg, tuberculosis), both patients received MMF 1 g twice daily. During the initial weeks of therapy, no substantial improvement in the lesions was noted, although the pruritus diminished. Within 5 to 6 weeks of therapy, all papulosquamous and oral reticulated lesions began to decrease. Complete remission was observed after about 20 weeks of therapy. Medication was discontinued, and no new lesions were observed in the woman and adolescent patient during a follow-up of 17 and 63 months, respectively. Treatment with MMF was well tolerated and had no side effects.

Conclusion.—Monotherapy with MMF may be considered safe and effective in the management of generalized, disseminated, cutaneous LP. It appears to be a promising therapeutic alternative, particularly in patients with LP who have refractory severe disease or contraindications to conventional therapy, including other immunosuppressive agents.

▶ Extensive LP can present a true treatment dilemma. In an effort to avoid long-term systemic corticosteroid therapy, I have had some success with systemic retinoids, either alone or in combination with phototherapy. Frieling et al suggest the use of MMF, an immunosuppressive agent whose use has been proposed for other cutaneous inflammatory disorders, including psoriasis, atopic dermatitis, and autoimmune blistering diseases. The drug specifically targets activated T-cells, which are thought to play a key role in the pathogenesis of LP.

B. H. Thiers, MD

3 Bacterial and Mycobacterial Infections

Duration of Antibiotic Therapy for Early Lyme Disease: A Randomized, Double-blind, Placebo-controlled Trial
Wormser GP, Ramanathan R, Nowakowski J, et al (New York Med College, Valhalla)
Ann Intern Med 138:697-704, 2003   3–1

Introduction.—The optimal duration of antibiotic therapy for patients with early Lyme disease and the need to treat for potential CNS involvement remain controversial. These issues were addressed in a placebo-controlled study comparing 10 days of doxycycline with both 10 days of doxycycline plus a single dose of IV ceftriaxone and 20 days of doxycycline only.

Methods.—This double-blind study included 180 patients with erythema migrans. Randomization was stratified by whether patients were asymptomatic or symptomatic so that the 3 treatment groups might have similar proportions of patients with dissemination of *Borrelia burgdorferi*. Patients were assessed for treatment efficacy and safety at 20 days, 3 months, 12 months, and 30 months. Evaluations included clinical examination and neurocognitive testing. Outcome was characterized as complete response, partial response, or failure.

Results.—The 3 treatment groups were similar in baseline demographic characteristics, clinical findings, and laboratory test results. Systemic illness was present in approximately three fourths of patients. In both on-study and intention-to-treat analyses, the complete response rate was similar for the 3 groups at all time points. Thirty-month complete response rates in the on-study analysis were 83.9% in the 20-day doxycycline group, 90.3% in the 10-day doxycycline group, and 86.5% in the doxycycline plus ceftriaxone group. In the only case of treatment failure at any time point, a patient in the 10-day doxycycline group was diagnosed with meningitis on day 18. A 2-week course of ceftriaxone resulted in improvement, and the results of neurocognitive testing were normal. Significantly more patients in the combination therapy group reported diarrhea.

Conclusion.—All 3 treatment groups had generally favorable outcomes. Thus, extending doxycycline treatment from 10 days to 20 days or adding ceftriaxone to a 10-day doxycycline course did not enhance the resolution of erythema migrans or associated systemic symptoms in early, uncomplicated Lyme disease.

▶ Various authorities have recommended antibiotic regimens of 10 to 30 days for the treatment of Lyme disease, while others have advocated enhancement of treatment with a parenteral agent such as ceftriaxone, which readily crosses the blood/brain barrier, and thus might provide additional benefit to patients in whom *Borrelia burgdorferi* has disseminated to the central nervous system at the time of presentation. Wormser et al compared 10- and 20-day regimens of doxycycline with or without a single IV dose of ceftriaxone to 20 days of oral doxycycline in the treatment of patients with early Lyme disease. They could discern no benefit either from extending the duration of therapy or from the addition of the second antibiotic.

B. H. Thiers, MD

A Newly Identified Tick-borne *Borrelia* Species and Relapsing Fever in Tanzania
Kisinza WN, McCall PJ, Mitani H, et al (Liverpool School of Tropical Medicine, England; Natl Inst for Med Research, Dar es Salaam, Tanzania; Fukuyama Univ, Hiroshima, Japan; et al)
Lancet 362:1283-1284, 2003   3–2

Background.—In central Tanzania, tick-borne relapsing fever from the spirochete *Borrelia duttonii* is a common cause of serious illness. A previously unidentified species of *Borrelia* was found during screening of *Ornithodoros* species ticks from infested houses for the presence of *B duttonii*. Whether this species infected the human population of a central Tanzanian village was investigated.

Methods and Findings.—Blood samples were obtained from 2 groups of children selected randomly during household surveys in Muungano during October and November of 2002. Thick blood smears were prepared and stained with Giemsa, then examined microscopically. *Borrelia* species were detected by polymerase chain reaction based on a flagellin gene. *Borrelia* species were identified in 11% of 54 febrile children and in 4% of 307 otherwise healthy children. Genotyping *Borrelia* from 17 infections revealed *B duttonii* and the unknown species.

Conclusion.—This newly identified species is a causal agent of tick-borne relapsing fever. The sensitivity of screening for *Borrelia* species infections can be increased by polymerase chain reaction use.

▶ Kisinza et al report a newly discovered, as yet unnamed species of *Borrelia* as a possible cause of tick-borne relapsing fever.

B. H. Thiers, MD

Ciprofloxacin Resistance in *Neisseria gonorrhoeae* in England and Wales in 2002
Fenton KA, for the GRASP Collaboration (Health Protection Agency, London; et al)
Lancet 361:1867-1869, 2003   3–3

Background.—National guidelines in the United Kingdom recommend ciprofloxacin as first-line treatment for gonorrhea. Anecdotal reports indicate that resistance of *Neisseria gonorrhoeae* to ciprofloxacin is increasing. Thus, a national surveillance program was undertaken to determine the incidence of gonococcal antimicrobial resistance to ciprofloxacin in England and Wales.

Methods.—The authors obtained 2200 to 2300 *N gonorrhoeae* isolates each year between 2000 and 2002 from 24 clinical laboratories in England and Wales. Antimicrobial resistance testing was performed at 1 of 2 central laboratories. Resistance to ciprofloxacin was defined as a minimum inhibitory concentration of 1 mg or more per liter. Susceptibility results were compared for the 3 years. Clinical data for the source patients were obtained from medical records.

Results.—The overall prevalence of ciprofloxacin-resistant *N gonorrhoeae* was 2.1% in 2000, 3.1% in 2001, and 9.8% in 2002. This 3-fold increase was independent of sex, recent sexual contact overseas, and residence inside or outside London.

Conclusion.—These findings of an increased prevalence of ciprofloxacin-resistant *N gonorrhoeae* are similar to those from regional and national surveillance programs in other countries and emphasize the urgent need to review and revise the UK's national guidelines regarding the treatment of gonorrhea.

▶ Three first-line options are included in the UK national guidelines for the treatment of gonorrhea: ciprofloxacin, ofloxacin, and ampicillin/probenecid; about 74% of the clinics in that country use ciprofloxacin as first-line treatment. Ideally, the chosen treatment regimen for gonorrhea should eliminate infection in at least 95% of the patients; ciprofloxacin clearly no longer meets that criterion in the UK. The findings demonstrate the propensity of bacteria to evolve to become resistant to commonly prescribed therapies.

B. H. Thiers, MD

Antibiotic Resistance Among Gram-Negative Bacilli in US Intensive Care Units: Implications for Fluoroquinolone Use
Neuhauser MM, Weinstein RA, Rydman R, et al (Univ of Houston; Rush Med College, Chicago; Cook County Hosp, Chicago; et al)
JAMA 289:885-888, 2003   3–4

Background.—The emergence of antibiotic resistance can be assessed with susceptibility data derived from national surveillance. The results of a national ICU surveillance study of aerobic gram-negative bacilli collected from 1990 to 1993 were presented in a previous report, which revealed an increasing incidence of ceftazidime-resistant *Klebsiella pneumoniae* and *Enterobacter* species in ICUs. National rates of antimicrobial resistance in ICUs between 1994 to 2000 were described.

Methods.—The institutions participating in this study represented 43 states in the United States plus the District of Columbia. These facilities provided antibiotic susceptibility results for 35,790 nonduplicate gram-negative aerobic isolates recovered from ICU patients from 1994 to 2000. Approximately 100 consecutive gram-negative aerobic isolates recovered from ICU patients were tested by each institution. Organisms were identified to the species level. Susceptibility tests were performed, and national fluoroquinolone consumption data were obtained.

Results.—The activity of most antimicrobial agents against gram-negative aerobic isolates was indicative of an absolute decrease of 6% or less over the study period. There was a steady decline in the overall susceptibility to ciprofloxacin, from 86% in 1994 to 76% in 2000. This decline was significantly associated with increased national use of fluoroquinolones.

Conclusions.—The increasing incidence of ciprofloxacin resistance among gram-negative bacilli is documented. This increased incidence has occurred in conjunction with the increased use of fluoroquinolones. Slowing this downward trend will require more judicious use of fluoroquinolones.

▶ One of the more predictable events in the evolution of antimicrobial therapy is that the incidence of antibiotic-resistant strains increases with the prevalence of antibiotic use. Thus, the article by Neuhauser et al is hardly surprising. Rarely does a day go by that I do not see patients who have been treated by their primary care physicians with expensive, potent, broad spectrum antibiotics for relatively simple skin infections that would readily respond to cheaper, more specific therapy. The overuse of antibiotics is leading us down a dangerous road toward the eventual emergence of organisms resistant to all available therapies.

B. H. Thiers, MD

Necrotizing Fasciitis: Clinical Presentation, Microbiology, and Determinants of Mortality
Wong C-H, Chang H-C, Pasupathy S, et al (Changi Gen Hosp, Singapore)
J Bone Joint Surg Am 85-A:1454-1460, 2003   3–5

Introduction.—Necrotizing fasciitis is a surgical emergency for which early recognition and prompt aggressive debridement of all necrotic tissue is crucial for survival. The clinical presentation and microbiological characteristics of necrotizing fasciitis were reviewed retrospectively, along with the determinants of mortality linked with this condition.

Methods.—The medical records of 89 consecutive patients admitted with necrotizing fasciitis between January 1997 and August 2002 were analyzed.

Results.—The paucity of cutaneous findings early in the disease course made it challenging to establish a diagnosis. Of the 89 patients, only 13 (14.6%) had a diagnosis of necrotizing fasciitis at the time of hospital admission. Preadmission treatment with antibiotics altered the initial clinical picture and frequently masked the underlying infection. The most common cause of necrotizing fasciitis was polymicrobial synergistic infection (n = 48, 53.9%), with streptococci and enterobacteriaceae being the most common isolates. Group-A streptococci was the most frequent cause of monomicrobial necrotizing fasciitis. The most common related comorbidity was diabetes mellitus (n = 63, 70.8%). Advanced age, 2 or more associated comorbidities, and delay in surgery of more than 24 hours were associated with an increased mortality rate; the association with delay in surgery was significant (*P* < .05; relative risk, 9.4).

Conclusion.—Early operative debridement was associated with a decreased mortality rate among patients with necrotizing fasciitis. A high index of suspicion is crucial because of the paucity of specific cutaneous findings early in the course of the condition.

▶ Because of the nonspecific cutaneous findings, the diagnosis of necrotizing fasciitis is typically difficult to make early in its course; in fact, Wong, et al noted that only 14.6% of patients in their series were diagnosed with that disorder at the time of admission. The usual presenting signs include the triad of exquisite pain, swelling, and fever. The presence of blisters filled with serous fluid is an important diagnostic clue. A high index of suspicion is important, as necrotizing fasciitis is a surgical emergency with early operative debridement being a critical factor in reducing mortality.

B. H. Thiers, MD

Antigens in Tea-Beverage Prime Human Vγ2Vδ2 T Cells In Vitro and In Vivo for Memory and Nonmemory Antibacterial Cytokine Responses
Kamath AB, Wang L, Das H, et al (Brigham and Women's Hosp, Boston; Harvard Med School, Boston; Univ of New Hampshire, Durham)
Proc Natl Acad Sci U S A 100:6009-6014, 2003   3–6

Background.—In humans, γδ T lymphocytes mediate innate immunity to microbes by means of T-cell receptor–dependent recognition of unprocessed antigens with conserved molecular patterns, such as alkylamines and organophosphates. One such alkylamine, ethylamine, is found in brewed tea as an intact molecule and in its precursor form, L-theanine. Tea has for centuries been promoted as a healthful and medicinal beverage, yet no in vivo data demonstrating an immunologic effect of tea on human tissue have been published. However, there is a significant body of evidence to support the role of γδ T cells in resistance to infection. This study demonstrates that priming of γδ T cells in vitro with alkylamine antigens results in their production of interferon γ in response to nonpeptide antigens, whole bacteria, and lipopolysaccharide.

Methods.—Eleven healthy non–tea-drinking subjects were asked to drink 5 to 6 cups of black tea, equivalent to approximately 600 mL per day, for either 2 or 4 weeks. The tea was prepared by steeping a tea bag for 5 minutes in 100 mL of water that had been brought to a boil. A second group of 10 healthy non-tea and non-coffee drinkers was asked to drink 5 to 6 cups of instant coffee, which contains caffeine but not L-theanine. Blood was sampled before and every week after the volunteers began drinking tea or coffee for 2 to 4 weeks, and peripheral blood mononuclear cells were isolated and frozen for later analysis.

Results.—The T cells of subjects in the tea-drinking group responded 5 times more rapidly to infectious organisms than did T cells from subjects in the instant coffee group.

Conclusion.—These findings provide evidence that consumption of tea, and perhaps vegetables and fruit containing alkylamine antigens or their precursors, may prime human $\gamma\delta$ T cells, which then may provide natural resistance to microbial infections and possibly tumors.

▶ Kamath et al showed that tea boosts the body's defenses against infection and contains a substance, L-theanine, that may form the basis of a drug to protect against disease. The investigators initially demonstrated that L-theanine primes the body's immune system to attack various invading microbes. In a second experiment, they observed that T cells from tea drinkers responded 5 times faster to infectious organisms than did T cells from drinkers of instant coffee, which does not contain L-theanine. L-theanine is related to a ubiquitous group of molecules called alkylamines which can be found in the blood, urine, breast milk, vaginal secretions, and amniotic fluid of healthy individuals. They are secreted by commensal and pathogenic bacteria but, more importantly, are found at high concentrations (mostly in precursor form) in tea and at lower concentrations in other edible plant products such as mushrooms, apples, and wine. Thus, alkylamine antigens or their precursors may act as a bridge between innate and acquired immunity. By priming the immune system, they may provide natural resistance to microbial infections and perhaps tumors, and this resistance may be enhanced by dietary intake of tea and other fruits and vegetables containing these substances. Claimed beneficial effects of tea have included a lower incidence of heart disease and cancer (possibly through the action of antioxidant flavonoids), reduction of osteoporosis, and relief of allergy symptoms. Other studies have claimed benefits in the prevention and repair of photodamage.[1,2]

B. H. Thiers, MD

References

1. Lu YP, Lou YR, Xie JG, et al: Topical applications of caffeine or (-)-epigallocatechin gallate (EGCG) inhibit carcinogenesis and selectively increase apoptosis in UVB-induced skin tumors in mice. *Proc Natl Acad Sci U S A* 99:12455-12460, 2002.
2. Katiyar SK, Bergamo BM, Vyalil PK, et al: Green tea polyphenols: DNA photodamage and photoimmunology. *J Photochem Photobiol B* 65:109-114, 2001.

Comparison of T-Cell–Based Assay With Tuberculin Skin Test for Diagnosis of *Mycobacterium tuberculosis* Infection in a School Tuberculosis Outbreak

Ewer K, Deeks J, Alvarez L, et al (Univ of Oxford, England; Inst of Health Sciences, Oxford, England; Leicestershire Health Authority, England; et al)

Lancet 361:1168-1173, 2003   3–7

Introduction.—The tuberculin skin test (TST) for latent tuberculosis infection can yield false-positive results, requires a return visit, and is further limited by operator-dependent variability in placement and reading of the test. A newly developed sensitive enzyme-linked immunospot (ELISPOT) assay detects T cells specific for *Mycobacterium tuberculosis* antigens that are absent from *M bovis* BCG and most environmental mycobacteria. An outbreak of tuberculosis at a secondary school provided an opportunity to compare the effectiveness of the ELISPOT assay with the TST.

Methods.—After a student with a chronic cough was found to have pulmonary tuberculosis, TST screening identified 69 cases of active tuberculosis and 254 cases of latent infection. A total of 963 students from the school were then invited to be tested for *M tuberculosis* infection with the ELISPOT assay; 595 children and their parents consented, and 550 (57% of those invited) had blood drawn and were interviewed by nurses. Samples used in the ELISPOT assays were processed and scored by 2 scientists who had no access to TST results or personal identifiers. Students were classified into 4 groups on the basis of degree of exposure to the index case.

Results.—Agreement between the TST and the ELISPOT was high (89% concordance), but ELISPOT correlated significantly more closely with *M tuberculosis* exposure, on measures of both proximity and duration of exposure to the index case, than did TST. Results of ELISPOT were not associated with BCG vaccination, whereas TST was significantly more likely to be positive in BCG-vaccinated than in nonvaccinated children. Both tests positively correlated with a history of household tuberculosis contact.

Conclusion.—Because there is no gold standard test for latent tuberculosis infection, the sensitivity and specificity of the ELISPOT assay or the TST could not be determined. However, a discordance of 11% in this study indicates that the tests are not equivalent, and the findings suggest that the ELISPOT assay is more accurate.

▶ There is no gold standard test for latent tuberculosis infection; thus, the sensitivity and specificity of the ELISPOT assay or the TST cannot be directly quantified.[1] However, in acknowledging that the likelihood of latent tuberculosis infection is determined by exposure to the causative organism, the authors were able to rank the tests according to their diagnostic accuracy. They concluded that the ELISPOT assay was more sensitive and specific than the TST. The latter is cheap, but related indirect costs associated with the need for return visits and trained staff to administer and read the test must be considered. In addition, improved tuberculosis control with a more accurate test such as the ELISPOT assay might ultimately yield significant cost savings. Whether the ELISPOT assay eventually replaces the TST in routine clinical practice cannot be predicted with certainty.

B. H. Thiers, MD

Reference

1. Jasmer RM, Nahid P, Hopewell PC: Clinical practice: Latent tuberculosis infection. *N Engl J Med* 347:1860-1866, 2002.

Activation and Regulation of Toll-like Receptors 2 and 1 in Human Leprosy

Krutzik SR, Ochoa MT, Sieling PA, et al (Univ of California, Los Angeles; Osaka Univ, Japan; Japan Science and Technology Corporation, Osaka; et al)
Nat Med April-Online:1-8, 2003   3–8

Introduction.—One mechanism by which the innate immune system recognizes the biochemical patterns of infectious invaders is through Toll-like receptors (TLRs). Previous investigations have shown the specificity of TLRs in mediating responses to defined bacterial ligands. When activated, TLRs trigger the release of cytokines and induce antimicrobial pathways. Leprosy, a disease with a clinical spectrum that correlates with the level of immune response to the pathogen, was selected to examine the innate immune response in human disease.

Methods.—Skin biopsy specimens were obtained from 20 patients, 10 with tuberculoid leprosy (T-lep) and 10 with lepromatous leprosy (L-lep). Those with T-lep are relatively resistant to the pathogen, with localized infection and lesions characterized by expression of the type-1 cytokines characteristic of cell-mediated immunity. Those with L-lep are relatively susceptible to the pathogen, with a systemically disseminated infection and lesions characterized by the type-2 cytokines characteristic of humoral responses. Human cell lines transiently expressing TLR homodimers (TLR1-10) or heterodimers (TLR2-TLR1, TLR2-TLR6, TLR2-TLR-10) were used to determine the role of TLRs in mediating cell activation by *Mycobacterium leprae*.

Results.—The TLR2-TLR1 heterodimers mediated cell activation by killed *M leprae*, an indication of the presence of triacylated lipoproteins. Thirty-one putative lipoproteins were detected in a genome-wide scan of *M leprae*, and ML1966 and ML0603 were chosen for further study. Both activated primary human monocytes obtained from healthy donors, as measured by the release of interleukin-12 (IL-12) p40. Activation was blocked by a TLR2-neutralizing antibody. Synthetic lipopeptides representing the 19-kd and 33-kd lipoproteins activated both monocytes and dendritic cells. Type-1 cytokines enhanced activation, whereas type-2 cytokines inhibited activation. The expression of TLR1 in monocytes and dendritic cells was enhanced, respectively, by interferon-γ and granulocyte-macrophage colony-stimulating factor, whereas TLR2 expression was downregulated by IL-4. Both TLR2 and TLR1 were more strongly expressed in lesions of localized T-lep than in those of disseminated L-lep.

Conclusion.—The Toll family of receptors, found in both insects and mammals, seems to be integral to the ability of the innate immune system to recognize and respond to microbial pathogens. In leprosy, the outcome of the immune response may be determined in part by the influence of the local cytokine environment on the regulated expression and activation of TLR2 and TLR1.

▶ The Toll receptors and TLRs include many highly conserved molecules that are involved in and crucial to the innate immune response to pathogens. For example, the mammalian TLR family includes members that recognize bacterial lipopeptides, lipopolysaccharides, CpG DNA sequences, and others. In this study, the putative role of TLR in the immune response to *M leprae* was examined with the use of human cells expressing TLR homo- or heterodimers. The data obtained suggested that the killed organisms were recognized by TLR2 homodimers, and also showed that the cellular activation response was dramatically increased in cells expressing both TLR1 and 2. This TLR2-TLR1–dependent response to *M leprae* was confirmed using appropriate knockout mice. The investigators also identified several *M leprae* lipopeptides that activated normal human monocytes in a TLR2-dependent manner. Of particular interest was the finding that TLR1 and 2 were expressed at a higher level in cells from T-lep than in those from L-lep lesions, and that monocyte activation by the *M leprae* lipopeptides was enhanced by Th1 cytokines, which are the hallmark of the T-cell response in T-lep. These data convincingly illustrate the cooperation between the innate and adaptive immune systems in host defense.

G. M. P. Galbraith, MD

4 Fungal Infections

Intraepidermal Neutrophils—A Clue to Dermatophytosis?
Meymandi S, Silver SG, Crawford RI (Univ of British Columbia, Vancouver, Canada)
J Cutan Pathol 30:253-255, 2003   4–1

Background.—Diagnosing dermatophytosis histopathologically can be challenging. Histopathologic criteria include the presence of neutrophils in the stratum corneum and alternating layers of compact orthokeratosis. Whether the presence of neutrophils in the stratum corneum is a sensitive and specific test for identifying dermatophytosis was examined.

Methods.—The medical records of 303 patients with spongiotic or psoriasiform dermatitides evaluated over a 35-month period were reviewed. Hematoxylin and eosin (H&E) and periodic acid-Schiff (PAS-D) staining had been performed for each patient. PAS-D results were negative in 295 patients; thus, they were given the diagnosis of other dermatitides. PAS-D results were positive in 8 patients; thus, they were given the diagnosis of dermatophytosis. The investigators selected 92 control subjects and all 8 case patients for further evaluation of the H&E stain to confirm the presence of dermatophytosis and the absence of neutrophils.

Results.—Of the 92 control subjects with negative PAS-D findings whose H&E stains were reviewed, 38 (41.3%) had neutrophils within the stratum corneum on H&E staining (Table 1). Of the 8 cases with positive PAS-D findings, 5 (62.5%) had neutrophils within the stratum corneum on H&E staining. Thus, the sensitivity of diagnosing dermatophytosis on the basis of finding neutrophils within the stratum corneum was 62%, and the specificity was 59%. The positive predictive value was 4%, and the negative predictive value was 98%, which yielded an overall accuracy of 59%.

TABLE 1.—Proportion of Cases With Neutrophils in Each Diagnostic Category of the Dermatophyte-Negative Controls

	Number of Cases	Neutrophils Present
Eczema	62	17 (27%)
Psoriasis	24	21 (87%)
Pityriasis rosea	6	0
Total	92	38 (41%)

(Courtesy of Meymandi S, Silver SG, Crawford RI: Intraepidermal neutrophils—A clue to dermatophytosis? *J Cutan Pathol* 30:253-255, 2003. Reprinted by permission of Blackwell Publishing.)

Conclusion.—Histopathologic diagnosis of dermatophytosis may be required when the clinical suspicion of dermatophytosis is high but potassium hydroxide and/or culture results are negative. Dermatophytosis must be differentiated histopathologically from both infectious and noninfectious causes, such as psoriasis, eczema, pityriasis rosea, and, less commonly, parapsoriasis, mycosis fungoides, lichen simplex chronicus, pityriasis lichenoides, pityriasis rubra pilaris, candidiasis, impetigo, and syphilis. The myeloperoxidase–hydrogen peroxidase system of neutrophils inhibits fungal growth; thus, neutrophils may play a role in the immune response to dermatophytes. Still, this does not mean that the presence of neutrophils is a key finding in the diagnosis of dermatophytosis. The results suggest the identification of neutrophils within the stratum corneum has low specificity and low sensitivity in the diagnosis of dermatophytosis. Indeed, 87% of the control subjects with psoriasis in this series had intracorneal neutrophils, and eczematous conditions are often characterized by intraepidermal neutrophils. With an overall accuracy of only 59%, the presence of intraepidermal neutrophils is not a reliable predictor of dermatophytosis.

▶ Criteria for the histopathologic diagnosis of inflammatory diseases of the skin have rarely been subjected to rigorous analysis. The authors of this article found that neutrophils in the stratum corneum had a sensitivity of 62% and a specificity of 59% for the diagnosis of dermatophytosis. Although the positive predictive value was only 4%, this may have been influenced by the geographic locality in which the study was conducted. The incidence of dermatophytosis in Vancouver, Canada, may be considerably less than in Charleston, South Carolina, where the climatologic conditions promote the growth of dermatophytes on human skin. Nevertheless, studies such as this demonstrate the gaps in our knowledge.

J. C. Maize, MD

Comparison of Diagnostic Methods in the Evaluation of Onychomycosis
Weinberg JM, Koestenblatt EK, Tutrone WD, et al (St Luke's-Roosevelt Hosp, New York; New York Med College)
J Am Acad Dermatol 49:193-197, 2003   4–2

Introduction.—Onychomycosis is the most common cause of dystrophic nails, but approximately half of dystrophic nails do not have a fungal origin. The infection needs to be diagnosed correctly, since long-term therapy with oral antifungal medication has potential side effects. Traditional diagnostic methods with potassium hydroxide (KOH) preparation and fungal culture often yield false-negative results. The sensitivity and specificity of KOH preparation for the diagnosis of onychomycosis were compared with those of 3 other methods: culture, nail plate biopsies (Bx) with periodic acid–Schiff (PAS) stain (Bx/PAS), and calcofluor white (CW) stain.

Methods.—Study participants were 105 patients with suspected onychomycosis. All were evaluated with the 4 diagnostic methods. On the basis of previous studies, CW was chosen as the gold standard for statistical analysis. Positive predictive values (PPVs) and negative predictive values (NPVs) were calculated for each method.

Results.—Ninety-three patients had at least 1 of the 4 diagnostic methods positive for the presence of organisms. When compared with the results of CW staining, the sensitivity was 80% for KOH, 92% for Bx/PAS, and 59% for culture; specificities for these 3 methods were, respectively, 72%, 72%, and 82%. The PPV was 88% for KOH, 89.7% for Bx/PAS, and 90% for culture; NPV results were 58% for KOH, 77% for Bx/PAS, and 43% for culture. Thirty-seven patients tested positive with all 4 methods, whereas 12 tested negative with all 4 methods.

Conclusion.—CW, a fluorescent brightener used in the textile and paper industries, selectively binds to cellulose and chitin, the major components in the cell walls of fungi. Thus, CW has been used in clinical microbiology and pathology as a nonspecific stain for fungi. In a previous study, CW had a sensitivity of 92%, a specificity of 95%, a PPV of 74%, and a NPV of 99% in the diagnosis of superficial fungal infection. This comparison of culture, Bx/PAS, and KOH suggests that Bx/PAS is the method of choice for the evaluation of onychomycosis.

▶ Weinberg et al demonstrate the importance of PAS staining of nail clippings to definitively rule out onychomycosis in patients with negative culture results. Unfortunately, a fluorescent microscope is required for using the CW stain, making this method impractical for most dermatologists' offices.

B. H. Thiers, MD

The Periodic Acid-Schiff Stain in Diagnosing Tinea: Should It Be Used Routinely in Inflammatory Skin Diseases?
Al-Amiri A, Chatrath V, Bhawan J, et al (Boston Univ)
J Cutan Pathol 30:611-615, 2003   4–3

Introduction.—Not all tinea infections exhibit the typical clinical and histopathologic characteristics and thus may be confused with other skin disorders. The presence of hyphal forms confirms the diagnosis, but because biopsy specimens stained with hematoxylin and eosin (H&E) may not reveal hyphae if few are present, the periodic acid–Schiff (PAS) stain may be needed. Cases of documented tinea were reviewed to determine whether PAS-staining should be routinely performed and whether certain histopathologic clues are suggestive of a dermatophyte infection.

Methods.—Two observers examined H&E-stained slides from 60 PAS-positive cases. One observer, aware of the diagnosis, searched for hyphal elements and recorded epidermal, dermal, and follicular changes in detail. The other observer, unaware of the diagnosis, recorded the same parameters in the 60 PAS-positive cases randomly mixed with slides from 21 nontinea cases.

Results.—Only 27 (45%) of the histologically confirmed tinea cases had been clinically identified as tinea, either as the primary consideration or in the differential diagnosis. Twenty-six distinct diagnoses had been offered for the remaining 33 cases, all but 1 of which had been submitted by dermatologists. The first observer noted spongiotic changes in 26 (43%) cases and papillary dermal edema in 14 (23%). Hyphae were detected in H&E sections of 41 (68%) cases, but PAS-stained sections were needed to identify hyphae in the remaining 19 (32%) cases. The blinded examiner found hyphae in only 27 (45%) of H&E-stained sections. The presence of hyphae was the only significant histologic difference between tinea and nontinea cases.

Discussion.—Dermatophytosis can have nonspecific or unusual histologic findings. Cases reviewed for this study frequently showed spongiotic changes, and in some instances the presence of psoriasiform dermatitis, subcorneal pustules, and folliculitis. An observer who knew that the diagnosis of dermatophytosis had been established was able to identify hyphae in only 68% of H&E-stained sections. The use of a PAS stain for biopsy specimens of inflammatory lesions may improve the detection of hyphae and avoid inaccurate diagnoses.

▶ Dermatopathologists rely on morphologic criteria for making their diagnoses. With regard to dermatophytosis, criteria that have been promulgated on the basis of retrospective analyses include the presence of neutrophils in the dermis and/or epidermis in inflammatory dermatoses in which the epidermis is not eroded or ulcerated, and the so-called "sandwich sign," in which fungal hyphae are found between 2 zones of cornified cells in the stratum corneum. Al-Amiri et al found that using these criteria prospectively was not helpful in diagnosing dermatophytosis. They did not examine the sensitivity or specificity of the criteria but noted that there were no specific findings or clues that were more prominent in tinea cases when compared with nontinea cases. On the basis of this study, the authors propose that a PAS stain should be considered for all biopsy specimens of inflammatory lesions to improve the detection of fungal hyphae that may be missed on routine H&E-stained slides. This to some extent represents hyperbolae because there are many inflammatory dermatoses that do not involve the epidermis; nevertheless, this study does indicate that the PAS stain is probably underused and, thus, dermatophytosis is probably underdiagnosed.

J. C. Maize, MD

Persistent and Recurrent Tinea Corporis in Children Treated With Combination Antifungal/Corticosteroid Agents
Alston SJ, Cohen BA, Braun M (Johns Hopkins Univ, Baltimore, Md; Univ of Maryland, Baltimore)
Pediatrics 111:201-203, 2003   4–4

Background.—Nondermatologists commonly prescribe combination antifungal/corticosteroid preparations to treat superficial fungal infections in patients of any age. Children younger than 4 years are frequently given the combination agent clotrimazole 1%/betamethasone diproprionate 0.05%. A series of children with recurrent or persistent tinea corporis, particularly tinea faciei, after treatment with a combination antifungal/corticosteroid cream is presented.

Methods.—All children examined for tinea corporis at the authors' clinic from January through June 2001 were included in a retrospective chart review. Treatment response was confirmed by telephone contact or follow-up appointment at least 1 month after the infection cleared.

Findings.—Six children, aged 4 to 11 years, were identified. All had been diagnosed clinically as having tinea corporis by their pediatrician and treated initially with clotrimazole 1%/betamethasone diproprionate 0.05% cream. Treatment duration ranged from 2 to 12 months. Patients' diagnoses were confirmed at the pediatric dermatology clinic by a positive potassium hydroxide preparation. One of several oral or topical antifungal agents was used to treat the patients, resulting in the clearing of all tinea infections.

Conclusions.—Tinea corporis treatment with combination topical antifungal/corticosteroid cream may prolong the course of therapy for months. These authors recommend that clinicians prescribe single-agent topical antifungal preparations for primary treatment of this condition. Clinicians may consider using low-potency topical corticosteroids for less than a week, no more than twice a day, only in children with severe symptoms.

▶ It is not surprising that treatment failures occur with clotrimazole/betamethasone diproprionate cream. Clotrimazole is fungistatic, and it is probable that an uninhibited inflammatory response is needed for this agent to be truly effective in clearing dermatophyte infections. Inflammation is suppressed by the strong topical corticosteroid in this combination drug; therefore, cure is less likely.

S. Raimer, MD

Two Hundred Ninety-Six Cases of Onychomycosis in Children and Teenagers: A 10-Year Laboratory Survey

Lateur N, Mortaki A, André J (Free Univ of Brussels, Belgium)
Pediatr Dermatol 20:385-388, 2003   4–5

Background.—The prevalence of onychomycosis has been estimated at 0.2% to 2.6% of the general pediatric population and is typically reported after puberty. Onychomycosis in adults is well described, but little information about onychomycosis in children is available. One laboratory's 10-year experience with onychomycosis in children is presented.

Methods.—From 1990 through 1999, the authors' laboratory processed 21,557 nail keratin samples from patients with onychopathy. The same laboratory technician performed all the direct examinations and cultures, and the same physician interpreted all the histopathologic specimens. Onychomycosis was defined as the presence of long, regularly septated hyphae on potassium hydroxide or histopathologic examination.

Results.—Of the 21,557 samples examined, 963 (4.5%) were from children. Of these 963 children, 296 (30.7%) had onychomycosis (166 boys and 130 girls, 6 weeks-17 years of age). The number of cases increased with age: 42.2% of patients were 12 to 17 years of age, whereas only 22.6% were younger than 6 years. In patients younger than 6 years, toenail involvement was twice as common as fingernail involvement. However, the toenails were involved in 77.3% of children older than 6 years. The causal agent could be identified in 189 patients (63.8%). Dermatophytes were the most common cause, typically *Trichophyton rubrum* (75.1% of cases). However, *Candida* species accounted for 19.6% of the infections and were particularly common in children younger than 6 years (44.2% of cases).

Conclusion.—Onychomycosis accounted for almost one third of nail diseases in these children. The clinical and microbiological characteristics of onychomycosis in children older than 6 years were similar to those in adults: the toenails were more commonly involved and *T rubrum* was the most common cause. In both adults and children, distal and lateral subungual onychomycosis was the predominant clinical type; family transmission was common, and about 50% of children with onychomycosis had a first-degree relative with tinea. In children younger than 6 years, onychomycosis was more likely to involve the fingernails, and *Candida* infections were prevalent.

▶ This study confirms that onychomycosis is rare in young children, although the incidence does increase near puberty. As in adults, *T rubrum* was the most common organism isolated. In children younger than 6 years with onychomycosis, more than 40% were infected with *Candida* species.

S. Raimer, MD

Primary Cutaneous Cryptococcosis: A Distinct Clinical Entity
Neuville S, and the French Cryptococcosis Study Group (nstitut Pasteur, Paris; et al)
Clin Infect Dis 36:337-347, 2003   4–6

Background.—The encapsulated yeast *Cryptococcus neoformans* produces disseminated meningitis in immunocompromised patients. Authorities disagree on whether cutaneous cryptococcosis is primary or only secondary to hematogenous dissemination. Cryptococcosis cases associated with skin lesions reported to the French National Registry were reviewed.

Methods and Findings.—Twenty-eight patients with primary cutaneous cryptococcosis (PCC), 80 with secondary cutaneous cryptococcosis, and 1866 with other forms of the disease were included in the review. Patients with PCC differed significantly from the other groups in living area (mostly rural), age (older), ratio of men to women (equal), and by the absence of underlying disease. PCC was characterized by absence of dissemination and, in

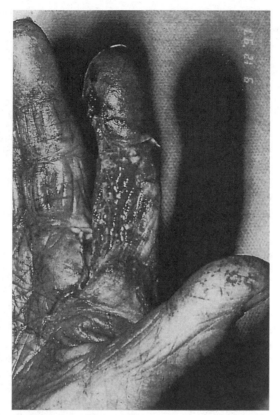

FIGURE 1.—Whitlow due to *Cryptococcus neoformans* complicated by extension with phlegmon of flexor fascia. (Courtesy of Neuville S, and the French Cryptococcosis Study Group: Primary cutaneous cryptococcosis: A distinct clinical entity. *Clin Infect Dis* 36:337-347, 2003. Published by the University of Chicago. © 2003 by the Infectious Diseases Society of America. All rights reserved.)

most cases, a solitary skin lesion on unclothed areas appearing as a whitlow or phlegmon; history of skin injury; participation in outdoor activities; or exposure to bird droppings (Fig 1). *Cryptococcus neoformans* serotype D was isolated in most patients with PCC.

Conclusion.—PCC appears to be a distinct epidemiologic and clinical entity. The prognosis of this condition is favorable, even in immunocompromised persons.

▶ Most cases of PCC represent hematogenous dissemination of the disease after systemic infection. The authors present a series of patients who appear to have true primary skin disease and suggest criteria for differentiating such patients from those whose skin disease is secondary to internal involvement.

B. H. Thiers, MD

Voriconazole Treatment for Less-Common, Emerging, or Refractory Fungal Infections

Perfect JR, Marr KA, Walsh TJ, et al (Duke Univ, Durham, NC; Fred Hutchinson Cancer Ctr, Seattle; Natl Cancer Inst, Bethesda, Md; et al)
Clin Infect Dis 36:1122-1131, 2003   4–7

Background.—The current therapies for refractory invasive fungal infections and for less-common and emerging fungal infections are inadequate. The use of voriconazole, a broad-spectrum triazole, has provided successful outcomes in the treatment of opportunistic infections, including aspergillosis, fluconazole-resistant candidiasis, and a variety of pediatric mycoses. In light of the clinical deficiencies of the present azoles and polyenes for the treatment of refractory and less-common fungal infections, the encouraging results of clinical studies of voriconazole provided the rationale for this multicenter, open-label, clinical study to determine the efficacy and safety of voriconazole for these difficult-to-treat fungal infections.

Methods.—This study investigated the efficacy, tolerability, and safety of voriconazole as salvage treatment in 273 patients with refractory fungal infections who were intolerant to treatment and as a primary treatment for 28 patients with infections for which no therapy has been approved. IV voriconazole was initiated at a loading dosage of 6 mg/kg every 12 hours for the first 24 hours, followed by 4 mg/kg every 12 hours for 3 or more days, after which patients could be switched to oral therapy at 200 mg twice daily.

Results.—Voriconazole was associated with a satisfactory global response in 50% of patients overall, including 47% of patients whose infections did not respond to previous antifungal therapy, and in 68% of patients whose infections had no approved antifungal therapy. In this population at high risk for treatment failure, the efficacy rates for voriconazole were 43.7% for aspergillosis, 57.5% for candidiasis, 38.9% for cryptococcosis, 45.5% for fusariosis, and 30% for scedosporiosis. Voriconazole was well tolerated, and discontinuation of therapy or dose reductions for treatment-related complications occurred in less than 10% of patients.

Conclusions.—Voriconazole appears to be an effective and well-tolerated treatment for patients with refractory or less-common invasive fungal infections.

▶ Although on the surface the response rates might not seem very impressive, it should be emphasized that the infections in approximately 75% of these patients had failed to respond to standard antifungal treatments, and that 82% of the patients had received more than 14 days of previous therapy. Thus, this was a select group of patients with unusually treatment-resistant disease.

B. H. Thiers, MD

5 Viral Infections (Excluding HIV Infection)

Therapeutic Use of IL-2 to Enhance Antiviral T-cell Responses In Vivo
Blattman JN, Grayson JM, Wherry EJ, et al (Emory Univ, Atlanta, Ga; Cornell Univ, New York)
Nat Med April:1-8, 2003   5–1

Introduction.—Experimental studies report that interleukin-2 (IL-2) has both positive and negative effects on T cells. Nevertheless, IL-2 is used to enhance T-cell responses to viral and tumor antigens. The design of therapy using IL-2 might be improved by defining the effects of the cytokine during the different phases of the antigen-specific T-cell response. Lymphocytic choriomeningitis virus (LCMV)-infected mice were used in a study that examined the effects of IL-2 therapy during the expansion, contraction, and memory phases of the T-cell response.

Methods and Findings.—IL-2 was administered to LCMV-infected mice 0 to 8 days after infection to investigate the effects of the cytokine on the generation of effector T-cell responses. Control animals received mock injections. Peak virus-specific CD4+ T-cell numbers were reduced by 80% in the IL-2-treated mice, and CD8+ T-cell numbers were similar in control and treated groups. Thus, during the expansion phase of the T-cell response to LCMV, IL-2 decreased the magnitude of the CD4+ T-cell response and did not enhance that of the virus-specific CD8+ T-cell response. In contrast, during the T-cell death phase (days 8-15), mice receiving IL-2 maintained higher numbers of virus-specific CD8+ T cells and control mice showed the expected 90% decrease. The effect of IL-2 was even greater on CD4+ T-cell responses, for LCMV-specific CD4+ T cells continued to increased in treated mice from days 8 to 30 and remained elevated 6 months after therapy was discontinued. Control mice again showed the excepted drop in these cells. IL-2 therapy was found to increase proliferation of virus-specific T cells and, in chronically infected mice, to decrease viral burden.

Conclusion.—IL-2 therapy can have different effects on T cells depending on the timing of administration. During T-cell expansion, IL-2 increased apoptosis by virus-specific CD8$^+$ cells and inhibited CD4$^+$ T-cell expansion. But when delayed until the contraction phase, IL-2 increased antigen-specific CD4$^+$ and CD8$^+$ T-cell numbers for several months. The administration of IL-2 to heighten T-cell responses could have a variety of clinical applications, including enhancing vaccination efficacy and treating patients with chronic viral infections or malignancy.

▶ The therapeutic use of IL-2 has met with varying degrees of success and is limited by the toxicity associated with high dosage. In addition, the complex effects of IL-2 on immune cells in vivo are not clearly understood. This elegant study used murine models of LCMV infection to determine the effects of low-dose IL-2 administration on T-cell function in acute and chronic infection. The data obtained showed that IL-2 administered early in acute LCMV infection did not enhance viral-specific T-cell proliferation, and in fact resulted in more rapid elimination of these cells after viral clearance. However, later administration of IL-2 during the T-cell death phase resulted in a dramatic increase in survival of virus-specific T cells and memory cells. Interestingly, IL-2 treatment of chronically infected mice resulted in both an increase in the virus-specific T-cell population and a decrease in viral load. The authors suggest that these findings support the rationale for therapeutic approaches using IL-2 in persistent infections such as hepatitis B and C, and HIV.

G. M. P. Galbraith, MD

Predisposing Factors and Clinical Features of Eczema Herpeticum: A Retrospective Analysis of 100 Cases
Wollenberg A, Zoch C, Wetzel S, et al (Ludwig Maximilian Univ, Munich)
J Am Acad Dermatol 49:198-205, 2003   5–2

Background.—Eczema herpeticum (EH), a widespread herpes simplex virus (HSV) infection of inflamed skin, usually occurs in patients with atopic dermatitis (AD). The clinical diagnosis is based on the finding of a monomorphic eruption of dome-shaped blisters and pustules in the eczematous lesions, along with the symptoms of a severe systemic illness. However, atypical variants with disseminated slits in tense erythematous plaques may also be seen. The use of topical corticosteroids may be a predisposing factor for EH. The clinical features and predisposing factors for EH were studied in a retrospective analysis.

Methods.—Data from 100 patients with EH treated between 1980 and 1996 were included in the study. A control group was comprised of 105 patients with AD.

Findings.—Fever and lymphopenia were found to be associated with EH. An increased erythrocyte sedimentation rate (ESR) was common in patients with EH and impetiginized patients in the control group. Primary HSV infection was the likely diagnosis in 20% of the patients with EH, and secondary HSV infection was suggested in 26%. Overall, 13 patients had a second EH, and 3 had a third. Compared with the control group, patients with EH had a significantly earlier AD onset and greater total serum IgE levels. More than three fourths of the patients with EH had not had corticosteroid therapy in the 4 weeks preceding EH onset.

Conclusions.—The characteristics of patients with EH are similar to those of patients with severe AD. Most EH cases occur in patients with untreated AD, which does not support the hypothesis that topical corticosteroid use plays a role in the development of EH.

▶ In this large retrospective placebo-controlled study, the authors noted that EH occurred more commonly in patients with AD whose IgE levels were higher (possibly correlating with disease severity) and whose disease presented earlier than in an atopic control population. The eczema of patients with EH often flared at the time of the infection, and patients often reported that close friends or relatives had had a recent HSV infection just before the development of their EH. Most patients had had no recent topical or systemic corticosteroid therapy. Lack of barrier function allowing invasion of epithelial cells by HSV, or other local factors, such as a defective innate immune system in the skin, may play a role in allowing cutaneous dissemination of HSV infection.

S. Raimer, MD

Valaciclovir as a Single Dose During Prodrome of Herpes Facialis: A Pilot Randomized Double-blind Clinical Trial

Chosidow O, for the Valaciclovir Herpes Study Group (Université Paris VI; Hôpital Tarnier-Cochin, Paris; Hôpital Pasteur, Nice, France; et al)

Br J Dermatol 148:142-146, 2003   5–3

Introduction.—Few randomized clinical trials have evaluated the use of valacyclovir (VACV) in recurrent herpes labialis. The results of a multicenter, double-blind, pilot clinical trial that assessed VACV as a single dose during the prodrome of herpes facialis were discussed.

Methods.—The study included 345 outpatients, divided into 3 groups, with a history of herpes labialis who were screened and selected randomly to treatment with a single dose of either VACV 500 mg, 1000 mg, or 2000 mg, administered during the prodrome of recurrent herpes facialis. Of the 345 patients evaluated, 96 (28%) had no recurrence after 6 months of follow-up; 249 (72%) were included in the intent-to-treat (ITT) population. The primary outcome measure was the rate of aborted episodes on day 3. All 3 treatment groups were similar at baseline.

Results.—No statistically significant between-group differences were noted in the rates of aborted lesions at day 3 in the ITT population, especially between the 500-mg and 2000-mg groups.

Conclusion.—A single VACV dose of 1000-mg or 2000-mg did not differ from that of a 500-mg dose regarding rates of aborted episodes on day 3. A single dose of VACV was not beneficial in preventing attacks of recurrent herpes facialis.

▶ Unfortunately, no placebo group was included, making the results difficult to interpret. However, other studies have shown that lesions do not develop in up to 30% of treated and untreated patients with prodromal symptoms. However, in unpublished controlled trials involving nearly 2000 patients, VACV treatment of recurrent herpes labialis was associated with less progression of lesions, less pain, and a shortening of the duration of lesions by about 1 day compared with that with placebo. The FDA has approved a 1-day course of VACV, given in two 2 g doses, for the treatment of labial herpes simplex virus infection.[1] Whether the modest benefit from this simple regimen is worth the cost is a patient-specific decision.

B. H. Thiers, MD

Reference

1. Valacyclovir (valtrex) for herpes labialis (letter). *Med Lett Drugs Ther* 44:95-96, 2002.

Shared Modes of Protection Against Poxvirus Infection by Attenuated and Conventional Smallpox Vaccine Viruses
Belyakov IM, Earl P, Dzutsev A, et al (NIH, Bethesda, Md)
Proc Natl Acad Sci U S A 100:9458-9463, 2003   5–4

Background.—The concern that smallpox could be used in a bioterrorism attack has raised the possible need for widespread vaccination in the United States, but the greater prevalence of immunocompromised persons today requires a safer smallpox vaccine. The vaccine currently licensed for use in this country, Dryvax (Wyeth strain), is associated with a risk of adverse effects and some mortality. In addition, there is significant risk attached to immunization of persons immunocompromised by AIDS, chemotherapy for cancer, or immunosuppression after organ transplant.

Because the prevalence of such immunosuppressed individuals was much less when universal smallpox vaccination was terminated in 1972, the morbidity and mortality rates from vaccination are likely to be higher now than during the smallpox eradication campaign. This study compared 2 more attenuated vaccinia virus–derived strains to the Wyeth strain in an effort to identify a better, safer smallpox vaccine.

Methods.—The modified vaccinia Ankara, NYVAC, and Wyeth strains of vaccinia virus were compared in a mouse model in which the animals were challenged via the respiratory route for protection against a lethal dose of pathogenic vaccinia virus. Whether a replication-defective virus such as MVA provides protection by means of the same immune response mechanisms as the replication-competent Wyeth strain was also investigated.

Results.—At sufficient doses, both the Ankara and NYVAC replication-deficient vaccinia viruses were safe in immunocompromised animals and provided protection equivalent to that of the licensed Wyeth strain vaccine against intranasal challenge of mice with pathogenic vaccinia virus. A similar variety and pattern of immune responses was involved in protection induced by modified vaccinia Ankara and Wyeth viruses. Antibody was essential in both for protection against disease, while neither effector CD4+ nor CD8+ T cells were necessary or sufficient. However, in the absence of antibody, T cells had a greater role in the control of sublethal infection of animals that were not immunized.

Conclusion.—These attenuated vaccinia viruses share properties with the existing vaccine strain. The findings reported here provide a basis for further investigation of these replication-deficient vaccinia viruses for use in safer vaccines against smallpox.

▶ The conventional smallpox vaccine is based on inoculation with the vaccinia virus, a relatively harmful virus that is a close cousin of the smallpox virus. Adverse events have occurred after vaccine administration, even leading to death in a few individuals. Unfortunately, none of the recently developed attenuated vaccinia virus–derived strains can be tested directly in humans for efficacy against smallpox, as challenge studies with variola virus cannot ethically be performed. Thus, the efficacy of candidate vaccines can be predicted only by the use of surrogate indicators in animal models, such as the level of different immune responses induced and their ability to protect against infection with other poxviruses.

Belyakov et al sought to produce weaker vaccinia virus strains that replicate poorly and could be incorporated into a safer smallpox vaccine. The investigators compared 2 replication-deficient vaccinia viruses and a conventional vaccinia virus to determine what level of immune protection they provided to mice. Inoculation with both weakened strains, as well as the regular vaccine, produced antibodies that protected the animals against a virulent strain of the vaccinia virus.

Both replication-deficient vaccinia virus strains may be tested as a smallpox vaccine in humans. Indeed, the similar modes of protection offered by the conventional and attenuated vaccines in mice suggest that the weakened virus might be used either as a replacement smallpox vaccine or as a primer to reduce the risk of adverse effects of the conventional vaccine.

B. H. Thiers, MD

Eczematous Skin Disease and Recall of Past Diagnoses: Implications for Smallpox Vaccination
Naleway AL, Belongia EA, Greenlee RT, et al (Marshfield Clinic Research Found, Wis; Ctrs for Disease Control and Prevention, Atlanta, Ga)
Ann Intern Med 139:1-7, 2003   5–5

Background.—Eczema vaccinatum may develop in persons with atopic dermatitis or eczema, regardless of disease severity or activity, whose close contacts receive smallpox vaccination. Current recommendations allow for a pre-exposure vaccination program to identify such persons and exclude them from participation. The prevalence of diagnosed atopic dermatitis and eczema in 1 population was determined, and the sensitivity of screening questions to identify such patients was assessed.

Methods and Findings.—Persons with a diagnosis of atopic dermatitis or eczema in 2000 and 2001 were identified from a population-based cohort in Wisconsin. The prevalence of atopic dermatitis or eczema diagnosis in that period was 0.8%. Thus, given the average household size of about 3, at least 2.4% would have been ineligible for smallpox vaccination because of active skin disease in themselves or members of their household. Fifty-nine percent of 94 adult respondents with atopic dermatitis correctly self-reported skin disease. Sixty percent of 133 household contacts of adults with atopic dermatitis correctly reported the presence of skin disease in their home. Seventy percent of 177 parents of children with atopic dermatitis reported their child's skin disease.

Conclusions.—Relying on a self-reported history of skin disease to identify dermatologic contraindications to smallpox vaccination will probably miss a substantial percentage of persons who should not receive the vaccination. A more effective prevaccination screening procedure is needed to minimize the risk for eczema vaccinatum.

▶ Naleway et al found that a self-reported dermatologic history failed to identify a considerable number of patients who should not receive smallpox vaccination. Although the question on eczema diagnosis was the single most sensitive screening question, a combination of questions about atopic dermatitis, eczema diagnosis, and history of rash provided the best recall.

B. H. Thiers, MD

Focal and Generalized Folliculitis Following Smallpox Vaccination Among Vaccinia-naive Recipients
Talbot TR, Bredenberg HK, Smith M, et al (Vanderbilt Univ, Nashville, Tenn)
JAMA 289:3290-3294, 2003   5–6

Introduction.—When smallpox vaccination was routine practice, severe and even fatal reactions occurred in a small number of patients. Less severe dermatologic reactions, such as generalized vaccinia and erythema multiforme, were also reported. To determine what adverse reactions might occur with the reintroduction of smallpox vaccination, healthy, vaccinia-naive adult volunteers were monitored for responses to vaccination.

Methods.—The volunteers, 148 healthy young men and women with a mean age of 23.6, were participants in a multicenter randomized trial investigating the safety and efficacy of 3 dilutions of smallpox vaccine. Both volunteers and study personnel were blinded to the specific vaccine dilution. Any focal or generalized papulovesicular eruptions that appeared after vaccination were characterized by clinical, virologic, and histopathologic characteristics.

Results.—Generalized follicular eruptions developed in 4 participants (2.7%) and similar focal eruptions in 11 (7.4%). Both types of eruptions appeared on various body sites, including the face, neck, back, and extremities. All lesions resolved without scarring. Fever occurred on postvaccination day 6 in 1 individual with a focal eruption. Viral cultures of sample lesions were negative for vaccinia, and a skin biopsy sample from a patient with a generalized rash showed suppurative folliculitis with no evidence of viral infection. No risk factors for the development of skin eruptions were identified; cases and noncases did not differ in dilution of the vaccine received, medication allergies, or the incidence of fever or lymphadenopathy.

Conclusion.—After smallpox vaccination, approximately 10% of the vaccinia-naive adult volunteers experienced generalized or focal eruptions diagnosed as folliculitis. This benign eruption may be confused with generalized vaccinia, but its lesions are distinct in that they develop in different stages, show no histopathologic evidence of viral infection, and heal without scarring.

▶ Unfortunately, a control population was not studied. However, the authors stress that the follicular eruptions noted in these patients were unlike any of their previous rashes, especially in severity and distribution.

B. H. Thiers, MD

Identification of Human Papillomavirus DNA in Cutaneous Lesions of Cowden Syndrome

Schaller J, Rohwedder A, Burgdorf WHC, et al (St Barbara Hosp, Duisburg, Switzerland; Ruhr Univ, Bochum, Switzerland; Ludwig Maximilian Univ, Munich, Germany; et al)
Dermatology 207:134-140, 2003   5–7

Introduction.—Cowden syndrome (CS), or multiple hamartoma syndrome, is a cancer-related genodermatosis inherited in an autosomal dominant pattern. One of the diagnostic criteria is facial papules that are considered to be trichilemmomas. These are benign hair follicle tumors that some investigators believe are induced by human papillomavirus (HPV). A variety of skin lesions from patients with CS were examined for HPV using both routine light microscopy and HPV DNA analysis.

Methods.—Skin lesions from patients with CS were classified histologically, then analyzed for HPV DNA by polymerase chain reaction with various primer sets. Positive amplicons were typed by direct sequencing.

Results.—The study included the examination of 29 biopsy specimens from 7 patients with CS. Only 2 of 29 tumors clinically suspected of being trichilemmomas were verified histologically. Additionally, 3 sclerotic fibromas that were also typical of CS were identified, along with 1 lesion of sebaceous hyperplasia. The remaining 23 specimens demonstrated histologic characteristics of HPV-induced tumors in various stages of development. It was possible to distinguish between a viral papilloma with HPV-induced ke-

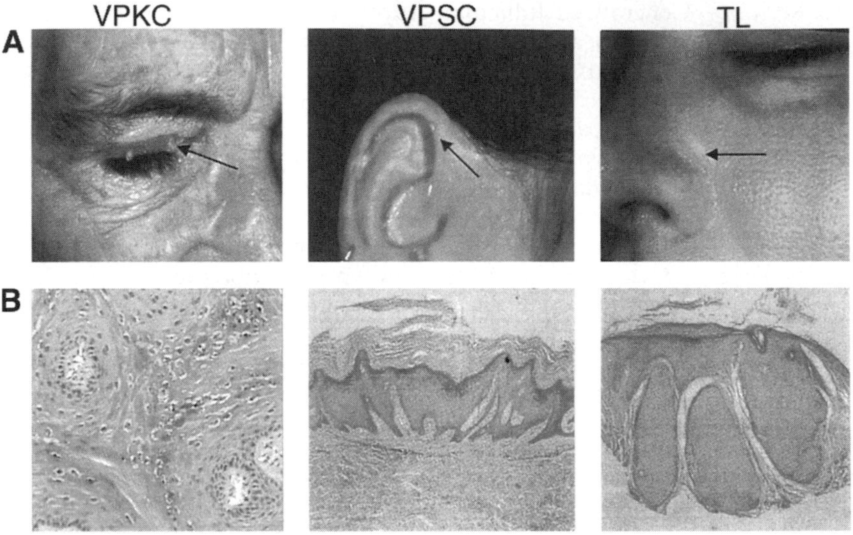

FIGURE 1.—Clinical (A) and histological (B) correlation of investigated tumors in CS: viral papilloma with keratinocyte changes (VPCK), viral papilloma with structural changes (VPSC), and trichilemmoma (TL). (Courtesy of Schaller J, Rohwedder A, Burgdorf WHC, et al: Identification of human papillomavirus DNA in cutaneous lesions of Cowden syndrome. *Dermatology* 207:134-140, 2003. Reproduced with permission of S. Karger AG, Basel.)

ratinocyte changes, a viral papilloma with structural changes, and a trichilemmoma (Fig 1; see color plate VI). Human papillomavirus DNA was detected in 19 of 29 cutaneous lesions. Tumors with no histologic signs of HPV induction were negative for HPV DNA. Two tumors, histologically classified as common warts, contained HPV types 27 and 28. All of the 17 other HPV types belonged to the group of epidermodysplasia-verruciformis (EV)–related types.

Conclusion.—Warty lesions that are challenging to diagnose clinically develop in patients with CS. In many of these lesions, EV-related HPV types can be detected. Classification is only possible by histologic and molecular-biological investigation.

▶ Many years ago, I heard a prominent dermatopathologist remark that he believed that the trichilemmomas associated with CS were really just old warts. Looks like he might have been right!

B. H. Thiers, MD

Childhood Indicators of Susceptibilty to Subsequent Cervical Cancer
Montgomery SM, Ehlin AGC, Sparén P, et al (Karolinska Institutet, Stockholm)
Br J Cancer 87:989-993, 2002   5–8

Background.—Common warts may indicate a susceptibility to cervical cancer, as human papillomavirus (HPV) causes both disorders. Childhood eczema may also be a marker of immune function relevant to HPV infection susceptibility. These childhood indicators of subsequent development of cervical cancer were investigated in 2 general population birth cohorts.

Methods.—Data were obtained from 2 British longitudinal birth cohort studies. After exclusions, 3654 persons enrolled in the 1958 National Child Development Study (NCDS) and 3941 in the 1970 British Cohort Study (BCS70) were included in the analysis. Odds ratios (ORs) were adjusted for cigarette smoking, number of cohabiting partners, and social class in early adult life.

Findings.—A total of 87 women reported having been diagnosed with cervical cancer. The ORs of childhood warts and eczema with cervical cancer were 2.5 and 3.27, respectively. The association between eczema and cervical cancer was independent of hay fever as a marker of atopy, which suggests that nonatopic eczema is important. Heavier smoking (compared with nonsmoking) had an OR of 8.26 for cervical cancer, and for 4 or more cohabiting partners (compared with 1 or none), the OR was 4.89 (Table 3).

TABLE 3.—The Risk of Cervical Cancer in the 1958 (NCDS) and 1970 (BCS70) Birth Cohorts Combined

		Adjusted*			Adjusted†	
	OR	95%CI	Sig (p)	OR	95% CI	Sig (p)
Common warts						
No	1.00			1.00		
Yes	2.47	1.15 5.32	0.020	2.50	1.14 5.47	0.022
Eczema						
No	1.00			1.00		
Yes	2.88	1.73 4.78	0.000	3.27	1.95 5.49	0.000
Cigarette smoking						
Non-smoker	1.00			1.00		
Moderate	2.17	1.58 4.66	0.000	2.42	1.40 4.19	0.002
Heavy	9.97	5.52 18.00	0.000	8.26	4.52 15.10	0.000
Number of cohabiting partners						
0/1	1.00			1.00		
2	2.09	1.27 3.42	0.003	1.66	1.01 2.75	0.047
3	5.02	2.35 10.73	0.000	3.91	1.79 8.52	0.001
4 or more	8.90	2.64 29.99	0.000	4.89	1.39 17.18	0.013
Social class						
Non-manual	1.00			1.00		
Manual	1.65	1.05 2.59	0.030	1.31	0.82 2.08	0.261
Not ascertained	1.31	0.46 3.73	0.609	1.14	0.39 3.29	0.813

*Adjusted for cohort.
†Adjusted for all measures shown and cohort.
(Courtesy of Montgomery SM, Ehlin AG, SParen P, et al: Childhood indicators of susceptibility of subsequent cervical cancer. *Br J Cancer* 87:989-993, 2002.)

Conclusions.—Common warts in childhood may indicate a later susceptibility to cervical cancer. Cigarette smoking and having multiple sexual partners are independent risk factors for the development of this cancer. Class II genes appear to be important in determining whether HPV infections are cleared. Defects in antigen presentation may lead to T-cell anergy, increasing the risk of persistent HPV infection. This, then, may be reflected in a greater susceptibility to common warts.

▶ One shortcoming of this study of 2 British cohorts is that cervical cancer was self-reported; nevertheless, there is compelling evidence that the incidence of this malignancy is increased in individuals who had either viral warts or "eczema" (which the authors surmised more likely represented either seborrheic dermatitis or atopic dermatitis) as children. Because cervical cancer is believed to be related to chronic cervical HPV infection, it is plausible that individuals susceptible to HPV infection in general may be more susceptible to cervical infection and possibly less able to clear chronic infections. The term "childhood eczema" needs to be better characterized before it can be used as a possible indicator.

S. Raimer, MD

Management of Women Who Test Positive for High-Risk Types of Human Papillomavirus: The HART Study
Cuzick J, Szarewski A, Cubie H, et al (Cancer Research UK, London; Royal Infirmary of Edinburgh, Scotland; City Hosp, Nottingham, England; et al)
Lancet 362:1871-1876, 2003   5–9

Background.—The primary cause of almost all cervical cancers is human papillomavirus (HPV). Testing for HPV in a cervical smear is more sensitive but less specific than cytology for identifying high-grade cervical intraepithelial neoplasia (CIN2+). The use of HPV testing as a primary screening tool requires efficient management of HPV-positive women with negative or borderline cytology. The detection rate and positive predictive values of HPV assay were compared with cytology. The best strategy for HPV-positive women was also defined.

Methods.—A total of 11,085 women, aged 30 to 60 years, were included in a multicenter screening. Those with borderline cytology and those positive for high-risk HPV with negative cytology were randomly assigned to immediate colposcopy or surveillance with repeat HPV testing, cytology, and colposcopy at 12 months.

Findings.—The sensitivity of HPV testing was 97.1% for detecting CIN2+ compared with 76.6% for borderline or worse cytology. However, specificities were 93.3% and 95.8%, respectively. At 12 months, surveillance was as effective as immediate colposcopy. In women positive for HPV at baseline who were assigned to surveillance, 45% of 164 with negative cytology and 35% of 23 with borderline cytology were HPV negative at 6 to 12 months. Neither these women nor women with an initially negative HPV test with borderline or mild cytology were found to have CIN2+.

Conclusions.—For women older than 30 years, HPV testing may be used as a primary screening method, with cytology reserved for the triage of those testing positive. Women who are HPV positive with normal or borderline cytology could be managed by repeat testing after 12 months. This approach may improve CIN2+ detection rates without increasing colposcopy referrals.

▶ Cuzick et al confirm that HPV testing is more sensitive than cytology for detecting CIN2+. They suggest that HPV testing could be a useful primary screening tool with cytology used to triage HPV-positive women. These proposals, if implemented, would shift cervical cancer screening from a morphology-based approach to one in which the search for a sexually transmitted virus becomes the focus of disease detection.[1] However, it should be emphasized that the results do not provide direct evidence that HPV testing would reduce cancer rates. A large randomized trial will be necessary to definitively establish such a benefit.

B. H. Thiers, MD

Reference

1. Franco EL: Are we ready for a paradigm change in cervical cancer screening? *Lancet* 362:1866-1867, 2003.

6 HIV Infection and Kaposi Sarcoma

Determinants of Survival Following HIV-1 Seroconversion After the Introduction of HAART

Porter K, for the CASCADE Collaboration (MRC Clinical Trials Unit, London)

Lancet 362:1267-1274, 2003   6–1

Background.—The efficacy of highly active antiretroviral therapy (HAART), introduced in 1996, relies on several variables, such as uptake and time of treatment initiation, adherence, previous treatments, and the presence of coinfections. Thus, survival improvements associated with HAART may not be uniform in all infected groups. Changes in the risk of AIDS and death among HIV-1 infected individuals and the prognostic importance of demographic factors since the introduction of HAART were investigated.

Methods.—Twenty-two cohorts of individuals from Europe, Australia, and Canada who had seroconverted were analyzed with the use of Cox models to estimate the effect of calendar year on time to AIDS and death. The effects of age at seroconversion, exposure category, sex, and presentation during acute HIV-1 infection before 1997, before the introduction of HAART; in 1997 and 1998, when the use of HAART was limited; and in 1999 to 2001, when HAART use was widespread, were compared.

Findings.—Twenty-six percent of 7740 patients who had seroconverted died. Compared with pre-1997 data, the hazard ratio for death declined to 0.47 (95% CI, 0.39-0.56) in 1997 and to 0.16 (95% CI, 0.12-0.22) in 2001. The proportion of person-time receiving HAART rose from 22% to 57% between 1997 and 2001. Compared with the pre-HAART period, in the period from 1999 to 2001, injectable drug users had a significantly greater mortality than did men infected by sex with other men. Before 1997, the risk of AIDS was greater in individuals aged 45 years or older at seroconversion than in individuals aged 16 to 24 years. However, between 1999 and 2001, little evidence of a difference in risk by age was observed. No such attenuation in the effect of age on survival was present.

Conclusions.—Since the introduction of HAART in 1996, the predicted survival rate for individuals with HIV-1 has continued to increase. The importance of age and exposure category as determinants of progression seems to have altered.

▶ This article confirms the effectiveness of HAART in improving the prognosis of HIV-infected persons. Interestingly, since the introduction of HAART, age at seroconversion seems to have become a less important prognostic factor for progression to AIDS, which is a somewhat surprising observation because reconstitution of immune functioning is somewhat more difficult in older people. In contrast, an increased risk of death was noted for users of injectable drugs after 1997. This may reflect decreased access to HAART in this group of patients and possibly poor adherence to recommended treatment regimens. Moreover, coinfections, such as with hepatitis C, that are more common in users of injectable drugs could also affect immune recovery and have prognostic implications.[1]

B. H. Thiers, MD

Reference

1. Greub G. Ledergerber B, Battegay M, et al: Clinical progression, survival, and immune recovery during antiretroviral therapy in patients with HIV-1 and hepatitis C virus coinfection: The Swiss HIV Cohort Study. *Lancet* 356:1800-1805, 2000.

Prognostic Importance of Initial Response in HIV-1 Infected Patients Starting Potent Antiretroviral Therapy: Analysis of Prospective Studies
Egger M, for the Antiretroviral Therapy (ART) Cohort Collaboration (Univ of Bern, Switzerland)
Lancet 362:679-686, 2003   6–2

Background.—Characteristics of patients with HIV-1—including high levels of HIV replication at baseline, older age, a history of AIDS, and infection though injection drug use—are associated with increased rates of clinical progression. In HIV-1 patients who are beginning highly active antiretroviral therapy (HAART), the prognosis is strongly associated with CD4 cell count at baseline. Thus, the characteristics of these patients at the initiation of HAART can be used to predict their probability of disease-free survival and overall survival. HIV-1 RNA concentrations fall quickly in many, but not all, patients, with significant increases in CD4 cell counts within months of the initiation of HAART. Whether the initial virologic and immunologic response to HAART is prognostic in patients with HIV-1 who begin HAART was investigated.

Methods.—Thirteen cohort studies from Europe and North America were analyzed. These studies included 9329 adult treatment-naive patients who were beginning HAART with a combination of at least 3 drugs. Clinical progression was modeled from month 6 after initiation of HAART, taking into account CD4 count and HIV-1 RNA measured at baseline and at 6 months.

Results.—During 13,408 person-years of follow-up, 152 patients died and 874 had AIDS develop or died. Compared with those of patients with a 6-month CD4 count of fewer than 25 cells/μL, adjusted hazard ratios for AIDS or death were 0.55 for 25 to 49 cells/μL; 0.62 for 50 to 99 cells/μL; 0.42 for 100 to 199 cells/μL; 0.25 for 200 to 349 cells/μL; and 0.18 for 350 or more cells/μL at 6 months. Compared with patients who had a 6-month HIV-1 RNA of 100,000 copies/mL or greater, adjusted hazard ratios for AIDS or death were 0.59 for 10,000 to 99,999 copies/mL; 0.42 for 500 to 9999 copies/mL; and 0.29 for 500 copies/mL or fewer. Baseline CD4 and HIV-1 RNA were not associated with progression after controlling for 6-month concentrations. The probability of progression at 3 years ranged from 2.4% for patients at lowest risk to 83% for patients at highest risk.

Conclusion.—The CD4 cell count and viral load 6 months after starting HAART, but not at baseline, are strongly associated with subsequent progression of disease. These findings should be included in guidelines as to when HAART should be modified.

▶ This large study demonstrates that in HIV-positive patients, the initial response to HAART therapy, but not the baseline CD4 cell count or viral load, determines the probability of subsequent disease progression. Thus, even patients who appear to have overwhelming infection at presentation deserve aggressive combination antiretroviral therapy.

B. H. Thiers, MD

Comparison of Sequential Three-Drug Regimens as Initial Therapy for HIV-1 Infection

Robbins GK, for the AIDS Clinical Trials Group 384 Team (Harvard Med School, Boston; et al)
N Engl J Med 349:2293-2303, 2003   6–3

Background.—The most effective sequencing of antiretroviral regimens for HIV-1 treatment has not been established. The effectiveness of several treatment strategies was investigated.

Methods.—A multicenter, randomized, partially double-blind trial was performed that included 620 patients who had not previously received antiretroviral treatment. A factorial design was used to compare pairs of sequential 3-drug regimens, beginning with 1 containing zidovudine and lamivudine or 1 containing didanosine and stavudine combined with nelfinavir or efavirenz. The patients were monitored for a median of 2.3 years.

Findings.—An initial 3-drug regimen that included efavirenz with zidovudine and lamivudine (but not efavirenz with didanosine and stavudine) appeared to prolong the time-to-failure of a second regimen, when compared with an initial regimen containing nelfinavir. The hazard ratio for failure of the second regimen was 0.71. In addition, that regimen (efavirenz, zidovudine, and lamivudine) delayed the second virologic failure (hazard ratio, 0.56) and significantly prolonged the time-to-failure of the first regimen (hazard ratio, 0.39) and the first virologic failure (hazard ratio, 0.34). Beginning with zidovudine and lamivudine combined with efavirenz (but not zidovudine and lamivudine combined with nelfinavir) appeared to prolong time-to-failure of the second regimen compared with an initial regimen including didanosine and stavudine (hazard ratio, 0.68). The former also significantly delayed the first and second virologic failures (hazard ratios, 0.39 and 0.47, respectively), and the failure of the first regimen (hazard ratio, 0.35). Initial use of zidovudine, lamivudine, and efavirenz was also associated with a shorter time to viral suppression.

Conclusions.—Different combinations of antiretroviral agents affect their efficacy. The combination of zidovudine, lamivudine, and efavirenz is more effective than other combinations for the initial treatment of HIV-1.

Comparison of Four-Drug Regimens and Pairs of Sequential Three-Drug Regimens as Initial Therapy for HIV-1 Infection

Shafer RW, for the AIDS Clinical Trials Group 384 Team (Stanford Univ, Calif; et al)

N Engl J Med 349:2304-2315, 2003   6–4

Background.—Whether HIV-1 treatment should begin with a 4-drug or 2 sequential 3-drug regimens is not clear. The efficacy of these 2 initial approaches was evaluated in a multicenter study.

Methods.—The study included 980 patients who were monitored for a median of 2.3 years. Initial treatment with 4-drug regimens containing efavirenz and nelfinavir combined with either didanosine and stavudine or zidovudine and lamivudine was compared with treatment involving 2 consecutive 3-drug regimens, the first containing efavirenz or nelfinavir.

Findings.—The occurrence of regimen failures did not differ between the group given the 4-drug regimen, including didanosine, stavudine, nelfinavir, and efavirenz, and the groups given the 3-drug regimen starting with didanosine, stavudine, and nelfinavir or didanosine, stavudine, and efavirenz. In addition, no significant difference was found between patients receiving the 4-drug regimen with zidovudine, lamivudine, nelfinavir, and efavirenz and those receiving the 3-drug regimens starting with zidovudine, lamivudine, and nelfinavir or with zidovudine, lamivudine, and efavirenz. A 4-drug regimen correlated with a longer time to first regimen failure than the 3-drug regimen of didanosine, stavudine, and nelfinavir (hazard ratio, 0.55); with that containing didanosine, stavudine, and efavirenz (hazard ratio, 0.63); and with that containing zidovudine, lamivudine, and nelfinavir (hazard ratio, 0.49). However, the 4-drug regimen was not superior to the 3-drug regimen containing zidovudine, lamivudine, and efavirenz in the longer time to first regimen failure.

Conclusions.—The duration of successful HIV-1 treatment did not differ between groups given a single 4-drug regimen and 2 consecutive 3-drug regimens. Initiating treatment with the 3-drug regimen containing zidovudine, lamivudine, and efavirenz appears to be the best approach.

▶ These 2 articles (Abstracts 6–3 and 6–4) collate the results of the AIDS Clinical Trials Group Study 384, a monumental undertaking with 6 treatment groups that examined initial treatment of HIV-I infection. Patients were treated with 1 of 2 four-drug regimens or 1 of 4 combinations of 2 consecutive 3-drug regimens. The article by Robbins et al (Abstract 6–3) shows that the zidovudine-lamivudine-efavirenz regimen is superior to the other 3 drug regimens for initial treatment. The article by Shafer et al (Abstract 6–4) demonstrates that a 4-drug regimen does not increase the duration of successful treatment. As a patient's best chance for successful treatment occurs with the first regimen that is used, these findings help guide the choice of regimen for the initial treatment of HIV infection. As noted by Skolnik,[1] determining what constitutes the best choice for initial therapy is a balancing act, with adherence another factor that must be considered. He also offers that clinical trials may be particularly ill suited to answer that question, as study populations often are not representative of the populations of patients that physicians see in everyday practice.

B. H. Thiers, MD

Reference

1. Skolnik PR: HIV therapy, what do we know and when do we know it? *N Engl J Med* 349:2351-2352, 2003.

Alternation of Antiretroviral Drug Regimens for HIV Infection: A Randomized, Controlled Trial

Martinez-Picado J, and the SWATCH Study Team (Hosp Germans Trias i Pujol, Badalona, Spain; et al)
Ann Intern Med 139:81-89, 2003   6–5

Background.—Triple-drug antiretroviral regimens are very effective in controlling HIV-1 infection, but viral resistance and other factors contribute to treatment failure. Computer simulations suggest that alternating antiretroviral therapy every few months while a patient's viral load remains suppressed may slow the development of resistant HIV mutations. Thus, the efficacy of standard care (ie, maintaining one therapy until it fails, then switching to another) was compared with that of alternating antiretroviral regimens in patients with HIV infection.

Methods.—One hundred sixty-one patients with HIV infection (126 men and 35 women; mean age, about 36 years) were enrolled in the SWATCH (SWitching Antiviral Therapy Combination against HIV-1) pilot study. All patients were naive to antiretroviral therapy. Patients were assigned in equal numbers to receive stavudine, didanosine, and efavirenz until virologic failure occurred (regimen A); to receive zidovudine, lamivudine, and nelfinavir until virologic failure occurred (regimen B); or to alternate between the 2 regimens every 3 months as long as their viral load was less than 400 copies/mL (regimen C). The following measurements were obtained: time to virologic failure, percentage of patients with undetectable plasma viremia during 48 weeks, CD4 and CD8 cell counts, adverse events, emergence of drug resistance, drug compliance, and quality of life.

Results.—During 48 weeks of treatment, none of the outcomes differed significantly between regimens A and B, and thus these data were pooled. Compared with the standard care regimens, regimen C was associated with significantly less virologic failure (1.2 vs 4.8 events per 1000 person-weeks). The proportion of patients with undetectable viral loads was also significantly higher in regimen C (87% vs 72% at week 24, 67% vs 58% at week 48). Among the 23 patients in regimens A or B who had treatment failure, 18 (79%) had drug resistance develop. Both groups had significant and similar increases in absolute CD4 and CD8 cell counts. The frequency of adverse events, drug adherence, and quality of life were also similar in the groups.

Conclusion.—Proactively switching antiretroviral regimens while viral load remains suppressed improved virologic outcomes in these patients with HIV infection, without compromising safety, adherence, or quality of life.

▶ The authors suggest that proactively switching and alternating antiretroviral regimens with drugs that have different resistance profiles might enhance the efficacy of antiretroviral therapy. In an editorial that accompanied this study, Saag[1] discussed intricacies in the study design and analysis that raised questions about the meaning and generalizability of the findings. These include the small number of patients studied, the less stringent HIV RNA end point than is used in more contemporary studies (400 copies/mL vs 50 copies/mL), the somewhat outdated drugs that were used in the various regimens, the lack of a genuine intention-to-treat analysis, and the fact that because of the design of the study, patients in the alternating therapy group received a 4-drug regimen rather than a 3-drug regimen for 1 week every 3 months, possibly conferring on them a subtle advantage. Given these caveats, the strategy of using a proactive switching regimen as part of routine practice should be avoided pending additional investigation.

B. H. Thiers, MD

Reference

1. Saag M: Is it time to proactively switch successful antiretroviral therapy? Carefully check your SWATCH. *Ann Intern Med* 139:148-149, 2003.

Impact of Highly Active Antiretroviral Therapy on the Presenting Features and Outcome of Patients With Acquired Immunodeficiency Syndrome–Related Kaposi Sarcoma
Nasti G, Martellotta F, Berretta M, et al (Italian Natl Cancer Inst, Aviano, Italy; Cuggiono Hosp, Italy; Luigi Sacco Hosp, Milan, Italy; et al)
Cancer 98:2440-2446, 2003   6–6

Introduction.—The incidence of Kaposi sarcoma (KS) fell sharply in patients with AIDS after the introduction of highly active antiretroviral therapy (HAART). Patients from 2 Italian HIV-positive cohorts were retrospectively studied to characterize the impact of HAART on the development, clinical presentation, and natural history of AIDS-related KS.

Methods.—A total of 211 patients met inclusion criteria and entered the study. All had a diagnosis of KS made in January 1996 (when HAART became widely available in Italy) or later. Fifty-one patients had been receiving treatment with HAART for at least 3 months at the time of KS diagnosis (KS-HAART group) and 160 started HAART after diagnosis (KS-naive group). Epidemiologic and HIV-related clinical data were obtained from databases and case report forms.

Results.—Most (190 of 211) patients were men and 59% were older than 35; the mean age at KS diagnosis was 37 years. The median CD4 cell count at the time of KS diagnosis was 86/μL; the median HIV viremia level was 89,000 copies/mL. At KS staging, only 17 patients had no poor-risk features. Fifty-one patients (24%) had an AIDS-defining disease before KS was diagnosed. At the time of KS diagnosis, patients already receiving HAART had a significantly more favorable immunologic and virologic status than those who had not had HAART. Cutaneous disease was more indolent and gastrointestinal tract involvement significantly less frequent among KS-HAART patients (14% vs 28% among KS-naive patients). The survival rate at 3 years was 75% overall and did not differ significantly in KS-HAART (64%) and KS-naive patients (78%). Thirty-three (70%) of all deaths were attributed to progression of KS.

Conclusion.—The improved immunologic and virologic status of patients already receiving HAART at the time of KS diagnosis appears to be associated with a less aggressive clinical presentation. However, the initiation of HAART before the development of KS does not appear to influence response to HAART or the natural history and outcome of KS.

▶ It has long been known that AIDS patients with KS experience improvement in their KS when effective antiretroviral treatment is initiated. The data offered by Nasti et al show that KS may nevertheless occur quite frequently, albeit with a rather indolent presentation, in patients already receiving HAART.

B. H. Thiers, MD

Efficacy of Enfuvirtide in Patients Infected With Drug-Resistant HIV-1 in Europe and Australia

Lazzarin A, Clotet B, Cooper D, et al (San Raffaele Vita-Salute Univ, Milan, Italy; Universitari Germans Trias i Pujol, Barcelona, Spain; National Ctr in HIV Epidemiology and Clinical Research, Sydney, Australia; et al)
N Engl J Med 348:2186-2195, 2003   6–7

Introduction.—Enfuvirtide (previously known as T-20) is a synthetic 36-amino-acid peptide that binds to the first heptad-repeat region (HR1) of envelope glycoprotein 41 of HIV-1, a protein that is important in the fusion of the virus with the cell membrane. Enfuvirtide has been shown in phase 1 and 2 clinical trials to decrease the plasma viral load. It is well tolerated when administered as a short-term monotherapy or as part of a long-term combination therapy in patients previously treated with multiple antiretroviral drugs. The efficacy and safety of 24 weeks of treatment with the fusion inhibitor enfuvirtide in combination with an optimized background antiretroviral regimen were compared with the same characteristics of the optimized background regimen alone in the T-20 vs Optimized Regimen Only Study 2 (TORO 2).

Methods.—All patients had previous treatment with each of the 3 classes of antiretroviral drugs, had documented resistance to each class, or both, and had plasma levels of HIV-1 RNA of at least 5000 copies/mL. Patients were selected randomly to treatment with either enfuvirtide (90 mg twice daily) plus a background regimen optimized with the help of resistance testing (enfuvirtide group) or the background regimen alone (control group).

Results.—Of the 512 patients selected randomly, 335 (65.4%) in the enfuvirtide group and 169 (33.0%) in the control group received a minimum of 1 dose of study medication and had at least 1 follow-up determination of plasma HIV-1 RNA. The median baseline plasma HIV-1 RNA level was 5.1 $\log_{10}$ copies/mL for both groups. The median CD4+ cell count was 98.0 and 101.5 cells/cubic mL in the enfuvirtide and control groups, respectively. Patients had a median of 7 years of previous treatment with a median of 12 antiretroviral drugs. For both groups, the background regimen consisted of a mean of 4 antiretroviral drugs. At 24 weeks, the least-squares mean change from baseline in the plasma viral load (intention-to-treat, last observation carried forward) was a reduction of 1.429 $\log_{10}$ copies/mL in the enfuvirtide group and a reduction of 0.648 $\log_{10}$ copies/mL in control subjects, a significant difference of 0.781 $\log^{10}$ copies/mL ($P < .001$). The mean increase in the CD4+ count was greater in the enfuvirtide group (65.5 cells/mm^3), compared with the control group (38.0 cells/mm^3; $P = .02$).

Conclusion.—The findings provide firm proof that HIV-1 glycoprotein 41 can be a viable target for the effective treatment of HIV-1 infection. The promising efficacy and tolerability profile of enfuvirtide indicates that the introduction of this new antiretroviral agent may represent a major advance in the care of previously treated patients.

Enfuvirtide, an HIV-1 Fusion Inhibitor, for Drug-Resistant HIV Infection in North and South America
Lalezari JP, Henry K, O'Hearn M, et al (Univ of California, San Francisco; Hennepin County Med Ctr, Minneapolis; Oregon Health and Science Univ, Portland; et al)
N Engl J Med 348:2175-2185, 2003   6–8

Introduction.—Enfuvirtide (T-20), an HIV-1 fusion inhibitor, binds to a region of the envelope glycoprotein 41 of HIV-1 involved in the fusion of the virus with the membrane of the CD4+ host cell. A randomized, open-label, phase 3 trial was performed to assess the effect of enfuvirtide in combination with an optimized antiviral regimen versus the effect of an optimized regimen alone on plasma HIV-1 RNA levels and CD4+ counts in patients who had previously received multiple antiretroviral drugs and who carried virus resistant to all 3 currently available classes of antiretroviral drugs.

Results.—Patients from 48 sites in the United States, Canada, Mexico, and Brazil with a minimum of 6 months of previous treatment with agents in 3 classes of antiretroviral drugs, virus resistant to drugs in all 3 classes, or both, and with at least 5000 copies of HIV-1 RNA/mL of plasma were randomly assigned in a 2:1 ratio to receive either enfuvirtide plus an optimized background regimen of 3 to 5 antiretroviral drugs (enfuvirtide group) or the optimized regimen alone (control group). The main efficacy end point was the change in the plasma HIV-1 RNA level from baseline to week 24.

Results.—Of 501 patients selected at random, 491 (98.0%) received a minimum of 1 dose of enfuvirtide and had at least 1 measurement of plasma HIV-1 RNA. Both groups were balanced regarding the median baseline HIV-1 RNA level (5.2 $\log_{10}$ copies/mL in both groups), median CD4+ cell count (75.5 cells/mm^3 in the enfuvirtide group and 87.0 cells/mm^3 in the control group), demographic characteristics, and previous antiretroviral therapy. At 24 weeks, the least-squares mean change from baseline in the viral load (intention-to-treat, last observation carried forward) was a reduction of 1.696 $\log_{10}$ copies/mL in the enfuvirtide group and a reduction of 0.764 $\log_{10}$ copies/mL in the control group ($P < .001$). The mean increases in CD4+ cell count were 76 and 32 cells/mL^3, respectively ($P < .001$). Reactions at the injection site were reported by 98% of patients who received enfuvirtide. More cases of pneumonia occurred in the enfuvirtide group than in the control group.

Conclusion.—Treatment with enfuvirtide produced improvement in virologic and immunologic responses, compared to that in control subjects. These findings are supported by those of a similar trial that was conducted in Europe and Australia (Abstract 6–7).

Injection Site Reactions With the HIV-1 Fusion Inhibitor Enfuvirtide
Ball RA, for the ISR Substudy Group (Greensboro Pathology Associates, NC; et al)
J Am Acad Dermatol 49:826-831, 2003   6–9

Introduction.—The most frequently occurring adverse event associated with enfuvirtide treatment is injection site reactions (ISRs) (Fig 1; see color plate VI), most of which are asymptomatic. In 2 large phase 3 trials (Abstracts 6–7 and 6–8), ISRs were found in 98% of patients. The literature has reported only 2 patients who have undergone biopsy for an ISR associated with enfuvirtide therapy. Punch biopsy specimens that were of insufficient depth and did not sample the reticular dermis and subcutaneous tissue were obtained in both cases. Given the variability in animal trials and the limitations of earlier samples in humans, biopsy specimens were obtained in 7 patients with HIV infection who received enfuvirtide. The pathologic characteristics of the ISRs were compared with those of other known de novo skin lesions and drug reactions.

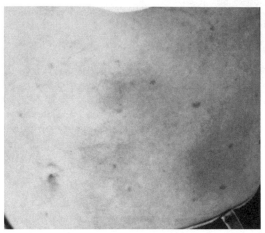

FIGURE 1.—Injection site reactions seen in a patient receiving enfuvirtide subcutaneously. (Reprinted by permission of the publisher from Ball RA, for the ISR Substudy Group: Injection site reactions with the HIV-1 fusion inhibitor enfuvirtide. *J Am Acad Dermatol* 49:826-831, 2003. Copyright 2003 by Elsevier.)

Findings.—All biopsy specimens showed an inflammatory response consistent with a localized hypersensitivity reaction. This was observed independent of the type of clinical lesion and included 1 patient with no clinical reaction. The pattern of inflammation resembled that of granuloma annulare (Fig 2; see color plate VII) and the recently characterized interstitial granulomatous drug reaction. Immunoperoxidase staining showed that the inflammatory and collagen changes were greatest in the areas where enfuvirtide was deposited.

Conclusion.—Some of the pathologic changes associated with enfuvirtide ISRs are discussed for the first time. These data provide valuable insights into the unusual pathogenic response to foreign antigens in HIV-infected patients.

▶ Enfuvirtide is the first in a novel class of antiretroviral drugs that inhibits the fusion of HIV with target cells in the host. The manufacturing process necessary to produce enfuvirtide is complex and protracted, a major factor in the initial cost of therapy, approximating $20,000 per year, more than twice that of the next most expensive antiretroviral agent. Its high cost and limited availability limits its use to a small subgroup of the 5% of the world's HIV-infected persons who live in industrialized nations. Side effects are a concern. The incidence of pneumonia (primarily bacterial) in the 2 studies was 8 times as frequent in the enfuvirtide groups as in the combined control groups. The reason for this finding is uncertain. A less serious side effect involves the skin. The drug is a large, 36-amino acid peptide that must be administered by subcutaneous injection twice daily, another reason for its low acceptance by the HIV-infected community. Development at the injection site of painful, pruritic subcutaneous nodules with histologic features of an interstitial granulomatous reaction was almost universal. However, few patients withdrew from the trials because of injection-site discomfort. Many HIV-infected patients have

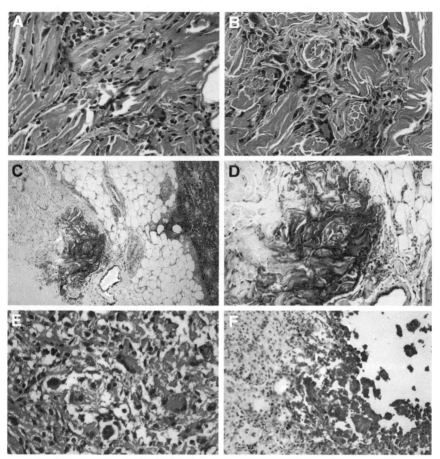

FIGURE 2.—Granuloma annulare-like changes in 2 patients with enfuvirtide-related injection site reactions. No. 1460 (**A**) and No. 1471 (**B**). **C** and **D**, Typical pattern of enfuvirtide deposition in interstitium and on surface of collagen fibers (No. 1204). **E**, Pools of eosinophilic material in association with foamy macrophages (No. 1247). **F**, Atypical pattern of extracellular and intracellular enfuvirtide deposition, included in foamy macrophages in subcutaneous tissue (No. 1247). **A, B,** and **E**, Hematoxylin-eosin stain; original magnifications ×200; **C, D,** and **F**, immunoperoxide stain; original magnifications: **C** and **F**, ×100; **D**, ×200.) (Reprinted by permission of the publisher from Ball RA, for the ISR Substudy Group: Injection site reactions with the HIV-1 fusion inhibitor enfuvirtide. *J Am Acad Dermatol* 49:826-831, 2003. Copyright 2003 by Elsevier.)

shown resistance to the 3 older classes of antiviral drugs. Likewise, resistance to enfuvirtide develops very quickly when it is the only effective antiretroviral drug in a regimen.[1,2]

B. H. Thiers, MD

References

1. Tashima KT, Carpenter CCJ: Fusion inhibition—A major but costly step forward in the treatment of HIV-1. *N Engl J Med* 348:2249-2250, 2003.

2. Kilby JN, Eron JJ: Novel therapies based on mechanisms of HIV-1 cell entry. *N Engl J Med* 348:2228-2238, 2003.

Slower Progression of HIV-1 Infection in Persons With GB Virus C Co-Infection Correlates With an Intact T-Helper 1 Cytokine Profile

Nunnari G, Nigro L, Palermo F, et al (Univ of Catania, Italy; Thomas Jefferson Univ, Philadelphia; Univ of Palermo, Italy; et al)
Ann Intern Med 139:26-30, 2003   6–10

Background.—Patients with both HIV-1 and hepatitis G virus (GBV-C) infection have a slower progression to AIDS. The clinical, virologic, and immunologic factors in HIV-1-seropositive patients with and without GBV-C coinfection were reported.

Methods.—Eighty asymptomatic HIV-1-seropositive patients examined were part of a prospective cohort study with an 8-year follow-up. Measures included GBV-C RNA levels; plasma HIV-1 viral load; CD4+ cell counts; and serum levels of interleukin (IL)-2, IL-4, IL-10, and IL-12.

Findings.—At baseline, 21% of the patients had detectable levels of plasma GBV-C RNA. During follow-up, IL-2 and IL-12 concentrations declined significantly in the patients without GBV-C but not in those with GBV-C. In addition, IL-4 and IL-10 concentrations increased significantly only in those without GBV-C. All variables measured differed significantly between the patients with and without GBV-C during follow-up.

Conclusions.—Patients with both HIV-1 and GBV-C infection maintained an intact T-helper 1 cytokine profile during the 8 years of follow-up, with lower plasma HIV-1 RNA levels and a better AIDS-free survival rate than patients without GBV-C coinfection. GBV-C may interfere immunologically with progression to AIDS by maintaining this intact T-helper 1 cytokine profile.

▶ Previous studies reviewed in the 2002 YEAR BOOK OF DERMATOLOGY AND DERMATOLOGIC SURGERY showed that coinfection with GBV-C is a positive prognostic indicator for patients with underlying HIV-1 infection, and GBV-C has been shown to inhibit HIV-1 replication in vitro.[1,2] Nunnari et al confirmed the prognostic benefits of GBV-C coinfection and suggest a second possible mechanism for this phenomenon (ie, maintenance of an intact Th1 cytokine profile and inhibited expansion of the Th2 response). Whether these findings represent a cause or consequence of delayed progression to AIDS is uncertain.

B. H. Thiers, MD

References

1. Tillmann HL, Heiken H, Knapik-Botor A, et al: Infection with GB virus C and reduced mortality among HIV-infected patients. *N Engl J Med* 345:715-724, 2001. (2002 YEAR BOOK OF DERMATOLOGY AND DERMATOLOGIC SURGERY, pp 179-181.)
2. Xiang J, Wunschmann S, Diekema DJ, et al: Effect of coinfection with GB virus C on survival among patients with HIV infection. *N Engl J Med* 345:707-714, 2001. (2002 YEAR BOOK OF DERMATOLOGY AND DERMATOLOGIC SURGERY, pp 178-179.)

Effect of Antiretroviral Therapy on Liver-Related Mortality in Patients With HIV and Hepatitis C Virus Coinfection
Qurishi N, Kreuzberg C, Lüchters G, et al (Univ of Bonn, Germany)
Lancet 362:1708-1713, 2003   6–11

Background.—Highly active antiretroviral therapy (HAART) has improved the prognosis of HIV infection, but HAART does not inhibit hepatitis C virus (HCV) replication. Treatment-related hepatotoxic effects are common. The effect of HAART in patients coinfected with HIV and HCV was clarified.

Methods.—Liver-related mortality and overall mortality rates were documented in 285 patients seen at one center between 1990 and 2002. Patients were stratified into 3 groups based on their antiretroviral treatment: 93 received HAART, available after 1995; 55 were treated with nucleoside analogs only, available after 1992; and 137 received no treatment.

Findings.—Liver-related mortality was 0.45 per 100 person-years in the HAART recipients, 0.69 in the recipients of antiretroviral treatment, and 1.7 in the untreated patients. Kaplan-Meier analysis of liver-related mortality confirmed that patients given antiretroviral therapy had a significant survival benefit. In a regression analysis, independent predictors of liver-related survival were HAART, antiretroviral therapy, CD4-positive T-cell count, serum cholinesterase level, and age. Five patients treated with nucleoside analogs alone and 13 given HAART experienced severe drug-related hepatotoxic effects. However, none of the patients died of treatment-related hepatotoxic effects.

Conclusions.—Antiretroviral treatment seems to significantly decrease long-term liver-related mortality rates, in addition to improving overall survival rates. The current data suggest that this survival benefit exceeds the associated risks of severe hepatotoxic effects.

▶ Circumstantial evidence indicates that antiretroviral therapy by itself does not inhibit HCV replication. Moreover, patients with positive findings for both HIV and HCV may be especially prone to severe and potentially life-threatening hepatotoxic side effects of antiretroviral drugs. The data presented by Qurishi et al demonstrate that HAART not only improves overall survival rates but also that it significantly reduces long-term liver-related mortality rates in HIV-infected patients. Thus, the survival benefit far outweighs the associated risk of severe hepatotoxicity. Interestingly, HAART did not reduce HCV loads: HCV viremia increased steadily over time in the cohort under observation. The authors concede that the mechanism underlying the reduced liver mortality rates observed in these patients is uncertain, as HAART did not seem to inhibit HCV replication.

B. H. Thiers, MD

Cardiovascular and Cerebrovascular Events in Patients Treated for Human Immunodeficiency Virus Infection

Bozzette SA, Ake CF, Tam HK, et al (Veterans Affairs San Diego Health Care System, Calif; Univ of California, San Diego, La Jolla; RAND Health, Santa Monica, Calif; et al)
N Engl J Med 348:702-710, 2003   6–12

Introduction.—Potent combination antiretroviral therapy has substantially improved survival of patients with HIV infection, but there are concerns about an increased risk of premature cardiovascular and cerebrovascular disease. Patients treated for HIV infection or AIDS at Veterans Affairs (VA) facilities between January 1993 and June 2001 were reviewed for trends in the rates of cardiovascular and cerebrovascular disease and the relation between disease risk and antiretroviral therapy.

Methods.—The retrospective cohort of patients was constructed from anonymous databases, augmented by the addition of information from VA death-benefit claims, Social Security records, and the National Death Index. Five outcomes were reported: admission for cardiovascular disease, admission for cardiovascular or cerebrovascular disease, admission for or death from cardiovascular or cerebrovascular disease, death from any cause, and admission for cardiovascular or cerebrovascular disease or death from any cause.

Results.—A total of 36,766 patients received care for HIV infection at VA facilities during the study period. For antiretroviral therapy, 70.2% of the patients received nucleoside analogues, 41.6% received protease inhibitors, and 25.6% received nonnucleoside reverse-transcriptase inhibitors. These therapies were given for median periods of 17 months, 16 months, and 9 months, respectively. Approximately 1000 patients were treated for at least 48 months with combination therapy with a protease inhibitor; a similar number received combination therapy with a nonnucleoside reverse-transcriptase inhibitor for at least 24 months. During the period between 1995 and 2001, there was a decrease in both admission rates for cardiovascular or cerebrovascular disease (from 1.7 to 0.9 per 100 patient-years) and the rate of death from any cause (from 21.3 to 5.0 per 100 patient-years).

Conclusion.—At least during the relatively short follow-up period, the risk of cardiovascular or cerebrovascular events among patients treated for HIV infection was not increased by the use of nucleoside analogues, protease inhibitors, or nonnucleoside reverse-transcriptase inhibitors. These newer antiviral drugs were associated with a decreased hazard of death from any cause.

▶ Abnormalities in glucose and lipid metabolism are associated with HIV infection and with several of the drugs used for its treatment. The report by Bozzette et al demonstrates the significant therapeutic benefits of the various antiretroviral therapies with no increase in mortality rate from cardiovascular or cerebrovascular events. This was a relatively short-term study; long-term follow-up is needed to confirm its findings.

B. H. Thiers, MD

Combination Antiretroviral Therapy and the Risk of Myocardial Infarction
Lundgren JD, for the Data Collection on Adverse Events of Anti-HIV Drugs (DAD) Study Group (Hvidovre Univ, Copenhagen; et al)
N Engl J Med 349:1993-2003, 2003   6–13

Introduction.—The metabolic side effects of combination antiretroviral therapy may increase a patient's risk for cardiovascular disease. To determine whether exposure to this therapy is independently associated with the risk of myocardial infarction, 11 cohorts including a total of 23,468 patients with HIV-1 infection were prospectively monitored.

Methods.—Patients were evaluated during regular visits to 188 outpatient clinics in 21 countries in Europe, the United States, and Australia. Enrollment took place between December 1999 and April 2001. Data on HIV-1 infection and risk factors for myocardial infarction were collected at enrollment and at least every 8 months thereafter. New cases of myocardial infarction had to meet standardized criteria to be included in the analysis; excluded were nonfatal myocardial infarctions not associated with clinical symptoms.

Results.—The median age of patients in the cohorts was 39 years; 75.9% were men and 26.2% had previously been found to have AIDS. Most patients (80.8%) had previous exposure to antiretroviral drugs. Many had cardiovascular risk factors, but only 1.5% had previous cardiovascular disease. Over a period of 36,199 person-years, 126 patients had a myocardial infarction. Greater length of exposure to combination antiretroviral therapy was associated with an increased incidence of myocardial infarction. Additional factors associated with myocardial infarction were older age, current or former smoking, a history of cardiovascular disease, male sex, elevated total serum cholesterol and triglyceride levels, and the presence of diabetes.

Conclusion.—In these cohorts of relatively young patients with HIV-1 infection, the absolute risk of myocardial infarction was low. Nevertheless, treatment with combination antiretroviral therapy was independently associated with a 26% relative increase in the rate of myocardial infarction per year of exposure during the first 4 to 6 years of use. The substantial benefits of the therapy, however, clearly outweigh this risk.

HIV Infection and Cardiovascular Disease—Is There Really a Link?

Sklar P, Masur H (Drexel Univ, Philadelphia; NIH, Bethesda, Md)
N Engl J Med 349:2065-2067, 2003   6–14

Background.—After the introduction of "highly active" combination antiretroviral drug regimens, clinicians noted unexpected cardiovascular events in relatively young patients with HIV infection. Several database reviews published between 1998 and 2003 appeared to validate the concern that HIV-infected patients, though surviving longer because of the new antiretroviral agents, were at increased risk for cardiovascular disease. Two studies published in *The New England Journal of Medicine* during 2003 reached contradictory conclusions, however.

Observations.—One study, a retrospective analysis based on data from the Veterans Affairs Medical System, found a decrease in the rate of admission for cardiovascular and cerebrovascular disease among patients with HIV infection. In addition, the use of any class of antiretroviral therapy was associated with a decreased hazard of death from any cause. The second study contained data from the prospective, multinational Data Collection on Adverse Events of Anti-HIV Drugs (DAD) Study. Its conclusions indicated a 26% relative increase in the rate of myocardial infarction per year of exposure to antiretroviral drugs during the first 4 years of antiretroviral therapy.

Discussion.—Both studies assessed large patient cohorts, but neither included an uninfected control group and both had relatively short follow-up periods. In the DAD Study, more than half the patients were current or former smokers and 21% had an elevated total cholesterol level. Cardiovascular risk thus preceded antiretroviral treatment in many cases. It is also possible that some cardiovascular events were a consequence of HIV infection, of antiretroviral therapy, or of a synergistic relation among all these risk factors. Studies in healthy volunteers have shown significant endothelial dysfunction after the administration of indinavir, and protease inhibitors are known to produce marked elevations in cholesterol and triglyceride levels. Overall, the weight of evidence suggests that patients with HIV infection who receive combination antiretroviral regimens are at increased risk for the development of premature atherosclerotic complications. Lifestyle changes and/or dietary and pharmacologic interventions may reduce the risk of the adverse consequences of antiretroviral therapy.

▶ As argued by Sklar and Masur, antiretroviral therapies are among the miracle drugs of recent decades. Clearly, their benefits markedly outweigh their risks. Future efforts should be directed at identifying those patients at highest risk for heart disease. Such individuals should be encouraged to take the appropriate drugs and make the appropriate lifestyle changes to decrease their risk for development of complications of premature atherosclerosis.

B. H. Thiers, MD

Short Postexposure Prophylaxis in Newborn Babies to Reduce Mother-to-Child Transmission of HIV-1: NVAZ Randomised Clinical Trial
Taha TE, Kumwenda NI, Gibbons A, et al (Johns Hopkins Univ, Baltimore, Md; Univ of Malawi, Blantyre; Univ of North Carolina, Chapel Hill; et al)
Lancet 362:1171-1177, 2003   6–15

Introduction.—Most women in sub-Saharan Africa are initially seen late for delivery and present with unknown HIV status. This limits the use of intrapartum nevirapine for prevention of mother-to-child transmission of HIV. The NPV/AZT trial (NVAZ) included infants born to women who arrived too late to the labor room to receive HIV counseling, testing, and administration of intrapartum nevirapine before delivery. The efficacy of short neonatal-only postexposure prophylaxis using nevirapine and zidovudine was compared with nevirapine alone in decreasing mother-to-child transmission of HIV-1.

Methods.—A total of 1119 infants of Malawian women with HIV initially seen within 2 hours of expected delivery were randomly assigned to treatment with either nevirapine alone or nevirapine and zidovudine. Both drugs were administered immediately after birth. One dose of nevirapine (2 mg/kg weight) was administered as a single dose. Infants in the nevirapine plus zidovudine group also received zidovudine twice daily for 1 wk (4 mg/kg weight). Infant HIV infection was ascertained at birth and at 6 to 8 weeks. The major outcome measure was HIV infection in infants at 6 to 8 weeks in those not infected at birth. The analysis was by intention to treat.

Results.—The overall incidence of mother-to-child transmission at 6 to 8 weeks was 15.3% in 484 infants who received nevirapine and zidovudine and 20.9% in 468 infants who received nevirapine only ($P = .03$). At 6 to 8 weeks, in babies who were HIV negative at birth, infections were discovered in 34 (7.7%) infants who had nevirapine and zidovudine and 51 (12.1%) who received nevirapine only ($P = .03$). This represents a protective efficacy of 36% after controlling for maternal viral load and other baseline factors. Adverse effects were mild and occurred at similar rates in both groups.

Conclusion.—Postexposure prophylaxis can offer protection against HIV infection to infants of women who missed opportunities to be counseled and tested before or during pregnancy. The nevirapine and zidovudine regimen is safe and easy to administer.

▶ Ideally, HIV-positive women should be counseled and treated prior to or during delivery. Unfortunately, especially in underdeveloped countries, many women present to the labor ward only hours before delivery, unaware of their HIV status and with little time for counseling, HIV testing, and, if necessary, antiretroviral therapy. Moreover, nevirapine must be given at least 2 hours or more prior to delivery in order to achieve protective concentrations of the drug in cord blood. Taha et al show that postexposure prophylaxis might protect babies of women who received suboptimal prenatal care. As safety data on alternative drugs become available, more effective antiviral agents may be used for the same purpose in the future. Extending the duration of the treatment regimen to prevent HIV transmission during breast-feeding should be the focus of future research.

B. H. Thiers, MD

Prevention of Virus Transmission to Macaque Monkeys by a Vaginally Applied Monoclonal Antibody to HIV-1 gp120
Veazey RS, Shattock RJ, Pope M, et al (Tulane Univ, Covington, La; St George's Hosp Med School, London; Population Council, New York; et al)
Nature Med 9:343-346, 2003   6–16

Background.—In persons at risk for sexually acquired HIV-1 infection, a topical microbicide applied to the vagina or rectum can decrease the probability of virus transmission. An effective microbicide may significantly decrease the global spread of HIV-1, especially if women can use this agent covertly. A microbicide may target the incoming virus and permanently deactivate it or reduce its infectivity. Alternatively, it may block receptors on susceptible cells near the transmission sites.

Methods and Findings.—The broadly neutralizing human monoclonal antibody b12 was administered vaginally to macaques to protect them from acquiring simian-human immunodeficiency virus (SHIV) infection through the vagina. Twelve animals received 5 mg b12 vaginally in saline or a gel and were then challenged vaginally with SHIV-162P4. Only 3 of the animals became infected. However, 12 of 13 animals given various control agents under similar conditions became infected. Decreased amounts of b12 were less effective than higher doses, suggesting a dose-dependent relation.

Conclusions.—These data support the concept of specific entry inhibitors as microbicides and offer a frame of reference for assessing other such inhibitors in the macaque model. Viral entry inhibitors may help prevent the sexual spread of HIV-1 among human beings.

▶ Veazey et al show that vaginal application of a monoclonal antibody against the viral surface glycoprotein gp120 can protect macaques against vaginal transmission of simian HIV-1 infection. In their study, only cell-free virus was used, and the efficacy of this antibody against cell-associated virus needs to be addressed. Moreover, although the antibody used in this study can neutralize many primary HIV-1 isolates from multiple genetic subtypes, it is not panreactive; thus, for it to be effective as a microbicide, it would have to be combined with other broadly neutralizing monoclonal antibodies.

B. H. Thiers, MD

Whole-Body Positron Emission Tomography in Patients With HIV-1 Infection

Scharko AM, Perlman SB, Pyzalski RW, et al (Univ of Wisconsin, Madison; Univ of Maryland, Baltimore)

Lancet 362:959-961, 2003   6–17

Introduction.—Positron emission tomography (PET) with fluorine-18-deoxyglucose (FDG-PET) identifies active lymphoid tissues during HIV-1 infection in humans. Fifteen patients with HIV-1 were evaluated by FDG-PET to examine anatomical correlates of HIV-1 infection in humans. Five representative patients were discussed.

> *Case 1.*—Patient was a recent seroconverter (exposure 10 weeks previously). He developed acute seroconversion illness at about 23 days of presumed HIV-1 exposure; 50 days later, PET scanning revealed high FDG uptake in the cervical lymph nodes and moderate uptake in the spleen. Weak FDG uptake was observed in axillary nodes. The patient was asymptomatic (Centers for Disease Control [CDC] stage A1). His CD4 count was 77 cells/µL.
>
> *Case 2.*—Patient had been diagnosed with HIV-1 eighty months earlier. He had stable CD4 counts (200 cells/µL) and was in excellent health without antiretroviral therapy (CDC stage A3). PET imaging revealed high FDG uptake in cervical and axillary lymph nodes and mild uptake in the spleen.
>
> *Case 3.*—Patient had been diagnosed with HIV-1 over 10 years previously. Her CD4 count was 330 cells/µL and her body weight loss was 11% (CDC stage B2). She was taking antiretroviral therapy with pneumocystis prophylaxis. PET imaging demonstrated high FDG uptake in cervical lymph nodes, weak axillary node uptake, moderate signals from the iliac lymph nodes, and a strong signal from the spleen. Unexplained signals in the hands and forearms were also seen.
>
> *Case 4.*—Patient had been diagnosed over 10 years previously. His CD4 count was 16 cells/µL. PET imaging revealed diffuse signals in the descending colon and a strong signal near the ileocecal junction. His CDC stage was C3.
>
> *Case 5.*—Patient had been diagnosed 18 months previously. His CD4 count was undetectable. He had severe wasting, neuropathy, herpes zoster reactivation, and thrush (CDC stage C3). PET imaging showed multiple signals in the esophagus, left lung, and ileocecal region. Biopsy of a pulmonary lesion verified metastatic lymphoma. Lymphoid tissue activation was observed only near the ileocecal junction, in ring-like structures. The patient died 17 days after PET imaging.

Conclusion.—Whole-body FDG-PET images from 15 patients with HIV-1 revealed distinct lymphoid tissue activation in the head and neck during acute disease, a generalized pattern of peripheral lymph-node activation at mid stages, and involvement of abdominal lymph nodes during late disease. Unexpectedly, HIV-1 progression was obvious by distinct anatomical correlates, indicating that lymphoid tissues are engaged in a predictable sequence.

Anatomical Loci of HIV-Associated Immune Activation and Association With Viraemia
Iyengar S, Chin B, Margolick JB, et al (Johns Hopkins Univ, Baltimore, Md)
Lancet 362:945-950, 2003   6–18

Introduction.—Lymphocyte activation associated with vaccination or infection can be measured by positron emission tomography (PET). The ability of PET to identify and measure the magnitude of lymph node activation among asymptomatic HIV-1-infected patients was examined.

Methods.—The PET response was evaluated in 8 HIV-1-uninfected persons who had received licensed killed influenza vaccine. Twelve patients recently infected with HIV-1 (less than 18 months since seroconversion) and 11 patients with chronic long-term HIV-1 who had stable viremia by reverse transcriptase-polymerase chain reaction (non-progressors) were recruited from an urban teaching hospital. Patients underwent PET with the use of ^{18}F-labelled fluorodeoxyglucose. The correlation of summed PET signal from nodes and viral load was examined via linear regression on log-transformed values.

Results.—Nodal activation was more localized after vaccination than after HIV-1 infection. In early and chronic HIV-1 disease, node activation was

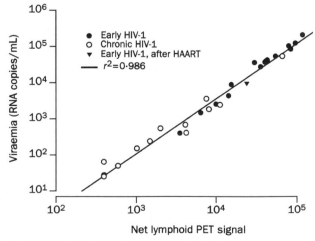

FIGURE 4.—Net lymphoid positron emission tomography signal versus plasma viremia. *Abbreviation: HAART,* Highly active antiretroviral therapy. (Courtesy of Iyengar S, Chin B, Margolick JB, et al: Anatomical loci of HIV-associated immune activation and association with viraemia. *Lancet* 362:945-950, 2003. Reprinted with permission from Elsevier Science.)

greater in the cervical and axillary chains, compared with the inguinal and iliac chains ($P < .0001$). Summed PET signal correlated with viremia across a 4-log range ($r^2 = 0.98$; $P < .0001$) (Fig 4). Non-progressors had a few persistently active nodes; most were surgically accessible.

Conclusion.—The anatomical restriction that was observed may reflect microenvironmental niche selection. The tight correlation of PET signal with viremia indicates that target-cell activation determines steady-state viral replication.

▶ The authors present data to indicate an association between pattern of lymphoid tissue activation and clinical staging of disease. They describe a nonrandom disease process that can be staged by discrete anatomical correlates. The patterns for tissue activation in HIV-disease that they define may provide fundamental insight into the disease process and lead to surgical or radiologic interventions to block disease progression.

B. H. Thiers, MD

Post-transplant Kaposi Sarcoma Originates From the Seeding of Donor-derived Progenitors

Barozzi P, Luppi M, Facchetti F, et al (Univ of Modena and Reggio Emilia, Italy; Univ of Brescia, Italy; Univ of Perugia, Italy; et al)

Nature Med 9:554-561, 2003   6–19

Introduction.—The posttransplant Kaposi sarcoma (KS) that develops in solid-organ (mainly kidney) transplant recipients may be caused by human herpesvirus 8 (HHV-8) activation in the recipient or by primary infection with HHV-8 transmitted by the donor. Various molecular and immunohistochemical methods were used to show that KS progenitor cells may be transmitted through solid grafts.

Methods.—Archival biopsy specimens from skin KS lesions that developed 9 to 40 months after renal transplantation in 6 HIV-negative female recipients of kidneys from male Italian donors and in 2 male recipients of kidneys from male donors of Arab and Jewish origin were studied. All 8 patients were found to have early to intermediate-stage KS.

Results.—The use of of molecular, cytogenetic, immunohistochemical, and immunofluorescence methods demonstrated that the HHV-8–infected neoplastic cells in posttransplant KS from 5 of the 8 renal transplant patients harbored either genetic or antigenic markers of their matched donors.

Conclusion.—The findings demonstrate that HHV-8–positive posttransplant KS maybe an example of a virus-associated tumor transmitted through transplantation. In addition to tumor cells of donor origin, it is possible that a proportion of tumor cells originate from the spread of HHV-8 to recipient endothelial precursor cells. The use of donor-derived HHV-8–specific T cells may be useful for the control of posttransplant KS.

▶ Barozzi et al report 5 patients with KS who may have received progenitor malignant cells from an organ transplant donor. The causative virus, HHV-8, is usually destroyed by the immune system, and the transplant patients' immunosuppressed state certainly made them more prone to proliferation of donor-derived progenitor cells. The possible usefulness of donor-derived HHV-8–specific cytotoxic T cells in the control of posttransplant KS should be explored. The findings reported here identify HHV-8–positive posttransplant KS as the second known example (in addition to posttransplant lymphoproliferative disease caused by Epstein-Barr virus–infected B cells) of a virus-associated tumor transmitted through transplantation.

B. H. Thiers, MD

7 Parasitic Infections, Bites, and Infestations

Sulfur for Scabies Outbreaks in Orphanages
Pruksachatkunakorn C, Damrongsak M, Sinthupuan S (Chiang Mai Univ, Thailand; Chiang Mai Orphanage Found, Thailand; Viengping Children's Home, Chiang Mai, Thailand)
Pediatr Dermatol 19:448-453, 2002   7–1

Introduction.—The current drug of choice for the management of scabies in young children is 5% permethrin cream; topical ivermectin is also effective. Neither agent, however, is available in Thailand, and the widely obtainable lindane gel carries a risk of CNS toxicity. At 2 large orphanages in Thailand, sulfur in petrolatum was chosen for mass treatment of children affected with scabies.

Methods.—Children included in the uncontrolled, open-label trial were diagnosed by clinical criteria or by the demonstration of eggs, mites, or fecal pellets by light microscopy. Those younger than 12 months were treated with 5% precipitated sulfur in petrolatum; a 10% preparation was applied in older children. The ointment was rubbed nightly on all body surfaces, with 4 applications on 3 consecutive days and repeated 1 week later. Hot water laundering of clothing and bedding was recommended. Staff members and treatment teams were treated simultaneously with 25% benzyl benzoate or donated 0.3% lindane. Follow-up was conducted at 2 and 4 weeks.

Results.—A total of 124 (87%) of 142 children and 7 (10%) of 73 orphanage staff members were infested with scabies. Frequently observed lesions were excoriated papulovesicular lesions (96%), discrete erythematous papulovesicular lesions (94%), and vesiculopustules (60%). Hands were the most common sites, and infants were most likely to have buttock and sacral area infestations. Overall, 47% of patients were cured at 2 weeks and 71% at 4 weeks (Table 2). Treatment failure tended to occur more often in toddlers and in index cases. The sulfur preparation caused mild facial edema in 3 preschool children. No diarrhea or other gastrointestinal symptoms were reported.

Conclusion.—Sulfur is a widely available and inexpensive choice for mass treatment of scabies. For the outbreak described here, the total cost was

TABLE 2.—Cure Rates of Children Treated With Sulfur

Class (Orphanage A + Orphanage B)	No. of Cases	Cured (%) 2 Weeks	Cured (%) 4 Weeks
Infant	34	20 (59%)	28 (82%)
Toddler	32	12 (38%)	17 (53%)
Preschooler	36	16 (44%)	27 (75%)
Total	102	48 (47%)	72 (71%)

(Courtesy of Pruksachatkunakorn C, Damrongsak M, Sinthupuan S: Sulfur for scabies outbreaks in orphanages. *Pediatr Dermatol* 19:448-453, 2002. Reprinted by permission of Blackwell Publishing.)

$194. Odor, messiness, and staining are inevitable disadvantages of the medication.

▶ There was an overall 72% cure rate without significant side effects when topical sulfur (5% or 10% ointment) was used to treat outbreaks of scabies in 2 orphanages in Thailand. Sulfur seems a reasonable choice when other agents are not available or cost prohibits their use. However, its smell, messiness, staining, the need for multiple applications, the cost of compounding, and the fact that it is less effective than permethrin or lindane make it less desirable when other agents are available.

S. Raimer, MD

Permethrin-Resistant Human Head Lice, *Pediculus Capitis,* and Their Treatment
Yoon KS, Gao J-R, Lee SH, et al (Univ of Massachusetts-Amherst; Seoul Natl Univ, Suwon, South Korea; Univ of Miami, Fla)
Arch Dermatol 139:884-1000, 2003   7–2

Background.—Pediculosis from the human head louse (HL) *Pediculus capitis* is the most common parasitic infestation among US children. Almost all nonprescription treatments available for this condition contain the natural botanical active ingredients, the pyrethrins, or the synthetic pyrethroid permethrin, as active ingredients. The pediculicidal activity of Ovide lotion and its active ingredient, 0.5% malathion, was compared with that of Nix and its active ingredient, 1% permethrin, in children with permethrin-resistant head lice.

Methods.—Lice were collected in 3 US regions and Yamburara, Ecuador, from otherwise healthy children. Lice were given a blood meal 3 to 6 hours after collection and exposed to products or active ingredients. The lice were then observed at regular intervals.

Findings.—DNA sequencing confirmed the presence of T929I and L932F mutations in permethrin-resistant lice from South Florida. Lice from Mathis, Texas, which included 13% with resistant genotypes, showed slight resistance to permethrin. South Florida lice exposed to permethrin died significantly more slowly than susceptible Ecuadorian lice. Compared with Nix and permethrin, Ovide and malathion killed permethrin-resistant lice faster.

Conclusions.—The presence of T929I and L932F mutations was confirmed in lice from South Florida resistant to the pediculicidal effects of permethrin and Nix, the leading permethrin-based head lice product. Malathion resistance was not documented in these lice populations. Ovide killed permethrin-resistant head lice about 10 times faster than did permethrin or Nix.

▶ This study provides additional evidence that permethrin-resistant head lice are present in the United States and that resistance is highly associated with the presence of kdr-type point mutations of T929I and L932F. The in vitro kill times were longer than in 3 previously reported studies.[1-3] Clinical trials to determine the length of application time required to kill lice in vivo would be helpful. Because resistance patterns change with extensive use of pediculicidal products, these studies would need to be repeated periodically. A concise review of head lice treatment has recently been published.[4]

S. Raimer, MD

References

1. Meinking TL, Serrano L, Hard B, et al: Comparative in-vitro pediculicidal efficacy of treatments in a resistant head lice population in the United States. *Arch Dermatol* 138:220-224, 2002.
2. Meinking TL, Entzel P, Villar ME, et al: Comparative efficacy of treatment for *Pediculus capitis* infestations: Update 2000. *Arch Dermatol* 137:287-292, 2001.
3. Pollack RJ, Kiszewski A, Armstrong P, et al: Differential permethrin susceptibility of head lice samples in the United States and Borneo. *Arch Pediatr Adolesc Med* 153:969-973, 1999.
4. Nash B: Treating head lice. *BMJ* 326:1256-1258, 2003.

Delayed Onset of Malaria—Implications for Chemoprophylaxis in Travelers

Schwartz E, Parise M, Kozarsky P, et al (Tel Aviv Univ, Israel; Ctrs for Disease Control and Prevention, Atlanta, Ga; Emory Univ, Atlanta, Ga)
N Engl J Med 349:1510-1516, 2003   7–3

Introduction.—Adherence to recommended antimalarial chemoprophylactic regimens may not prevent late-onset illness in travelers, for most available agents are blood-stage schizonticides that do not affect the liver stage of the parasite. The extent of this problem was investigated among Israeli and American travelers.

Methods.—Malaria surveillance data were reviewed to determine the traveler's destination, the infecting species, the type of chemoprophylaxis used, and the incubation period. Only civilian residents of Israel and the United States were included in the analyses.

Results.—Returning Israeli travelers reported 307 cases of malaria for the period from 1994 through 1999. *Plasmodium vivax* accounted for 50.8% of

TABLE 3.—Types of Chemoprophylaxis Against Malaria

Type and Agent*	Characteristics

Blood-stage (suppressive) prophylaxis
  Mefloquine
  Doxycycline
  Chloroquine
	Prevents primary infection; completely prevents only
	  P. falciparum and *P. malariae* infection; should be
	  continued for 4 wk after the traveler has left the area
	  of endemic disease

Liver-stage (causal) prophylaxis
  Primaquine
	Prevents primary infection and late-onset illness;
	  completely prevents all types of malaria; can be
	  discontinued after the traveler has left the area of
	  endemic disease

*The agents listed are examples of those that may be used for chemoprophylaxis.
(Reprinted by permission of *The New England Journal of Medicine* from Schwartz E, Parise M, Kozarsky P, et al: Delayed onset of malaria—Implications for chemoprophylaxis in travelers. *N Engl J Med* 349:1510-1516, 2003. Copyright 2003, Massachusetts Medical Society. All rights reserved.)

cases, *P falciparum* for 44.0%, and *P ovale* for 1.6%. In 134 (44.7%) cases, the illness developed more than 2 months after the traveler's return and, in 108 cases, occurred despite use of a prophylactic antimalarial regimen. Infection with *P vivax* or *P ovale* accounted for almost all of these cases. From 1992 through 1998, 2822 assessable cases of malaria occurred among travelers from the United States. The onset of malaria was late in 35.0% of these cases; 62.2% of travelers with late-onset of disease had appropriately taken an antimalarial agent. Late-onset infections were cause by *P vivax* in 811 cases, *P ovale* in 66, *P falciparum* in 59, and *P malariae* in 51.

Discussion.—Late-onset of disease is common among American and Israeli travelers infected with malaria, most of whom have used a nationally recommended antimalarial regimen. More effective prevention of malaria in travelers will require the use of agents that act on the liver phase of the parasites (Table 3).

Two Worlds of Malaria
Wellems TE, Miller LH (Natl Inst of Allergy and Infectious Diseases, Bethesda, Md)
N Engl J Med 349:1496-1498, 2003   7–4

Introduction.—Because parasites delivered by mosquitoes infect the liver before beginning the cycles of infection in red cells that cause the disease, travelers who receive antimalarial drugs that are effective only against bloodstream parasites may experience relapses from liver stages of plasmodium parasites (Figure; see color plate VIII). Improvements need to be made in prophylactic regimens and in the diagnosis and treatment of travelers' malaria.

Observations.—In the study by Schwartz et al (Abstract 7–3), of 3122 cases of malaria, 1121 (36%) occurred between 2 months and 4½ years after the traveler's return. Most of these cases consisted of *Plasmodium vivax* and *P ovale* malaria caused by hypnozoites that were unaffected by prophylaxis with blood-stage antimalarial drugs. Late cases of *P falciparum* and

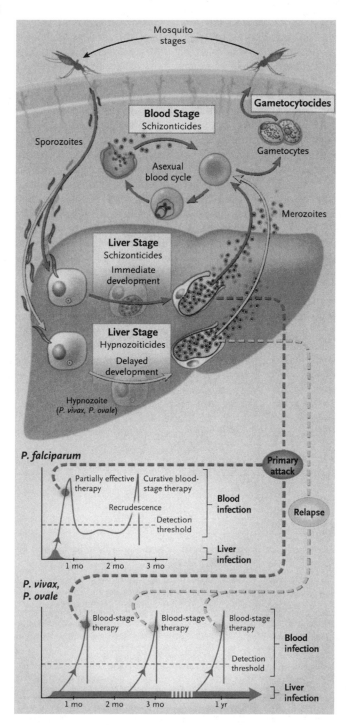

(Continued)

P malariae were probably caused by blood-stage parasites that were drug-resistant or had survived incomplete prophylaxis. Because *P falciparum* progresses through the liver in about a week and then moves into the bloodstream, antimalarial drugs that are effective against blood-stage forms will clear *P falciparum* infection after the liver-stage transition has been completed. The drugs need to be taken, however, for a full 4 weeks after leaving the endemic area.

Discussion.—Chloroquine, an inexpensive drug that acts promptly on blood-stage parasites, once met the needs of the 2 worlds of malaria: children in malarious regions and travelers from industrialized countries. But with the development of chloroquine-resistant strains, this drug now provides reliable prophylaxis only in limited regions. Decisions about prophylaxis must include the changing regional risks and the limitations and contraindications of alternatives to chloroquine. Sulfadoxine-pyrimethamine has replaced chloroquine in some countries in Africa, but drug resistance to this combination is spreading. The development of new drugs to prevent and treat malaria remains a challenge.

▶ Most malaria cases reported by Schwartz et al (Abstract 7–3) were detected within 2 months after exposure, and the majority probably can be attributed to inadequate prophylaxis. However, approximately one third of these cases occurred 2 months to 4½ years after the traveler's return from an endemic area. These patients likely had infections caused by liver-stage organisms that were unaffected by prophylaxis with blood-stage antimalarial agents. The findings stress the need for drugs that act on the liver phase of malaria parasites to allow for more effective disease prevention.

B. H. Thiers, MD

FIGURE.—Life cycle and courses of infections from malaria parasites in humans. Plasmodium parasites transmitted by anopheline mosquitoes always develop through a first stage of growth and division in the liver. Sporozoites enter individual hepatocytes and produce 10,000 to 30,000 merozoites that emerge to invade red cells. In all malarial infections, this bloodstream phase (asexual blood cycle) is responsible for the signs, symptoms, and complications of malaria; gametocytes in red cells and the liver infection itself cause no disease. Most infections produce a primary attack of malaria within two to four weeks after the mosquito bite occurs. Drugs may act as blood-stage schizonticides, liver-stage schizonticides, as blood-stage schizonticides, hypnozoiticides, or gametocyticides, depending on the parasite stages they attack. *Plasmodium falciparum,* the species responsible for the most malignant form of malaria, completes the liver stage of infection in about a week and can be prevented from causing disease by one month of effective blood-stage prophylaxis with schizonticides after exposure to mosquitoes. Surviving *P falciparum* parasites can, however, give rise to recrudescence if the treatment of or prophylaxis against the blood stage is only partially effective. In *P vivax* and *P ovale* infections, some sporozoites do not develop immediately but remain latent in the liver as hypnozoites for months to years before becoming activated to produce relapses of malaria. These relapses are not prevented by a course of antimalarial prophylaxis that kills blood-stage but not liver-stage parasites. (Reprinted by permission of *The New England Journal of Medicine* from Wellems TE, Miller LH: Two worlds of malaria. N Engl J Med 349:1496-1498, 2003. Copyright 2003, Massachusetts Medical Society. All rights reserved.)

Forecasting, Warning, and Detection of Malaria Epidemics: A Case Study
Hay SI, Were EC, Renshaw M, et al (Univ of Oxford, England; Ministry of Health, Nairobi, Kenya; UNICEF ESARO, UN Complex Gigiri, Nairobi, Kenya; et al)
Lancet 361:1705-1706, 2003   7–5

Introduction.—A malaria early warning system (MEWS) based on seasonal climate forecasting and monitoring and case surveillance might prevent and contain malaria epidemics. The 2002 malaria emergency in western Kenya was studied to determine whether a MEWS would have been an effective control strategy.

Methods.—The highlands of western Kenya have seasonal mesoendemic malaria transmission, with outbreaks occurring in June and July after long periods of rain. A role of the MEWS is to detect whether a seasonal resurgent outbreak is usual or may become a true epidemic. A joint United Nations Children's Fund (UNICEF) and Division of Malaria Control team was sent to 4 highland districts to examine the extent of the emergency and investigate how existing surveillance mechanisms and available data might have assisted in preparations for an epidemic.

Results.—A Greater Horn of Africa Climate Forum forecast, published in February 2002, indicated a 40% likelihood of normal conditions and a 35% likelihood of higher than average rainfall. There was exceptional rainfall, however, in some areas in May 2002. Estimates from satellite and meteorologic station data indicated average rainfall in April and May for 2 of the districts, both of which had normal resurgent outbreaks. True epidemics occurred in the other 2 districts during June and July, as predicted by their excessive rainfall in May. Early detection of epidemics was not possible using other health information and management systems.

Discussion.—Malaria remains a leading cause of death in 65 of 70 Kenyan administrative districts. Some aspects of a MEWS might benefit the western highlands of Kenya. Throughout the country there is poor access to, and use of, insecticide-treated nets; emerging antimalarial drug resistance, poor case management, and inadequate prescription practices by healthcare providers are additional obstacles. Better use of a MEWS and better planning for the annual resurgent outbreak would improve epidemic preparedness in Kenya.

▶ Normal seasonal increases in rainfall lead to concomitant resurgent outbreaks of malaria in endemic areas. Exceptionally high rainfall conditions lead to true malaria epidemics. The authors demonstrate that monitoring climatologic conditions can increase epidemic preparedness in malaria-prone areas.

B. H. Thiers, MD

Evidence of *Plasmodium falciparum* Malaria Resistant to Atovaquone and Proguanil Hydrochloride: Case Reports

Färnert A, Lindberg J, Gil P, et al (Karolinska Inst, Stockholm; Sahlgrenska Univ Hosp, Östra, Gothenburg, Sweden; Uppsala Univ, Sweden; et al)
BMJ 326:628-629, 2003   7–6

Background.—Several countries have begun using the combination of atovaquone and proguanil hydrochloride (Malarone; GlaxoSmithKline, NC) to treat *Plasmodium falciparum* malaria. A few treatment failures have been reported but have been attributed to suboptimal dosing, reinfection, or a point mutation in the cytochrome b gene. Two patients in whom treatment failed because of atovaquone and proguanil-resistant *P falciparum* are described.

Case Reports.—In September 2000, an 18-month-old boy, his 4-year-old brother, and their mother were given diagnoses of *P falciparum* malaria. All 3 had used chloroquine and proguanil as chemoprophylaxis during a trip to the Ivory Coast. All 3 patients were treated with the atovaquone and proguanil combination and had adequate drug concentrations in the blood. The mother's infection cleared without recurrence. The older boy's symptoms and parasites cleared initially, but 4 weeks later the symptoms and parasites recurred; he was successfully treated with mefloquine. The younger boy did not respond to the atovaquone and proguanil combination, and treatment was switched to mefloquine, which was successful. Genetic analyses showed a mutation associated with resistance to atovaquone in the older boy and the mother, and all 3 patients had double or triple mutations associated with resistance to proguanil and cycloguanil.

Conclusion.—Antimicrobial resistance was found in 2 of these 3 patients with *P falciparum* malaria who were treated with the atovaquone and proguanil combination. These results suggest that careful surveillance is needed with this combination drug to monitor the spread of antimicrobial resistance.

Effect of Intermittent Treatment With Amodiaquine on Anaemia and Malarial Fevers in Infants in Tanzania: A Randomised Placebo-controlled Trial

Massaga JJ, Kitua AY, Lemnge MM, et al (Natl Inst for Med Research, Amani, Tanzania; Natl Inst for Med Research, Dar es Salaam, Tanzania; Univ of Copenhagen)

Lancet 361:1853-1860, 2003   7–7

Background.—Falciparum malaria remains a major cause of morbidity in children in sub-Saharan Africa. Chemoprophylaxis with most affordable agents active against *Plasmodium falciparum* is ineffective because of drug resistance. In Tanzania, most strains of *P falciparum* are resistant to chloroquine and sulfadoxine/pyrimethamine. Whether presumptive intermittent treatment with amodiaquine and daily iron supplementation can prevent malarial fevers and anemia in infants was examined.

Methods.—The subjects were 291 infants 12 to 16 weeks old. Subjects were randomly assigned in equal numbers to receive daily oral iron supplementation (2.5 mL/day), intermittent amodiaquine (given over 3 days every 2 months in 10-, 10-, and 5-mg/kg doses), amodiaquine plus iron, or placebo. After 6 months of therapy, the incidences of malarial fever and anemia were compared among the groups.

Results.—Intermittent amodiaquine alone reduced the incidence of a first or only malarial episode by 64.7% compared with placebo; reductions associated with iron supplementation alone and amodiaquine plus iron were 13.0% and 63.9%, respectively. Amodiaquine plus iron and amodiaquine alone were equally effective in preventing anemia (reductions of 74.4% and 71.2% compared with placebo, respectively), and each was more effective than iron supplementation alone (reduction of 59.0% compared with placebo). There were no episodes of rebound during 4 months of follow-up, nor were there any hematologic or clinical adverse events.

Conclusion.—In Tanzania, where malaria is holoendemic, presumptive intermittent treatment with amodiaquine at 3, 5, and 7 months of age significantly reduced the incidences of malarial fever and anemia. Iron supplementation had protective effects on anemia but did hot have a significant additive effect on preventing malaria fever beyond that provided by amodiaquine therapy. This approach to prevention of malaria in areas where resistance to chloroquine and sulfadoxine/pyrimethamine is high holds great promise in controlling malaria among infants in endemic areas.

▶ Drug-resistant strains remain a serious obstacle to the prophylaxis and treatment of malaria. The combination of atovaquone and proguanil has been 1 of the main new developments in malaria chemotherapy but, as noted by Färnert et al (Abstract 7–6), resistance is already being observed. The report by Massaga et al (Abstract 7–7) documents the efficacy of intermittent treatment with amodiaquine in areas where resistance of *P falciparum* to sulfadoxine/pyrimethamine is frequent. Resistance to antimalarial therapy is directly correlated with frequency of use; to prevent the same fate from befalling amodiaquine, its prescription should be reserved for sulfadoxine/pyrimethamine-resistant cases.

B. H. Thiers, MD

Enhanced T-Cell Immunogenicity of Plasmid DNA Vaccines Boosted by Recombinant Modified Vaccinia Virus Ankara in Humans

McConkey SJ, Reece WHH, Moorthy VS, et al (Univ of Oxford, England; Imperial College, London; Walter Reed Army Inst of Research, Silver Spring, Md; et al)
Nat Med 9:729-735, 2003 7–8

Background.—Malaria is an increasingly uncontrolled public health problem, and 1 to 3 million deaths per year are attributable to *Plasmodium falciparum* infection. A preventive vaccine is likely to be one of the most effective methods for controlling malaria. In animal models, effective immune responses against malignancies and severe infectious pathogens, including *P falciparum*, are mediated by T cells. In contrast to most traditional vaccination strategies, which have focused on the humoral arm of the immune system, efforts to develop a vaccine for the pre-erythrocytic stages of malaria have been directed primarily at induction of cellular immunity. Findings were presented of a series of sequential small clinical trials that were designed to evaluate a large number of diverse vaccination regimens incorporating the prime-boost strategy in an effort to rapidly identify a highly immunogenic regimen.

Methods.—The study group comprised 63 healthy malaria-naive adult volunteers. The volunteers were immunized with plasmid DNA and modified vaccinia virus Ankara (MVA) vaccines recombinant for a pre-erythrocytic malaria antigen, thrombospondin-related adhesion protein (TRAP), individually and with the use of heterologous prime-boost immunization regimens at a range of doses. The sequential trials were designed to investigate the number of priming vaccinations and boosting vaccinations required and to incorporate dose-ranging studies.

Results.—A heterologous prime-boost regime of DNA administered either IM or epidermally and followed by intradermal recombinant MVA induced high frequencies of interferon-γ–secreting, antigen-specific T-cell responses to TRAP. The responses observed in this study were 5-fold to 10-fold higher than T-cell responses induced by the DNA vaccine or recombinant MVA vaccine alone and provided partial protection manifest as delayed parasitemia after sporozoite challenge with a different strain of *P falciparum*.

Conclusion.—Heterologous prime-boost immunization such as that described in this report may provide a basis for preventive and therapeutic vaccination in humans.

▶ Malaria is a serious public health concern, and a preventive vaccine is likely to be among the most effective means for its control. Existing lines of evidence implicate T lymphocytes in the immunologic control of pre-erythrocytic malaria infection in humans. McConkey et al found that a 1-2 punch of a malaria DNA sequence followed by intradermal injection of a recombinant modified vaccinia virus spurs the human immune system to mount a powerful immune response against the malaria organism, characterized by high frequencies of interferon-γ–secreting, antigen-specific T cells. The response with this combined approach was greater than with either the DNA vaccine or the recombinant modified vaccinia virus vaccine alone and produced partial protection against clinical infection. This approach may yield better vaccines not only against malaria, but against other infectious and neoplastic conditions as well.

B. H. Thiers, MD

8 Disorders of the Pilosebaceous Apparatus

Inflammatory Events Are Involved in Acne Lesion Initiation
Jeremy AHT, Holland DB, Roberts SG, et al (Univ of Leeds, England; Leeds Gen Infirmary, England)
J Invest Dermatol 121:20-27, 2003   8–1

Background.—The microcomedone is the earliest subclinical acne lesion. Hyperproliferation of the follicular epithelium is a characteristic feature of the microcomedone. Inflammatory cells at the periphery of such lesions have been reported. Whether inflammatory events occur before or after the hyperproliferative changes was investigated.

Methods.—Punch biopsy specimens of clinically normal follicles from uninvolved skin and early inflamed lesions were obtained from the interscapular region of the backs of adolescent patients with acne. Control follicles were also obtained from persons without acne. Cellular, vascular, and proliferative markers were analyzed by means of immunohistochemical methods.

Findings.—No microcomedonal features were documented in follicles from uninvolved skin. Epithelial proliferation was similar to that in control subjects and was significantly less than in inflamed lesions. Increased numbers of CD3+ and CD4+ T cells were noted in the perifollicular and papillary dermis, although levels were not comparable to those in papules. In addition, macrophages were greatly increased in number, similar to those in papules. No changes were seen in blood vessel numbers or vascular intercellular adhesion molecule 1 expression. However, E-selectin expression was increased to concentrations occurring in papules, and vascular adhesion molecule 1 levels were upregulated. Perifollicular upregulation of concentrations of the proinflammatory cytokine interleukin-1 (IL-1) was also noted. Aberrant integrin was expressed in the epidermis around the uninvolved follicles and inflamed lesions. However, the basement membrane was still intact.

Conclusions.—Inflammatory events are not secondary events but precede and play a causal role in the hyperproliferative changes in acne lesions. The increase in IL-1 activity before hyperproliferation around uninvolved follicles supports the recently proposed notion of the "keratinocyte activation cycle," in which keratinocytes are activated by release of IL-1, with activation markers K6 and K16 expressed subsequently.

▶ For years, inflammation in acne has been considered to be a secondary event that is preceded by hyperproliferation and hypercornification of the follicular duct. This study suggests that inflammation may be a primary event, which would validate the use of topical anti-inflammatory therapies for this disorder.

S. Raimer, MD

The Response of Skin Disease to Stress: Changes in the Severity of Acne Vulgaris as Affected by Examination Stress
Chiu A, Chon SY, Kimball AB (Stanford Univ, Calif)
Arch Dermatol 139:897-900, 2003   8–2

Introduction.—There is growing evidence that psychological stress may influence the course of a number of dermatologic disorders, including acne vulgaris. Stressful events have been shown to provoke or worsen breakouts of acne, and treatments such as biofeedback have proven effective. To demonstrate the association between stress and acne, stress levels were assessed and changes in disease severity were graded in a volunteer sample of university students.

Methods.—The 22 students recruited for the study had a mean age of 22 years. Nineteen (12 women and 7 men) completed the questionnaires and had acne severity graded according to the Leeds technique. A single observer graded acne severities on 2 occasions: once during a nonexamination period (at least 1 month before any examination) and later during an examination period (within 3 days before to 7 days after an examination). Students completed the Perceived Stress Scale questionnaire and reported on their sleep and diet quality at both visits. They were allowed to continue on oral and topical therapies (excluding isotretinoin) during the study.

Results.—There was a strong correlation between an increase in stress and an increase in acne severity. Persons reporting the greatest stress during examination periods also showed the greatest exacerbations in acne severity. The mean Leeds score increased from 0.97 in nonexamination periods to 1.33 during examination periods. Worsening perceived diet quality was also significantly associated with acne exacerbation, although to a lesser degree than stress. An association between worsened sleep quality and acne exacerbation was close to significant.

Conclusion.—This study of university students showed a significant association between stress experienced during examination periods and worsened acne.

► The authors found a high correlation between increasing stress and changes in acne severity. This correlation remained significant even after controlling for changes in diet and sleep habits.

B. H. Thiers, MD

Body Dysmorphic Disorder in Patients With Acne
Uzun Ö, Basoğlu C, Akar A, et al (Gülhane Military Med Academy School of Medicine, Ankara; GATA Haydarpasa Eğitim Hastanesi Psychiatry Clinic, Istanbul, Turkey)
Compr Psychiatry 44:415-419, 2003   8–3

Introduction.—Patients with body dysmorphic disorder (BDD) are preoccupied by the presence of an imagined or exaggerated physical anomaly. One survey found a high diagnostic rate of BDD (11.9%) among patients seeking treatment from dermatologists. Individuals with BDD and acne may request aggressive therapy for minimal lesions. The prevalence of BDD and its related demographic characteristics were investigated in a sample of Turkish patients with mild acne.

Methods.—The study included 159 outpatients (82 male, 77 female) who were seen at a dermatology clinic in Ankara, Turkey. All had acne that was graded as mild on the Cook scale. Patients completed a self-report questionnaire that covered sociodemographic and dermatologic treatment variables, dissatisfaction with appearance, and 16 items that included the DSM-IV criteria for BDD. Those who reported dissatisfaction with their appearance were individually examined by a psychiatrist.

Results.—Of the 159 patients, 57 (35.8%) expressed dissatisfaction with some aspect of their appearance, but only 14 (8.8%) of the 159 fulfilled the criteria for BDD. Eight acne patients with BDD were male (57.1%) and 6 (42.9%) were female, a sex proportion similar to that in the non-BDD group. Patients with BDD were significantly older and had a higher level of education than those without BDD. None of the patients with BDD had consulted a psychiatrist; 3 of 14 were found to have current comorbid psychiatric disorders (a rate not different from that of acne patients without BDD).

Conclusion.—BDD is apparently more prevalent in patients with acne than in the general population. All patients in this series also reported dissatisfaction with other parts of their body. Dermatologists should screen their acne patients for BDD.

► The results are compromised by possible selection bias (the data were recorded at a university hospital), the small number of patients with BDD, and a lack of an appropriate control population.

B. H. Thiers, MD

Effect of Antibiotics on the Oropharyngeal Flora in Patients With Acne

Levy RM, Huang EY, Roling D (Univ of Pennsylvania, Philadelphia)
Arch Dermatol 139:467-471, 2003   8–4

Background.—Persons with acne are generally an otherwise healthy group of individuals who are often exposed to antibiotics for long periods. The effects of long-term antibiotic use on cutaneous microbial environments have been well documented in this patient population. However, the effects on noncutaneous surfaces, such as the oropharynx, have not been well studied. The prevalence and resistance patterns of *Streptococcus pyogenes* and *Staphylococcus aureus* in the oropharynx of patients with acne were investigated in a cross-sectional study.

Methods.—The study included 105 patients. Forty-two patients were using oral tetracyclines or topical antibiotics, and 63 were not. The presence of *S pyogenes* and *S aureus* in the oropharynx was assessed by culture. Resistance patterns to tetracycline antibiotics were determined by agar disk diffusion.

Findings.—Ten percent of patients not using antibiotics had positive *S pyogenes* cultures, compared with 33% of those using antibiotic therapy. Eighty-five percent of *S pyogenes* cultures from antibiotic users were resistant to at least 1 tetracycline antibiotic, compared with 20% from nonusers. *S aureus* cultures were positive in 29% of those not using antibiotics and in 22% of those using antibiotics. Resistance patterns of *S aureus* did not differ significantly.

Conclusions.—Antibiotic treatment in patients with acne is associated with *S pyogenes* colonization and resistance in the oropharynx. Further study of the clinical and long-term significance of this finding is warranted.

▶ This study was the first to look at the effect of antibiotics on the oropharyngeal flora of patients with acne. When compared with acne patients on no antibiotic therapy, 20% more of those on either oral tetracycline or on a topical antibiotic had *S pyogenes* in their oropharynx. The transfer of resistant organisms from the skin to the oropharynx was suggested as a possible explanation for resistant organisms being present in this location in patients using only topical antibiotics. Slightly fewer antibiotic-treated patients (22%) versus untreated patients (29%) grew *S aureus*; however, 44% of these organisms isolated from antibiotic-treated patients were resistant to at least 1 tetracycline.

Patients in this study were all asymptomatic, so it is difficult to assess the clinical relevance of the increased incidence of *S pyogenes* in the oropharynx for antibiotic-treated patients or for their household contacts. The increased incidence of potentially pathogenic streptococcal bacteria supports the avoidance of long-term antibiotic therapy whenever possible. There was no increase in the numbers of *S aureus* in the oropharynx of antibiotic-treated patients, and it is doubtful that tetracycline therapy for acne has contributed significantly to the problem of staphylococcal resistance. Staphylococcal organisms, even those resistant to numerous antibiotics, are more likely to be sensitive to tetracycline at the present time than they were in the 1970s. It would be interesting to know whether concomitant therapy with benzoyl peroxide, which has been shown to decrease the resistance of *Propionibacterium acnes*, would affect the oropharyngeal flora or the resistance pattern of organisms in acne patients being treated with antibiotics.

S. Raimer, MD

Effects of Subantimicrobial-Dose Doxycycline in the Treatment of Moderate Acne

Skidmore R, Kovach R, Walker C, et al (Univ of Florida, Gainesville; West Virginia Univ, Morgantown; Covance Inc, Princeton, NJ; et al)
Arch Dermatol 139:459-464, 2003   8–5

Background.—Minocycline and other chemically modified tetracyclines may inhibit matrix metalloproteinases (MMPs) and downregulate connective tissue destruction in inflammatory diseases, independent of their antimicrobial activity. The effects of subantimicrobial dose (SD) doxycycline hyclate in patients with moderate acne were investigated.

Methods.—The study included 51 adults with moderate facial acne who were enrolled in a multicenter, double-blind, randomized, placebo controlled trial. Patients received SD doxycycline, 20-mg tablets twice daily, or placebo for 6 months. Forty patients completed treatment.

Findings.—At 6 months, patients receiving active treatment, compared with those receiving placebo, had a significantly greater percent decrease in the number of comedones, inflammatory and noninflammatory lesions combined, and total inflammatory lesions. Doxycycline recipients also had significantly more improvement, as determined by the clinician's global assessment. Microbial counts did not differ significantly between groups. In addition, no evidence of change was noted in antibiotic susceptibility or colonization by potential pathogens. Patients tolerated doxycycline treatment well.

Conclusions.—Twice-daily treatment with SD doxycycline can significantly decrease the number of inflammatory and noninflammatory lesions in persons with moderate facial acne. This treatment was tolerated well, had no detectable antimicrobial effect on skin flora, and did not increase the number or severity of resistant organisms.

▶ It is generally acknowledged that subtherapeutic doses of antibiotics should be avoided as they may promote the emergence of resistant organisms. In this study, treatment of acne with 20 mg of doxycycline twice daily for 6 months appeared to have no effect on *Propionibacterium acnes* or other skin microflora and did not result in the emergence of organisms resistant to doxycycline. Only 21 patients completed the active treatment arm of the study. The study dosage resulted in a reduction of about 50% in inflammatory acne lesions, which was better than placebo. Patients, however, are generally not satisfied with a 50% decrease in inflammatory lesions, and in this study, they judged themselves to be little improved according to their self-assessment scores. Combination therapy with topical agents likely would result in greater improvement. Antibiotics remain a mainstay in the treatment of moderate to severe acne, although the recent emergence of resistant organisms should encourage the development of and our use of additional alternative nonantibiotic regimens. In the meantime, a direct comparison of the clinical effectiveness of standard versus subtherapeutic doses of doxycycline for the treatment of acne would be helpful.

S. Raimer, MD

Isotretinoin and Antidepressant Pharmacotherapy: A Prescription Sequence Symmetry Analysis
Hersom K, Neary MP, Levaux HP, et al (Quintiles Late Phase, San Francisco; Hoffmann-La Roche, Inc, Nutley, NJ; Univ of Iowa, Iowa City)
J Am Acad Dermatol 49:424-432, 2003   8–6

Introduction.—Isotretinoin is indicated for the treatment of patients with severe, recalcitrant nodular acne. Spontaneous reports have indicated a possible relationship between isotretinoin treatment and depression. Depression has been reported in patients with acne and is often seen in adolescents.

TABLE 1.—Antidepressants Included in the Isotretinoin and
Minocycline Analyses

Therapeutic Class	Antidepressant
SSRIs	Citalopram
	Fluoxetine
	Fluvoxamine
	Paroxetine
	Sertraline
Secondary and tertiary amine tricyclics	Amitriptyline
	Clomipramine
	Doxepin
	Imipramine hydrochloride
	Imipramine pamoate
	Trimipramine
	Amoxapine
	Despiramine
	Nortriptyline
	Protriptyline
Other antidepressants*	Bupropion
	Maprotiline
	Mirtazapine
	Nefazodone
	Trazodone
	Venlafaxine
	Amitriptyline hydrochloride/perphenazine
	Amitriptyline/chlordiazepoxide

*Monoamine oxidase inhibitors were not included because of their primary use in chronic depression.
(Reprinted by permission of the publisher from Hersom K, Neary MP, Levaux HP, et al: Isotretinoin and antidepressant pharmacotherapy: A prescription sequence symmetry analysis. *J Am Acad Dermatol* 49:424-432, 2003. Copyright 2003 by Elsevier.)

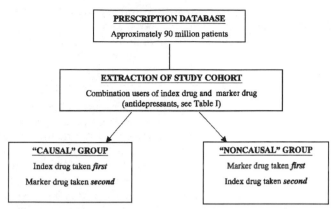

FIGURE 1.—Study population selection process. This figure provides the study design that develops the 2 groups that were analyzed. The "causal" group includes patients who filled their isotretinoin prescriptions first, and the "noncausal" group includes patients who filled their antidepressant prescriptions first. (Reprinted by permission of the publisher from Hersom K, Neary MP, Levaux HP, et al: Isotretinoin and antidepressant pharmacotherapy: A prescription sequence symmetry analysis. *J Am Acad Dermatol* 49:424-432, 2003. Copyright 2003 by Elsevier.)

The possible association between isotretinoin use and onset of depression was examined retrospectively.

Methods.—A large database was searched to review pharmacy claims. The order of first-documented isotretinoin and antidepressant dispensings (Table 1) was evaluated in incident users (Fig 1). A total of 2821 patients aged 12 to 49 years who filled isotretinoin prescriptions between June 1, 1999, and March 31, 2000, were included. The ratio of the number of patients who filled isotretinoin prescriptions first versus second was determined, with adjustments for variations in physician prescribing patterns. A ratio significantly greater than 1.0 indicates a depression-invoking association. Similar analyses of minocycline were conducted.

Results.—Adjusted ratios for all antidepressants and by class were not significantly greater than 1.0, with similar results observed for minocycline.

Conclusion.—These findings do not support a relationship between the use of isotretinoin and the onset of depression. Findings for minocycline, which is a commonly used antibiotic for the treatment of acne, were similar.

▶ This cleverly done study adds to the growing body of evidence that casts doubt on the purported association between isotretinoin use and depression.

B. H. Thiers, MD

Pulsed-Dye Laser Treatment for Inflammatory Acne Vulgaris: Randomised Controlled Trial

Seaton ED, Charakida A, Mouser PE, et al (Imperial College, London; Univ of Wales, Swansea, England)
Lancet 362:1347-1352, 2003   8–7

Introduction.—Because acne often improves after exposure to sunlight, artificial visible light sources have been investigated as treatment for this condition. Anecdotal reports suggest that a single low-fluence pulsed-dye laser (PDL) exposure can produce long-term improvement in inflammatory acne. The validity of these reports was tested in a randomized trial.

Methods.—The study included patients between 18 and 45 years old who had mild to moderate inflammatory facial acne. Thirty-one were assigned to PDL and 10 to sham treatment. After a washout period for previous treatments, a single PDL or sham treatment was administered. Patients were assessed after 2, 4, 8, and 12 weeks for acne severity, lesion counts, and adverse events.

Results.—Most patients had a long history of acne and had been treated previously with oral antibiotics (90%), oral isotretinoin (30%), and topical agents. Acne severity was reduced after 12 weeks from a mean of 3.8 to a mean of 1.9 (on the Leeds revised grading system) in the PDL group. Improvement was slight, however, in the sham group (from a mean of 3.6 to 3.5). Total lesion counts were reduced by 53% in the PDL group in contrast to 9% in the control group; reductions in inflammatory lesion counts in the PDL and the sham treatment groups were 49% and 10%, respectively. Two patients reported pain during laser treatment, but few additional adverse effects were noted. Most of the benefits of PDL were seen by the 4-week assessment.

Conclusion.—Patients with inflammatory acne responded well to PDL treatment and experienced no serious adverse side effects. The improvement came rapidly, in contrast to conventional pharmacologic treatment methods, and the laser was also effective in patients with acne-associated scarring. Lower laser fluences (1.5 vs 3.0 J/cm^2) may lessen discomfort in individuals with deeply pigmented skin.

▶ In a commentary that accompanied this article, Webster observed that although most patients had a significant decrease in lesions, the majority was not rendered acne-free. He concluded that the response to the PDL seemed to be similar to that achieved with topical benzoyl peroxide. The mechanism of action of a single low-fluence laser treatment, as well as its true utility, can only be determined by additional studies on larger numbers of patients.[1]

B. H. Thiers, MD

Reference

1. Webster GF: Laser treatment of acne. *Lancet* 362:1342, 2003.

Nonablative Radiofrequency for Active Acne Vulgaris: The Use of Deep Dermal Heat in the Treatment of Moderate to Severe Active Acne Vulgaris (Thermotherapy): A Report of 22 Patients
Ruiz-Esparza J, Gomez JB (Univ of California, San Diego; Instituto Dermatologica de Jalisco, Guadalajara, México)
Dermatol Surg 29:333-339, 2003   8–8

Introduction.—Acne vulgaris can have a profound impact on the quality of life of affected persons. Physical methods, including chemical peeling, laser ablation, and surgery, are usually directed at the sequelae (scars) of acne rather than at the active disease. Heat therapy has historically been used in the treatment of microorganism-induced diseases. Heat and its effect were assessed in 22 patients in the active stage of moderate to severe acne vulgaris.

Methods.—Ten females and 12 males (ages 16-28 years) with moderate to severe, scarring, cystic, active acne vulgaris underwent treatment that used a new nonablative radiofrequency unit that delivered a concomitant spray of cryogen for epidermal sparing. One and 2 sessions were performed in 20 and 2 patients, respectively, at an average fluence or energy delivery of 72 J/cm^2. Nine patients were on concomitant medical therapy (oral antibiotics or topical agents). Follow-up ranged from 1 to 8 months. Treatment response was assessed via patient questionnaires and active acne lesion counts.

Results.—Eighteen (82%) patients had an excellent response, 2 (9%) had a modest response, and 2 (9%) had no response. The Student's *t*-test on active lesion counts before treatment and after treatment was less than 0.009004. No side effects were observed, and no downtime was caused by the procedure. Only topical anesthesia (ELA-Max 5%) was required.

Conclusion.—This novel use of 1 session of deep dermal heat in the treatment of moderate to severe active acne vulgaris appears to be safe and effective. Multiple sessions after a 4-month waiting period may be beneficial for patients who do not respond to the first session. This therapy may be an important future treatment option for patients with active acne vulgaris.

▶ In the absence of histologic examination, the mechanism of action of nonablative radiofrequency when used for the treatment of acne vulgaris remains unknown. Clinical improvement may reflect destruction of sebaceous glands or inhibition of their function.

B. H. Thiers, MD

Interaction of Spironolactone With ACE Inhibitors or Angiotensin Receptor Blockers: Analysis of 44 Cases
Wrenger E, Müller R, Moesenthin M, et al (Otto-von-Guericke Univ, Magdeburg, Germany)
BMJ 327:147-149, 2003   8–9

Introduction.—The addition of low-dose spironolactone (25-50 mg/d) to standard treatment was reported in a randomized study to substantially reduce (30%) the risk of mortality in patients with severe congestive heart failure. Follow-up showed the incidence of serious hyperkalemia to be similarly low in placebo (1%) and spironolactone (2%) groups. A case series of life-threatening hyperkalemia in 44 patients who were receiving spironolactone plus angiotensin (AT)-converting enzyme (ACE) inhibitors or AT_1 receptor blockers was reported.

Results.—Patients were seen at a nephrology unit during the period from January 1999 until December 2002. The mean patient age was 76 years, and the mean dosage of spironolactone was 88 mg daily. Diabetes mellitus was present in 35 of 44 patients. Common symptoms on admission were severe dehydration, muscle weakness and paralysis, vomiting, and bradyarrhythmia. The estimated creatinine clearance was below normal in all patients; the mean plasma potassium concentration was 7.7 mmol/L. Thirty-seven patients were started on hemodialysis, and 7 were given conventional potassium-lowering treatment. Two patients died of complications and 6 had to be kept on chronic dialysis treatment. Surviving patients were treated with ACE inhibitors, β-receptor blockers, and loop diuretics; spironolactone was not reintroduced.

Discussion.—The combination of spironolactone and ACE inhibitors or AT_1 receptor blockers can lead to hyperkalemia, arrhythmia, or death. Most patients had been treated with a larger dosage of spironolactone than the 25 to 50 mg/d recommended by a randomized evaluation study. Patients with heart failure who are taking spironolactone and ACE inhibitors or AT_1 receptor blockers need to be monitored carefully, especially when the risk factors of reduced renal function, diabetes mellitus type 2, and advanced age are present. Spironolactone dosage in such cases should be no more than 25 mg/d or every other day.

▶ Spironolactone is used not uncommonly in dermatology, primarily for the treatment of acne and female androgenetic alopecia. The adverse drug interaction reported by Wrenger et al emphasizes the importance of taking a complete medication history from all our patients.

B. H. Thiers, MD

Stress Inhibits Hair Growth in Mice by Induction of Premature Catagen Development and Deleterious Perifollicular Inflammatory Events Via Neuropeptide Substance P-Dependent Pathways
Arck PC, Handjiski B, Peters EMJ, et al (Humboldt Univ, Berlin; Univ of Hamburg, Germany)
Am J Pathol 162:803-814, 2003   8–10

Background.—Whether stress can cause clinically relevant hair loss remains a matter of debate. Evidence suggests neuropeptide substance P (SP) is involved in the stress response. A murine model was used to examine the effects of stress on hair growth, and to explore whether SP is involved in stress-induced hair loss.

Methods.—Female CBA/J and C57BL/6 mice aged 6 to 8 weeks were studied; these mice have a profound response to stress and at this age are in the telogen stage of the hair cycle. Depilation was used to induce anagen. During late anagen (ie, day 14 after depilation), some of the mice were exposed to sound stress for 24 hours. Other mice were given an intraperitoneal injection of SP to mimic the effects of stress, and some mice were left as controls (no stress, no SP injection). Another set of animals was similarly treated, except they were given a specific SP receptor antagonist, neurokinin-1, every other day beginning on day 2. All animals were killed on day 16 after depilation, and hair follicle cycling was examined by quantitative histomorphometry. Major histocompatibility complex class II (MHC-II)-positive cell clusters (evaluated by immunohistochemistry), mast cell expression (evaluated by Giemsa staining), and apoptosis (evaluated by TUNEL staining) were also determined.

Results.—Sound stress promoted premature catagen development, as most hair follicles of stressed mice were in early catagen, whereas most hair follicles of nonstressed mice were still in anagen VI (Fig 2, A and B; see color plate IX). Accordingly, perifollicular MHC-II–positive cell clusters, mast cell degranulation, and intrafollicular apoptosis were significantly increased in stressed mice. Stress also significantly increased the number of SP-positive

FIGURE 2

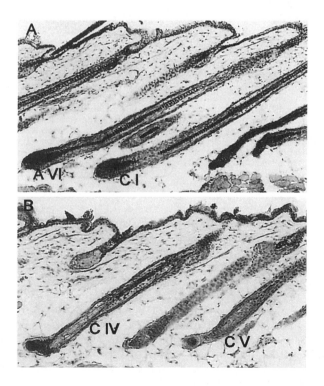

(Continued)

FIGURE 2 (cont.)

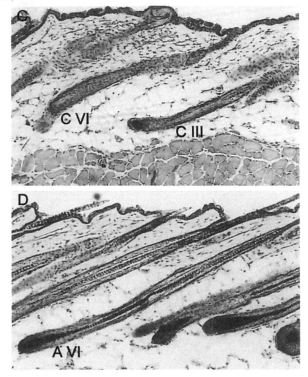

FIGURE 2.—The effect of stress on the hair cycle stage is depicted in **A-D. A,** A representative area of control mice 16 days after depilation with the majority of hair follicles (HFs) in anagen VI (*AVI*). **B,** Mirrors the effect of stress on the hair cycle stage on day 16 after depilation with HFs in catagen IV (*CIV*) or catagen V (*CV*). **C,** HF of stressed mice that received injection of substance P (SP), which mimicked the effect of stress on the vulnerability of hair follicles toward catagen progression with HFs in catagen III to VI (*CIII-VI*). **D,** A representative example of mice exposed to stress and treated with the neurokinin-1 receptor antagonist (NK1-RA), in which the majority of HFs were scored as anagen VI, similar to the nonstressed control group. (Courtesy of Arck PC, Handjiski B, Peters EMJ, et al: Stress inhibits hair growth in mice by induction of premature catagen development and deleterious perifollicular inflammatory events via neuropeptide substance P-dependent pathways. *Am J Pathol* 162:803-814, 2003. Copyright American Society for Investigative Pathology.)

nerve fibers in the dermis and subcutis. All of these effects were mimicked by the injection of SP (Fig 2, C; see color plate X). Most of these stress-induced changes were absent in the animals pretreated with neurokinin-1 receptor antagonist (Fig 2, D; see color plate X).

Conclusion.—In this murine model, psychoemotional stressors altered hair follicle cycling in vivo, causing the normal duration of hair growth to terminate prematurely. This effect and the accompanying upregulation of apoptosis and deleterious inflammatory events could be mimicked by injection of the stress-related neuropeptide SP. Most of these effects were effectively counteracted by coadministration of a specific SP receptor antagonist. The mechanisms described may offer a rationale for the pharmacologic treatment of hair loss in humans.

Intermittent Foot Shock Stress Prolongs the Telogen Stage in the Hair Cycle of Mice

Aoki E, Shibasaki T, Kawana S (Nippon Med School, Tokyo)
Exp Dermatol 12:371-377, 2003   8–11

Background.—Physical and emotional stress can significantly affect skin diseases and cutaneous function. The skin appears to have its own local stress response system, and some evidence suggests stress can influence the hair growth cycle. The effects of intermittent physical stress on the hair cycle were examined in a murine model.

Methods.—Areas of the dorsal skin in 10 female C57BL/6 mice aged 8 weeks were depilated. Four weeks later, when all hair follicles in the area were in telogen, half the animals were given 2 weeks of intermittent foot shocks via a floor grid, whereas the other 5 animals served as controls. After 2 weeks, macroscopic and histologic changes in the hair cycle were examined. Skin concentrations of the stress-related neuropeptide corticotropin-releasing factor (CRF) and its receptor, as well as plasma concentrations of corticosterone were measured.

Results.—Macroscopically and histologically, the test areas in control mice stained black (indicating anagen), whereas most of the areas in the stressed mice were pink (indicating telogen) (Fig 1, E). CRF-positive keratinocytes were present in the telogen follicles and epidermis of the stressed mice but were not present in the telogen follicles of the controls. In both groups, CRF receptor–positive cells were seen only in the sebaceous glands. Plasma corticosterone levels in the stressed mice were significantly higher than those in the controls (approximately 28 vs 11 µg/dL).

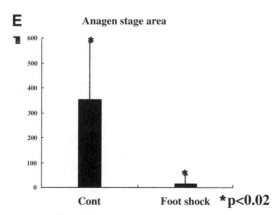

FIGURE 1.—E, In the stressed mice, the anagen stage area was significantly smaller after 2 weeks of foot shock exposure than in the controls (*P* < .02). (Courtesy of Aoki E, Shibasaki T, Kawana S: Intermittent foot shock stress prolongs the telogen stage in the hair cycle of mice. *Exp Dermatol* 12:371-377, 2003. Reprinted by permission of Blackwell Publishing.)

Conclusion.—Intermittent foot shock inhibits the induction of the anagen stage in mice. Corticosterone may be involved in the prolongation of the telogen stage.

▶ These authors used a murine animal model to study hair cycle changes; mice are commonly used for hair experiments because they display a highly synchronized hair cycle. While the applicability of the findings to human hair loss can be debated, the findings are certainly provocative and provide a possible pathophysiologic basis for stress-induced hair loss and telogen effluvium.

B. H. Thiers, MD

Transplants From Balding and Hairy Androgenetic Alopecia Scalp Regrow Hair Comparably Well on Immunodeficient Mice
Krajcik RA, Vogelman JH, Malloy VL, et al (Orentreich Found for the Advancement of Science Inc, Cold Spring-on-Hudson, NY)
J Am Acad Dermatol 48:752-759, 2003   8–12

Introduction.—Both the athymic (nude) mouse and the severe combined immunodeficient (SCID) mouse are used in studies of male-pattern baldness, or androgenetic alopecia (AGA). In seeking to optimize the procedure of grafting AGA hair follicles to immunodeficient mice, investigators found, contrary to some previous reports, that miniaturized hair follicles of a balding scalp could successfully regenerate and produce terminal anagen hairs when removed from the human scalp.

Methods.—Tissue from patients was removed by 2-mm, full-thickness, punch excisions from both balding and hairy areas of the scalp, then prepared and transplanted into the subcutaneous tissue of the nude and SCID mice. Hair follicles from 2 men with frontal balding were used in study I; a woman with frontal balding was the donor source for hair follicles in study II. Hair was allowed to grow undisturbed for 22 weeks in study I. Growing hairs were cut at the level of the epidermis at 6.5, 9, 13.5, 18, and 22 weeks in study II.

Results.—In study I, nearly 50% of the grafts gave rise to viable follicles after the postoperative effluvium period of about 7 weeks. The combined mean diameter of the hairs from the balding scalp, which was 24 μm before transplantation, increased to 99 μm at 22 weeks. Terminal hairs showed a 38% reduction from baseline values (from a mean diameter of 151 to 93 μm). Thus, balding hairs were significantly thicker and terminal hairs were significantly thinner relative to baseline. In study II, the mean diameter of balding hairs was 26 μm and that of terminal hairs was 108 μm before grafting. Balding hairs increased more than 300% in maximum diameter by 22 weeks, whereas terminal hairs decreased 50% in diameter. The calculated mean volume growth per week of balding-area hairs was double that of hairs from the nonbalding scalp.

Conclusion.—Balding, miniaturized follicles were found to quickly regenerate when removed from the human scalp and transplanted into mice. This finding applied equally to men and women with AGA.

▶ Krajcik et al found that the miniaturized hair follicles of a balding scalp had a remarkable ability to regenerate and produce terminal androgen hairs when removed from their natural human milieu. This suggests the importance of extrinsic factors in the pathogenesis of AGA. The findings contrast with those of Van Neste et al, who reported that the hair growth rates of hair follicles from human male and female donors transplanted onto female nude mice were less than growth rates recorded in situ on patients' scalps.[1] The divergent findings may be ascribed to different characteristics of the pretransplantation hairs used in the 2 studies.

B. H. Thiers, MD

Reference

1. Van Neste D, De Brouwer B, Dumortier M: Reduced linear hair growth rates of vellus and of terminal hairs produced by human balding scalp grafted onto nude mice. *Ann N Y Acad Sci* 642:480-482, 1991.

Topical Nitrogen Mustard in the Treatment of Alopecia Areata: A Bilateral Comparison Study
Bernardo O, Tang L, Lui H, et al (Univ of British Columbia, Vancouver, Canada)
J Am Acad Dermatol 49:291-294, 2003   8–13

Introduction.—A study published in 1985 reported positive results when patients with alopecia areata (AA) were treated with topical nitrogen mustard. Because these results have never been confirmed, a controlled study of topical nitrogen mustard was conducted in 10 patients with AA.

Methods.—The patients were 5 men and 5 women who ranged in age from 23 to 53 years. The duration of AA ranged from 1 to 17 years, and all patients had more than 50% scalp involvement at study entry. For a period of 16 weeks, patients applied 0.02% mechlorethamine in Aquaphor to the left or right half of the scalp daily. When hair regrowth appeared, the application frequency was reduced to 3 times per week. The hair-growth index was used to determine outcome; the minimum score was 0 and the maximum was 300, indicating a full half-head of hair.

Results.—Six patients completed the 16 weeks of treatment. In 1 patient, the hair-growth index on the treated side increased from 10 to 150, with considerable regrowth of hair. Four of the remaining 5 patients showed little change in the hair-growth index, and 1 experienced worsening of AA on both sides of the head. Contact hypersensitivity developed in 1 patient who completed therapy. Complete blood cell counts, performed at baseline and at 4 and 16 weeks, remained normal in all patients.

Discussion.—In this small series, 1 of 6 patients with AA responded positively to topical nitrogen mustard. Longer treatment may have yielded better results, but there is concern that topical nitrogen mustard may be a carcinogen or tumor promoter.

▶ I have observed little benefit from the use of topical nitrogen mustard in a few patients with alopecia totalis. Admittedly, this subset of patients is characteristically refractory to any form of therapy.

B. H. Thiers, MD

9 Collagen Vascular and Related Disorders

Development of Autoantibodies Before the Clinical Onset of Systemic Lupus Erythematosus
Arbuckle MR, McClain MT, Rubertone MV, et al (Univ of Oklahoma, Oklahoma City; NIH, Bethesda, Md; US Army Ctr for Health Promotion and Preventive Medicine, Washington, DC)
N Engl J Med 349:1526-1533, 2003   9–1

Background.—Systemic lupus erythematosus (SLE) is almost always accompanied by the production of autoantibodies, and it has been shown that autoantibodies contribute directly to the pathologic changes of SLE. Autoantibodies are central to the pathogenesis of the disorder, so their development must coincide with or precede clinical disease. The prevalence of SLE autoantibodies among patients with confirmed SLE has been established; however, little is known of the autoimmune history of patients before the diagnosis of SLE. The onset and progression of autoantibody development before clinical diagnosis of SLE were investigated.

Methods.—This study utilized the Department of Defense Serum Repository, which contains about 30 million specimens prospectively collected from over 5 million armed forces personnel. Serum samples obtained from 130 persons before they received a diagnosis of SLE were evaluated along with samples from matched controls.

Results.—At least 1 SLE autoantibody tested was present before the diagnosis (up to 9.4 years earlier; mean, 3.3 years) in 115 of the 130 patients (88%). Antinuclear antibodies were present in 78% of patients (at a dilution of 1:120 or more); anti–double-stranded DNA antibodies in 55%; anti-Ro antibodies in 47%; anti-La antibodies in 34%; anti-Sm antibodies in 32%; antinuclear ribonucleoprotein antibodies in 26%; and antiphospholipid antibodies in 18%. Antinuclear, antiphospholipid antibodies, anti-Ro, and anti-La autoantibodies were present earlier than anti-Sm and antinuclear ribonucleoprotein antibodies (a mean of 3.4 years before the diagnosis vs 1.2 years).

Anti–double-stranded DNA antibodies, with a mean onset of 2.2 years after the diagnosis, were found later than antinuclear antibodies and earlier than antinuclear ribonucleoprotein antibodies. The earliest available serum sample was positive in many patients; thus, these measures of the average time from the first positive antibody test to the diagnosis are underestimates of the time from the development of the antibodies to the diagnosis. Among the 130 initial matched control subjects, 3.8% were positive for 1 or more autoantibodies.

Conclusion.—Autoantibodies are usually present many years before the diagnosis of SLE. The appearance of autoantibodies in patients with SLE often follows a predictable course, with a progressive accumulation of specific autoantibodies before the onset of SLE.

Autoantibodies in Systemic Lupus Erythematosus—There Before You Know It
Shmerling RH (Harvard Med School, Boston)
N Engl J Med 349:1499-1500, 2003   9–2

Introduction.—The antinuclear antibody (ANA) has been closely associated with systemic lupus erythematosus (SLE), but positivity for ANA is also found in other rheumatic and nonrheumatic diseases. Furthermore, most positive results are of uncertain significance, and many autoimmune diseases have no known association with autoantibodies. The role of autoantibodies in the diagnosis of SLE was examined.

Observations.—Knowledge of why and how pathogenic autoantibodies develop might clarify the origin of the disease, explain why certain organs are targeted, and suggest how autoimmune disease could be prevented or treated. However, the diversity of the biological actions of autoantibodies presents a challenge. It appears that SLE develops when an individual genetically predisposed to the disease is exposed to 1 or more environmental triggers. However, more than a single trigger may be required, and the first, least specific autoantibodies (ie, antinuclear, antiphospholipid, anti-Ro, and anti-La antibodies) may be involved in subsequent, more specific antibody formation (including anti-Sm, anti-nuclear ribonucleoprotein, and

---

TABLE—Specific Antinuclear Antibodies

Anti-ds-DNA (anti–double-stranded (DNA), specific for SLE, associated with activity of SLE and lupus nephritis
Anti-SM (anti-Smith), specific for SLE, correlation with disease activity uncertain
Anti-RNP (also called anti-snRNP, or anti–small nuclear ribonucleoprotein), present in SLE, correlates with myositis, esophageal dysmotility, Raynaud's phenomenon, sclerodactyly, interstitial lung disease; a defining auto-antibody in mixed connective-tissue disease
Anti-Ro, associated with SLE, Sjögren's syndrome, neonatal lupus, photo-sensitive rash, subacute cutaneous lupus erythematosus
Anti-La, present in SLE (may be associated with reduced risk of nephritis), Sjögren's syndrome, neonatal lupus

anti–double-stranded DNA antibodies). The diagnosis of SLE in a patient with features suggestive of the disease may be supported by a positive ANA test result, especially if the more specific autoantibodies are present (Table). Screening asymptomatic individuals for ANA is unlikely to improve clinical outcomes because no preventive treatment is available and a positive result in such cases does not mean that SLE will develop.

Discussion.—When an individual tests positive for ANA, autoimmune disease might be present or develop in the future, or it might be a false-positive test result. Thus, the tests must be ordered selectively so as not to increase the number of worried patients.

▶ Arbuckle et al (see Abstract 9–1) show that autoantibodies are often present for many years before the diagnosis of SLE. However, as observed by Shmerling (Abstract 9–2), most persons who have a positive test result for ANA or other autoantibodies never develop the disease. In the absence of clinical features, it remains impossible to predict which persons with positive serologic findings will go on to have SLE. Although it is tempting to assume that early treatment of patients with SLE would improve their prognosis, exposing all patients with positive serologic findings to potentially toxic immunosuppressive agents certainly seems unwarranted.

B. H. Thiers, MD

Prevalence and Correlates of Accelerated Atherosclerosis in Systematic Lupus Erythematosus

Roman MJ, Shanker B-A, Davis A, et al (Cornell Univ, New York; State Univ of New York, Stony Brook)
N Engl J Med 349:2399-2406, 2003   9–3

Background.—Systemic lupus erythematosus (SLE) has been associated with premature myocardial infarction. However, the prevalence of underlying atherosclerosis and its relationship to traditional risk factors for cardiovascular disease and lupus-related variables have not been well documented.

Methods.—This case-control study included 197 patients with SLE and 197 matched control subjects. Carotid US, echocardiography, and a risk factor assessment for cardiovascular disease were performed. Clinical and serologic features, inflammatory mediators, and disease treatment were also assessed.

Findings.—Patients and control subjects had similar risk factors for cardiovascular disease. The prevalence of atherosclerosis was 37.1% in the patient group and 15.2% in the control group. In a multivariate analysis, factors independently associated with the presence of plaque included older age, the presence of SLE (odds ratio, 4.8), and a higher serum cholesterol level. Compared to patients without plaque, those with plaque were older, had a longer disease duration and more disease-related damage, were less likely to have multiple autoantibodies, and were less likely to have been treated with prednisone, cyclophosphamide, or hydroxychloroquine. Multivariate analyses including patients with lupus identified longer disease duration, greater damage-index score, lower incidence of cyclophosphamide use, and absence of anti-Smith antibodies as independent predictors of plaque.

Conclusions.—Atherosclerosis occurs prematurely in patients with SLE. This complication appears to be independent of traditional risk factors for cardiovascular disease. The clinical profile of these patients with lupus and atherosclerosis suggests that disease-related factors play a role in atherogenesis. Trials of more focused, effective anti-inflammatory treatment for patients with SLE are needed.

Premature Coronary-Artery Atherosclerosis in Systemic Lupus Erythematosus

Asanuma Y, Oeser A, Shintani AK, et al (Vanderbilt Univ, Nashville, Tenn; Tulane Univ, New Orleans, La)
N Engl J Med 349:2407-2415, 2003   9–4

Background.—Premature coronary artery disease (CAD) is known to be a major cause of morbidity and mortality in patients with systemic lupus erythematosus (SLE). However, few data are available on the prevalence, extent, and causes of coronary artery atherosclerosis in this patient population.

Methods.—Sixty-five patients with SLE and 69 control subjects with no history of CAD were included in the study. The groups were comparable in age, race, and ratio of women to men. Electron-beam CT was conducted to screen for the presence of coronary artery calcification. The extent of calcification was determined by using the Agatston score.

Findings.—Coronary artery calcification was found in 20 patients and in 6 of the control subjects. The mean calcification scores were 68.9 and 8.8, respectively. Patients with SLE did not have increased concentrations of total, high density lipoprotein, or low density lipoprotein cholesterol. However, triglyceride and homocysteine levels were increased in the patients. Measures of disease activity were comparable in patients with SLE with and without coronary artery calcification. However, patients with calcification tended to be older and male.

Conclusions.—The prevalence of coronary artery atherosclerosis in patients with SLE is increased, and age at onset is lower. Detecting this complication early may enable more effective treatment.

▶ These articles (Abstracts 9–3 and 9–4) demonstrate that coronary-artery atherosclerosis is more prevalent among patients with lupus than in the general population and cannot be predicted by the measurement of traditional risk factors of markers of disease activity. This confirms the results of a previous retrospective study that found that the risk of adverse cardiovascular outcomes is increased by a factor of 7 to 17 in patients with lupus when compared with a control group with similar baseline cardiovascular risk factors as defined in the Framingham study.[1] The possibility that more vigorous therapy might decrease the likelihood and burden of atherosclerosis in patients with lupus and perhaps even in those with other chronic inflammatory diseases is suggested by the negative correlation between atherosclerosis and aggressive therapy. Hahn has observed that traditional risk factors such as hypertension, hyperglycemia, obesity, and hyperlipidemia are frequently treated inadequately in patients with SLE, and should be managed as aggressively as disease-related activity in order to prevent atherosclerosis in these individuals.[2]

B. H. Thiers, MD

References

1. Esdaile JM, Abrahamowicz M, Grodzicky T, et al: Traditional Framingham risk factors fail to fully account for accelerated atherosclerosis in systemic lupus erythematosus. *Arthritis Rheum* 44:2331-2337, 2001.
2. Hahn BH: Systemic lupus erythematosus and accelerated atherosclerosis. *N Engl J Med* 349:2379-2380, 2003.

Myocardial-Tissue-Specific Phenotype of Maternal Microchimerism in Neonatal Lupus Congenital Heart Block

Stevens AM, Hermes HM, Rutledge JC, et al (Univ of Washington Seattle; Children's Hosp, Seattle; Hosp for Joint Diseases, NY)
Lancet 362:1617-1623, 2003   9–5

Background.—Neonatal lupus syndrome (NLS) is an autoimmune disorder that develops in utero. Its most serious complication is inflammation of the atrioventricular node, resulting in congenital heart block. Maternal cells that pass into the fetus during pregnancy can persist in the child for many years after birth. The presence of maternal cells in NLS tissue was investigated in a blinded, case-control study.

Methods.—Maternal cells were quantified in heart-tissue samples from males with NLS and control subjects. X and Y chromosomes were labeled with the use of fluorescence in situ hybridization. A newly developed technique was used to identify and characterize maternal cells simultaneously. In this technique, multiple phenotypic markers could be detected concurrently with fluorescence in situ hybridization in the same cells of a tissue section.

Findings.—Maternal cells were identified in all 15 sections of NLS heart tissue. Maternal cells comprised 0.025% to 2.2% of the total cells in this tissue. However, maternal cells were detected in only 2 of 8 control sections, comprising 0% to 0.1% of total cells. The hemopoietic cell marker CD45 was expressed in very few maternal cells. Most such cells expressed sarcomeric α actin, a marker specific for cardiac myocytes.

Conclusions.—Differentiated tissue-specific maternal microchimerism may occur in newborn infants. The immune response may target semiallogeneic maternal cells, or maternal cells may contribute to a secondary process of tissue repair.

▶ During pregnancy, maternal cells may travel into the fetus and their persistence in low concentrations can create a state of microchimerism that can last for years after birth, even in otherwise healthy children. Because these persistent maternal cells are semiallogeneic, they might serve as effector cells or target cells and may thus play a role in autoimmune disease. NLS occurs in a small proportion of children born to mothers with specific anti-Ro and anti-La antibodies. Ample evidence indicates that these autoantibodies play an important part in the pathogenesis of the congenital heart block associated with this disorder. The data presented by Stevens et al demonstrate that maternal cells transferred in utero to the fetus can differentiate into cardiac myocytes, and that the resulting tissue microchimerism may contribute to the pathogenesis of heart disease or repair of cardiac injury in NLS.[1]

B. H. Thiers, MD

Reference

1. Meyer O: Neonatal cutaneous lupus and congenital heart block. It's not all antibodies. *Lancet* 362;1596-1597, 2003.

Drug-Induced, Ro/SSA-Positive Cutaneous Lupus Erythematosus
Srivastava M, Rencic A, Diglio G, et al (Johns Hopkins Med Institutions, Baltimore, Md)
Arch Dermatol 139:45-49, 2003   9–6

Purpose.—An index case and a review of the clinical and immunopathologic findings of drug-induced Ro/SSA-positive cutaneous lupus erythematosus (CLE) were presented.

> *Case Report.*—Man, 58, white, was seen with a history of hypercholesterolemia and hypertension and new skin lesions. He had recently added 40 mg/d of pravastatin to his drug regime. He began experiencing myalgias after initiating pravastatin, and 6 weeks later he had a symptomatic, subacute CLE (SCLE)–like cutaneous eruption develop. Clinical and laboratory analyses demonstrated elevated levels of creatine kinase, alanine aminotransferase, aspartate aminotransferase, lactate dehydrogenase, and aldolase. There was no evidence of inflammatory myopathy.
>
> The pravastatin dose was halved and prednisone was initiated. The muscle and cutaneous disease improved, but muscle enzymes remained elevated. Serologic studies were positive for Ro/SSA. Pravastatin was discontinued and sunblock and avobezone were prescribed. Within 2 weeks all muscle symptoms resolved and within 8 weeks the skin rash had disappeared.

Study Design.—A retrospective review was performed of patients who had serologic testing for anti-Ro/SSA antibodies from July 1991 to March 2002 at the Division of Immunodermatology at the Johns Hopkins Hospital.

Findings.—Of the 120 patients with anti-Ro/SSA antibodies, 70 had clinical and immunopathologic confirmation of CLE. Of the 70 patients with confirmed CLE, 15 had a history of new drug exposure. The disease-associated drugs included hydrochlorothiazide, angiotensin-converting enzyme inhibitors, calcium channel blockers, interferons, and statins. The most common presentations were photodistributed diffuse erythema and SCLE–like lesions, without evidence of significant systemic disease. All biopsy specimens demonstrated interface dermatitis and fine granular immunoglobulin G deposition along the basement membrane and in the lower epidermis. Most patients experienced improvement of clinical lesions within 8 weeks of discontinuation of drug treatment and a decrease of Ro/SSA titers within 8 months of discontinuation.

Conclusion.—Many medications, especially antihypertensive drugs, are associated with Ro/SSA-positive CLE. The clinical and immunopathologic presentations of this drug-induced CLE variant do not seem to differ from idiopathic CLE. The disease usually resolves after discontinuation of the drug. It is important for physicians to appropriately diagnose patients with drug-induced CLE because drug discontinuation is essential for successful resolution. All patients treated with these medications should be informed of this risk.

▶ The results stress the importance of taking a complete drug history in patients with SCLE. In contrast, classic drug-induced lupus erythematosus often lacks cutaneous involvement and presents as a systemic disease associated with circulating antihistone antibodies and a relatively low incidence of nephritis. Implicated drugs include procainamide, hydralazine, isoniazid, and minocycline.

B. H. Thiers, MD

Low-Dose Thalidomide Therapy for Refractory Cutaneous Lesions of Lupus Erythematosus
Housman TS, Jorizzo JL, McCarty MA, et al (Wake Forest Univ, Winston-Salem, NC)
Arch Dermatol 139:50-54, 2003   9–7

Introduction.—Thalidomide has anti-inflammatory and immunomodulatory properties that inhibit the production of tumor necrosis factor–α. It may be efficacious in the treatment of cutaneous manifestations of lupus erythematosus (LE). A retrospective medical record review of one of the largest modern series of patients with refractory cutaneous manifestations of LE was performed to evaluate the extent of clinical response, the duration of therapy before documented clinical improvement, and the incidence of adverse events (including peripheral neuropathy) with low-dose thalidomide therapy at 100 mg/d.

Methods.—The medical records of 29 patients with LE seen between 1998 and 2000 were examined. Twenty-eight patients had failed standard therapy with antimalarial drugs. In addition to demographic data, information was obtained from dermatology clinical medical records regarding all cutaneous manifestations of LE, results from histopathologic examination, diagnostic laboratory results while patients were receiving thalidomide therapy, and thalidomide dosing and response. Also investigated was the incidence of adverse effects. Patients were categorized as having either no response, partial response, or complete response. Partial response was considered as either 75% or greater or less than 75% improvement. The rate of adverse effects, including peripheral neuropathy, was ascertained.

Results.—Of 23 patients who took thalidomide for 1 month or more, 17 (74%) experienced complete resolution of the cutaneous manifestation of LE, 3 patients (13%) had 75% or greater partial improvement, and 3 (13%) had less than 75% partial clinical improvement. Most patients who had a complete or partial response to thalidomide therapy did so within 8 weeks of initiation of treatment. Five patients (22%) had documented sensory, axonal neuropathy during thalidomide treatment. Symptoms were reported by patients as follows: 6 (26%) reported parethesias; 4 (17%), drowsiness/fatigue; 3 (13%), dizziness; 2 (9%), nausea or headache; and 1 (4%), weight gain or constipation.

Conclusion.—It is recommended that thalidomide be considered as a treatment for antimalarial drug-resistant interface lesions in patients with LE.

▶ Although thalidomide is effective, its toxicity limits its usefulness as a therapy for cutaneous LE. The incidence of neurologic symptoms in these patients was significant, despite the low doses that were used.

B. H. Thiers, MD

Discoid Lupus Erythematosus in Children: Clinical, Histopathologic, and Follow-up Features in 27 Cases

Moises-Alfaro C, Berrón-Pérez R, Carrasco-Daza D, et al (Natl Inst of Pediatrics, Mexico City, Mexico)
Pediatr Dermatol 20:103-107, 2003   9–8

Background.—Discoid lupus erythematosus (DLE) is characterized by coin-shaped, dark to erythematosus scaly lesions. Also common in DLE are keratinous plugs, whitish depressed areas, and telangiectases. Systemic lupus erythematosus (SLE) is diagnosed in 5% to 10% of adults with DLE. Only 29 children with DLE have been reported in the English language literature. The clinical and histopathologic features, follow-up, and risk factors for SLE in 27 children with DLE were reported.

Methods.—The retrospective review included data from 27 children with DLE who were diagnosed clinicopathologically between 1971 and 1999 at 1 center in Mexico City. Cutaneous lesions were localized in 15 patients and disseminated in 12. The status of 13 patients was followed through 2001.

Findings.—At a mean follow-up time of 36 months, SLE developed in 7 (26%) patients, 4 of whom were younger than 10 years. Neither localized nor disseminated lesions appeared to be associated with the development of SLE. SLE developed in 3 of 4 patients with a positive family history of rheumatoid disease. Hyperpigmentation was significantly more frequent in patients younger than 10 years. The female predominance among children less than 10 years old was 5:1.

Conclusions.—The onset of DLE before a child is 10 years old does not indicate an increased risk of SLE development. Whether lesions are localized or disseminated does not appear to affect outcomes.

▶ The children were seen during a 30-year period at the National Institute of Pediatrics in Mexico City. Clinical, histopathologic, and serologic features were recorded. After a mean follow-up time of 36 months, 26% of them had SLE.

S. Raimer, MD

The Use of Topical Tacrolimus (FK506/Protopic) in Cutaneous Manifestations of Autoimmune Diseases
Graf J, Webb A, Davis J (Univ of California, San Francisco)
J Clin Rheumatol 9:310-315, 2003   9–9

Introduction.—Many of the cutaneous manifestations of autoimmune diseases such as systemic lupus erythematosus (SLE) are refractory to treatment. In such cases, the skin lesions may progress to disfiguring atrophy, scarring, and alopecia. Corticosteroids, commonly used as topical treatment, have undesirable side effects. The 3 patients reported here were treated with a topical preparation of tacrolimus, a potent immunomodulating medication.

Case Report 3.—A white woman, 64, had a 2-year history of nonpruritic erythematous macular/papular eruptions, occurring first on the face and subsequently on the hands, toes, elbows, trunk, and back. Serologic screening, positive for antinuclear antibody at 1:320, was negative for double-stranded DNA, extractable nuclear antigen, SSA, SSB, Jo-1, and Scl-70 antibodies. Treatment with hydroxychloroquine (HCQ) was started at 400 mg orally per day. The patient discontinued HCQ after 2 months because of improvement, but a significant recurrence appeared over her hands and back 6 months later. These lesions became pruritic, continued to spread, and failed to respond to HCQ. The patient received a diagnosis of amyopathic dermatomyositis and was treated with prednisone and methotrexate. Notable improvement came only when topical tacrolimus (0.1% twice daily) was added to a regimen of methotrexate (20 mg orally per week) and prednisone (5 mg/d). The topical therapy produced no side effects.

Discussion.—Toxicity limits the use of topical steroids in patients with autoimmune skin diseases. Tacrolimus, approved recently for use in both adults and children with atopic dermatitis, appears to have no systemic side effects and only minimal adverse events at the site of application. In this small series of patients with slightly different manifestations of autoimmune skin diseases, topical tacrolimus produced improvement with a low incidence of side effects.

▶ All patients were on multiple systemic agents; thus, it is difficult to ascribe their improvement exclusively to the topical tacrolimus.

B. H. Thiers, MD

Histopathologic Findings in Lupus Erythematosus Tumidus: Review of 80 Patients
Kuhn A, Sonntag M, Ruzicka T, et al (Heinrich-Heine-University, Düsseldorf, Germany; Univ of Witten-Herdecke, Wuppertal, Germany)
J Am Acad Dermatol 48:901-908, 2003   9–10

Background.—Cutaneous lupus erythematosus (LE) can be categorized as acute, subacute, or chronic. LE tumidus (LET) is a subtype of chronic cutaneous LE characterized by erythematous, succulent, urticaria-like, nonscarring plaques in sun-exposed areas and extreme photosensitivity. Many clinicians, however, do not consider LET a separate entity. Thus, in a review of 80 cases of LET, the histopathologic features of LET were described and LET was differentiated from discoid LE (DLE) and subacute cutaneous LE (SCLE).

Methods.—The medical records of 80 patients with LET seen between 1984 and 2000 were reviewed. The diagnosis of LET was based on the presence of standard histopathologic features in combination with extreme photosensitivity on provocative phototesting. Histopathologic findings from 53 patients with primary skin lesions of LET and from 27 patients with UV-induced skin lesions of LET (91 lesions total) were compared with those in UV-induced lesions from 10 patients with DLE and from 10 patients with SCLE.

Results.—Primary skin lesions of LET contained a moderate to dense, relatively well-circumscribed dermal infiltrate in a perivascular and periadnexal distribution. The infiltrate consisted of lymphocytes and, occasionally, neutrophils, and sometimes extended into the subcutis. All specimens contained abundant interstitial mucin deposits between collagen bundles. The follicular plugging and atrophy commonly seen in DLE and SCLE were absent, and only a few specimens had mild to moderate acanthosis or slight parakeratosis. Importantly, neither vacuolar degeneration of the dermoepidermal junction nor basement membrane thickening, which are characteristic of DLE and SCLE, were detected in LET. The histopathologic findings in UV-induced lesions of LET were virtually identical to those in the primary skin lesions. Ten percent of patients with LET had antinuclear antibodies with a titer greater than 1:160, with titers as high as 1:640.

Conclusion.—The histopathologic features in primary skin lesions and UV-induced lesions of LET are nearly identical and can be clearly differentiated from those of DLE and SCLE. Furthermore, patients with LET generally have a better prognosis than patients with other forms of chronic cutaneous LE; no patients with LET in a recently reported series had 4 or more of the American Rheumatism Association criteria for systemic LE. LET must be differentiated from polymorphous light eruption (PLE), reticular erythematous mucinosis (REM), and Jessner's lymphocytic infiltration of the skin. LET can be differentiated from PLE because PLE specimens have no mucin deposits in the reticular dermis. LET can be differentiated from REM clinically because REM lesions are typically confined to the central aspect of the chest or the upper portion of the back and are most common in young to middle-aged women. Jessner's lymphocytic infiltrate of the skin is found on the face, and the lesions have a patchy perivascular and sometimes periadnexal infiltrate that tends to arrange itself around cutaneous appendages and blood vessels but occasionally extends into the subcutaneous fat.

▶ Kuhn et al report the largest group of patients with LET to date. A major difficulty is that there are no characteristic laboratory findings, such as in SCLE, to define this subset of disease. Therefore, the gold standard for diagnosis is the finding of the characteristic clinical lesions described by the authors and the extreme photosensitivity noted on provocative phototesting. To some observers, these criteria may be soft. The redeeming feature of this study is the consistency of the histopathologic findings, which seem to indicate a homogeneous group of patients. Because (1) only about 10% of patients demonstrated a positive antinuclear antibody with a titer greater than 1:160, (2) there were no other cutaneous or systemic findings of LE vis-a-vis the American Rheumatism Association criteria for systemic LE, and (3) there were no epidermal findings on histopathologic examination, such as basement membrane thickening or a macular interface change, an argument might be made that so-called LET is actually not an expression of LE. The burden of proof is certainly on those who advocate it as a clinical entity.

J. C. Maize, MD

Raynaud's Phenomenon in Children: A Retrospective Review of 123 Patients

Nigrovic PA, Fuhlbrigge RC, Sundel RP (Harvard Med School, Boston)
Pediatrics 111:715-721, 2003   9–11

Background.—Few data are available on Raynaud's phenomenon (RP) in children. The clinical presentation and disease associations of RP in children and adolescents were reported.

Methods and Findings.—One hundred thirty-two patients younger than 19 years were included in the systematic chart review. Approximately 70% of these patients did not have a recognized underlying connective tissue disorder. Approximately 80% of patients with primary or secondary RP were female. The mean age of onset was similar in the primary and secondary RP groups (Fig 1). Biphasic or triphasic color changes were not as common as monophasic changes and were equally common in the primary and secondary RP groups. Only the presence of antinuclear antibodies and abnormal nailfold capillaries predicted secondary RP. At some time, at least 21% of patients with primary or secondary RP had antiphospholipid antibodies.

Conclusions.—As in adulthood, RP in childhood and adolescence mainly affects girls. It is often unassociated with connective tissue disease. In this series, antiphospholipid antibodies were surprisingly common, the implications of which are not clear.

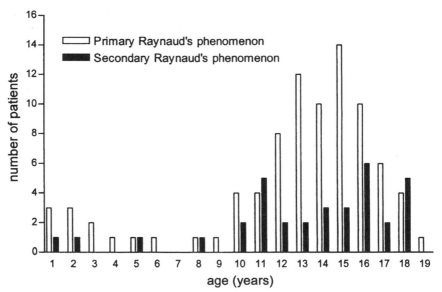

FIGURE 1.—Age of onset of primary and secondary RP (n = 119). (Courtesy of Nigrovic PA, Fuhlbrigge RC, Sundel RP: Raynaud's phenomenon in children: A retrospective review of 123 patients. *Pediatrics* 111:715-721, 2003. Copyright 2003. Reprinted with permission from *Pediatrics*.)

▶ This study is the first to attempt to define the clinical presentation of RP in children. Nigrovic et al document that most cases of RP in children are primary, as they are in adults. Predictors of underlying connective tissue disease identified in this study include a positive antinuclear antibody, a positive precipitin panel, and abnormal nailfold capillaries. This series also confirms that the number of color phases does not distinguish primary from secondary RP in children. Only a minority of patients, even those with secondary RP, had triphasic changes. The data also document that antiphospholipid antibodies are surprisingly common in children with RP. Any causative role for these antibodies remains to be determined.

S. Raimer, MD

The Handheld Dermatoscope as a Nail-Fold Capillaroscopic Instrument
Bergman R, Sharony L, Schapira D, et al (Rambam Med Ctr, Haifa, Israel)
Arch Dermatol 139:1027-1030, 2003   9–12

Introduction.—Capillary microscopy of the nail fold can detect local vascular changes in patients with connective tissue diseases (CTDs) such as scleroderma and dermatomyositis. Such capillary abnormalities are diagnostic and may help to differentiate primary Raynaud phenomenon (RP) from RP associated with scleroderma or mixed CTD. The handheld dermatoscope was evaluated for its potential as a capillaroscopic instrument in patients referred for evaluation of CTDs.

Methods.—The handheld dermatoscope is a relatively simple tool that involves the application of immersion oil to the skin and offers a magnification power of 9.3-fold. Study participants were 106 patients with clinical diagnoses of scleroderma, dermatomyositis, systemic lupus erythematosus, mixed CTD, or RP without evidence of CTD. A control group consisted of 170 randomly selected healthy persons. A single investigator viewed all nail folds through the ocular piece of the dermatoscope and recorded parameters indicative of a scleroderma-dermatomyositis (SD) pattern. Two or more findings in at least 2 nail folds were required for the definition of an SD pattern.

Results.—A capillary pattern typical of SD was found in 19 (70.4%) of 27 patients with scleroderma, 7 (63.6%) of 11 patients with dermatomyositis, and 4 (50%) of 8 with mixed CTD. Such a pattern occurred in only 1 (4.5%) of 22 patients with systemic lupus erythematosus and only 2 (5.3%) of 38 patients with RP but no evidence of CTD. None of the controls showed an SD pattern.

Discussion.—Capillaroscopy requires special equipment and often involves a referral to a specialized center. Many practicing dermatologists already have a dermatoscope, which, when used with the same immersion oil applied to pigmented lesions, can aid in the clinical diagnosis of CTDs. A

strict definition of an SD pattern will yield maximum sensitivity and specificity.

▶ In our institution, capillaroscopy is performed by the Division of Rheumatology. Substitution of the dermatoscope, which is ubiquitous in dermatology offices, can yield savings to the patient in both time and dollars.

B. H. Thiers, MD

Treatment of Cutaneous Calcinosis in Limited Systemic Sclerosis With Minocycline
Robertson LP, Marshall RW, Hickling P (Royal Cornwall Hosp, Truro, England; Univ of Bristol, England; Derriford Hosp, England)
Ann Rheum Dis 62:267-269, 2003   9–13

Introduction.—The tetracyclines, including minocycline, have other actions and effects in addition to their antibacterial properties. They also chelate calcium and iron, can affect osteoclast function, inhibit collagenases,
and are important inhibitors of neutrophil matrix metalloproteinase function. Calcinosis is observed in approximately 25% of patients with limited
cutaneous systemic sclerosis (lcSSc). Because of its calcium chelating properties, minocycline was used for the treatment of painful, ulcerating dermal
calcinosis in patients with lcSSc.

Methods.—Patients with lcSSc who had cutaneous calcinosis that caused
pain, ulceration, or both, were given minocycline 50 or 100 mg daily regularly in an open-label fashion between November 1994 and April 2000.
During routine follow-up, the appearance of the calcium deposits was examined clinically and radiographically. The extent of patient discomfort and
the size and frequency of ulceration were documented. Also noted were de-
mographics, disease duration, clinical characteristics, and antinuclear antibody titers.

Results.—Of 9 patients who were treated, 8 had positive antinuclear antibody titers and 5 were positive for anticentromere antibodies. Eight patients had definite improvement and 7 continued to receive treatment. The
frequency of ulceration and the degree of inflammation associated with the
calcium deposits diminished with therapy. The size of the calcium deposits
also decreased, yet less than expected. Improvement was seen as early as 1
month after treatment commenced (mean, 4.8 months). The mean duration
of treatment was 3.5 years. An unexpected consequence of treatment was
the darkening of the calcium deposits to a blue-black color.

Conclusion.—Minocycline may be effective in controlling cutaneous calcinosis in patients with lcSSc. Only a low dose is needed and seems to be well
tolerated. The mechanism of action may be primarily through the inhibition
of matrix metalloproteinases and anti-inflammatory effects. The calcium
binding properties and antibacterial actions of minocycline may also have a
role.

▶ As the authors readily admit, a double-blind placebo-controlled study would be necessary to confirm the efficacy of minocycline for the treatment of cutaneous calcinosis in patients with systemic sclerosis. If proven effective, the mode of action would presumably relate to properties of the drug separate from its antibacterial activity, such as its ability to chelate calcium, its influence on osteoclast function, its ability to inhibit collagenases and neutrophil matrix metalloproteinases, or its anti-inflammatory actions and ability to suppress neutrophil activity.

B. H. Thiers, MD

Aggressive Management of Juvenile Dermatomyositis Results in Improved Outcome and Decreased Incidence of Calcinosis
Fisler RE, Liang MG, Fuhlbrigge RC, et al (Harvard Med School, Boston)
J Am Acad Dermatol 47:505-511, 2002   9–14

Introduction.—Patients with juvenile dermatomyositis (JDM), the most common pediatric myopathy, benefit from corticosteroid therapy, but calcium deposition remains a problem in more than one third of cases. Some studies suggest that the incidence and severity of calcinosis may be reduced by early, aggressive treatment. The medical records of 35 children with JDM were reviewed to determine the effect of aggressive management on outcome and the presence of calcinosis.

Methods.—Twenty-one girls and 14 boys met criteria for inclusion in the study. The mean age at onset of symptoms was 7.6 years and the average time from onset of symptoms to treatment was 6.6 months. Management was individualized according to severity of weakness and muscle enzyme abnormalities. Thirty-one patients received pulse IV methylprednisone (IVMP; 30 mg/kd daily) or high-dose prednisone; 23 patients who did not respond within 6 weeks were started on methotrexate. Patients who had calcinosis were compared with those without calcinosis.

Results.—Creatine kinase levels were abnormal in 30 patients, aldolase levels in 27, and von Willebrand factor antigen levels in 29. The mean time to achieve normalization of muscle enzymes after diagnosis and treatment was 15.5 months. Clinical remission was achieved by 26 patients at the time of analysis. The mean time to achieve remission was 25.7 months. One patient (3%) had multiple, discrete calcifications at follow-up and 3 (12%) had transient calcinosis. There were no cases of severe, diffuse calcinosis. Onset of calcinosis was associated with a longer time to diagnosis and treatment (30.6 months vs 6 months for patients without calcinosis), longer duration of elevated muscle enzymes (34 vs 12.6 months, respectively), and longer disease duration (42.8 vs 22.2 months, respectively. Patients with and without calcinosis did not differ in age at disease onset, peak enzyme values, or use of IVMP therapy.

Conclusion.—Children with JDM who are treated intensively to suppress muscle inflammation have an excellent prognosis. Combination therapy with IVMP, methotrexate, or cyclosporine can achieve rapid control of disease and an early tapering of oral corticosteroids. Toxicity was minimal in this series of patients.

▶ In this retrospective study of 35 patients with juvenile dermatomyositis, induction of remission and prevention of subsequent calcinosis cutis was possible in most children diagnosed and treated aggressively soon after symptoms began. Faster normalization of muscle inflammation appeared to result in fewer long-term sequelae.

S. Raimer, MD

Abnormal Vitamin B₆ Status Is Associated With Severity of Symptoms in Patients With Rheumatoid Arthritis

Chiang E-PI, Bagley PJ, Selhub J, et al (Tufts Univ, Boston; New England Med Ctr, Boston)
Am J Med 114:283-287, 2003   9–15

Background.—Plasma vitamin B_6 levels are low in patients with rheumatoid arthritis (RA). Such patients also have increased plasma homocysteine responses to a methionine load. Whether these abnormalities correlate with clinical and biochemical indicators of disease status was investigated.

Methods.—Thirty-seven patients with RA were included in the cross-sectional study. Vitamin B_6 status was determined with the plasma pyridoxal 5'-phosphate concentration and with the homocysteine response to a methionine load test. Joint counts, the Health Assessment Questionnaire disability score, and biochemical markers of acute-phase response were used to determine clinical disease activity.

Findings.—Plasma pyridoxal 5'-phosphate concentrations correlated inversely with the erythrocyte sedimentation rate, C-reactive protein level, disability score, morning stiffness, and degree of pain. Increased homocysteine concentrations after a methionine load were associated with the erythrocyte sedimentation rate, C-reactive protein concentration, disability score, degree of pain and fatigue, and the number of painful and swollen joints.

Conclusions.—In this series of patients with RA, markers of vitamin B_6 status correlated with disease activity and severity, synovial burden, and pain. These findings suggest that impaired vitamin B_6 status results from inflammation.

▶ Previous studies have demonstrated that low plasma pyridoxal 5'-phosphate levels in patients with RA are inversely associated with high TNF-α production by peripheral blood mononuclear cells; this suggests that the decline in pyridoxal 5'-phosphate is associated with the degree of inflammation. Other studies have confirmed that the low vitamin B₆ status is not caused by lower intake or excessive catabolism of the vitamin but more likely results from the inflammatory process. Low plasma pyridoxal 5'- phosphate levels, increased plasma homocysteine levels, and chronic inflammation all have been associated with an increased incidence of cardiovascular disease, and may contribute to the increased risk of heart problems in patients with RA. An article reviewed in the 2003 YEAR BOOK OF DERMATOLOGY AND DERMATOLOGIC SURGERY demonstated the beneficial effect of methotrexate in reducing cardiovascular mortality in patients with RA, possibly through its anti-inflammatory properties.[1]

B. H. Thiers, MD

Reference

1. Choi HK, Hernán MA, Seeger JD, et al: Methotrexate and mortality in patients with rheumatoid arthritis: A prospective study. *Lancet* 359:1173-1177, 2002. (2003 YEAR BOOK OF DERMATOLOGY AND DERMATOLOGIC SURGERY, pp 301-302.)

Antinuclear Antibodies Following Infliximab Treatment in Patients With Rheumatoid Arthritis or Spondylarthropathy

De Rycke L, Kruithof E, Van Damme N, et al (Ghent Univ Hosp, Belgium)
Arthritis Rheum 48:1015-1023, 2003   9–16

Background.—Rheumatoid arthritis (RA) and spondylarthropathy (SpA) are the 2 most frequent types of autoimmune arthritis and have a prevalence of 1% to 2%. The standard therapy for RA includes a combination of disease-modifying antirheumatic drugs and nonsteroidal anti-inflammatory drugs. For SpA, the standard therapy is treatment with nonsteroidal anti-inflammatory drugs, eventually in combination with sulfasalazine for peripheral arthritis or methotrexate for psoriatic arthritis. However, this approach often results in only partial control of the inflammation and structural damage. In recent years, there have been new insights into the cellular and molecular mechanisms of RA and SpA, and new therapies have been developed on the basis of these insights. The effects of infliximab treatment on antinuclear antibodies (ANAs), anti–double-stranded DNA (anti-dsDNA), antinucleosome, antihistone, and anti-extractable nuclear antigen (anti-ENA) antibodies were investigated in patients with RA and SpA.

Methods.—Serum samples were obtained from 62 patients with RA and from 35 patients with SpA treated with infliximab and tested at baseline and at week 30 (RA group) or week 34 (SpA group). ANAs were tested by indirect immunofluorescence on HEp-2 cells. Anti-dsDNA antibodies were detected by indirect immunofluorescence on *Crithidia luciliae* and by enzyme-linked immunosorbent assay with further isotyping with γ, μ, and α chain-specific conjugates at various time points. Enzyme-linked immunosorbent assay was used to test antinucleosome antibodies, and anti-ENA antibodies were detected by line immunoassay.

Results.—Initial testing identified 32 of the 62 patients with RA and 6 of the 35 patients with SpA as having positive findings for ANAs. After infliximab treatment, 51 of the 62 patients with RA and 31 of the 35 patients with SpA had positive findings for ANAs. At baseline, none of the patients with RA or SpA had anti-dsDNA antibodies. After infliximab therapy, 7 patients with RA and 6 patients with SpA had positive findings for anti-dsDNA antibodies. All 7 patients with RA with anti-dsDNA–positive findings had IgM and IgA anti-dsDNA antibodies. Among the patients with SpA, 3 of the 6 patients with anti-dsDNA–positive findings had IgM and IgA anti-dsDNA antibodies, and 2 had IgM anti-dsDNA antibodies only. The IgM anti-dsDNA antibodies appeared before the IgA anti-dsDNA antibodies in both RA and SpA. No IgG anti-dsDNA antibodies or lupus syndromes were noted during the observation period. Some patients had antinucleosome, antihistone, or anti-ENA antibodies after infliximab treatment, but the number of patients was not statistically significant.

Conclusions.—Treatment with infliximab may induce ANAs, particularly IgM and IgA anti-dsDNA antibodies, in patients with RA and SpA. However, this study found no anti-dsDNA IgG antibodies or lupus symptoms in patients with RA or SpA, and the development of antinucleosome, antihistone, or anti-ENA antibodies was not statistically significant. However, further follow-up is necessary because the findings of this study do not exclude the potential induction of clinically significant lupus in the long-term.

▶ ANAs have previously been detected in patients with RA treated with infliximab, and the authors found the same phenomenon in patients with SpA. Although the absence of IgG anti-dsDNA antibodies and other lupus-specific autoantibodies or clinical features of lupus is reassuring, long-term observation remains mandatory. The mechanism underlying the induction of IgM and IgA anti-dsDNA antibodies in patients undergoing infliximab therapy is unknown.

B. H. Thiers, MD

Treatment of Rheumatoid Arthritis by Selective Inhibition of T-Cell Activation With Fusion Protein CTLA4Ig

Kremer JM, Westhovens R, Leon M, et al (Ctr for Rheumatology, Albany, NY; Universitaire Ziekenhuizen Leuven, Belgium; Free Univ of Brussels, Belgium; et al)
N Engl J Med 349:1907-1915, 2003   9–17

Introduction.—Cytokines such as tumor necrosis factor alpha (TNF-α) and interleukin-1 (IL-1) are therapeutic targets in rheumatoid arthritis, but drugs that block TNF-α fail to bring substantial improvement to approximately 60% of patients. Because T cells play an important role in the disease, a fusion protein directed against them (cytotoxic T-lymphocyte-associated antigen 4-IgG1 [CTLA4Ig]) was evaluated for the treatment of rheumatoid arthritis. The efficacy of CTLA4Ig was assessed in a randomized double-blind study.

Methods.—The study included those patients who had active rheumatoid arthritis that failed to respond adequately to methotrexate therapy. Participants in the study were divided into 3 groups. Group 1 (n = 105) received 2 mg of CTLA4Ig per kilogram of body weight, group 2 (n = 115) received 10 mg of CTLA4Ig per kilogram of body weight, and group 3 (n = 119, control group) received placebo. Methotrexate therapy continued during the study. The extent of response to treatment was assessed at 6 months with the use of American College of Rheumatology (ACR) criteria: 20% (ACR 20), 50% (ACR 50), or 70% (ACR 70). Patients completed a survey designed to assess health-related quality of life and were asked to report adverse events.

Results.—Patients treated with the higher dose of CTLA4Ig were more likely to have an ACR 20 response (60%) than were patients who received placebo (35%). Both CTLA4Ig groups had significantly higher rates of ACR 50 and ACR 70 responses than did the placebo group. Group 2 (10 mg of CTLA4Ig per kilogram of bodyweight) had clinically important and statistically significant improvements in all 8 subscales of the Medical Outcomes 36-Item Short-Form General Health Survey. The active treatment was well tolerated, with rates of adverse events similar or lower than in the placebo group. No antibody responses to the fusion protein were detected.

Conclusion.—Treatment with CTLA4Ig significantly improved the signs and symptoms of disease and health-related quality of life in patients who had symptomatic rheumatoid arthritis despite ongoing methotrexate therapy. Response to the drug was dose-dependent.

▶ Current biological agents block the activity of a single cytokine (eg, TNF-α) released by macrophages. CTLA4Ig, the first in a new class of molecules known as costimulation blockers, acts early in the inflammatory cascade and directly inhibits the activation of T cells as well as the secondary activation of other important cells, such as macrophages and B cells. It appears to prevent T-cell activation by interfering with the interaction between antigen-presenting cells and T cells. CTLA4Ig has also been tested in psoriasis patients with modestly beneficial results.[1,2]

B. H. Thiers, MD

References

1. Abrams JR, Lebwohl MG, Guzzo CA, et al: CTLA4Ig-mediated blockade of T-cell costimulation in patients with psoriasis vulgaris. *J Clin Invest* 103:1243-1252, 1999.
2. Abrams JR, Kelley SL, Hayes E, et al: Blockade of T lymphocyte costimulation with cytotoxic T lymphocyte-associated antigen 4-immunoglobulin (CTLA4Ig) reverses the cellular pathology of psoriatic plaques, including the activation of keratinocytes, dendritic cells, and endothelial cells. *J Exp Med* 192:681-694, 2000.

Sjögren's Syndrome–Associated Myelopathy: Response to Immunosuppressive Treatment
Vincent TL, Richardson MP, Mackworth-Young CG, et al (Imperial College, London; Univ College, London)
Am J Med 114:145-148, 2003   9–18

Introduction.—A study published in 1986 described signs and symptoms of multiple sclerosis in 20 patients with Sjögren's syndrome and claimed that

20% of patients with the syndrome have CNS complications. Subsequent studies, however, found no association between Sjögren's syndrome and CNS disease. More recently, 18 cases of patients with transverse myelitis and Sjögren's syndrome were reported; 7 of 16 patients with a documented response to treatment showed improvement after receiving corticosteroids with or without other immunosuppressive agents. The 3 patients reported here had primary Sjögren's syndrome complicated by acute myelitis.

> *Case Reports.*—Three women, aged 36 to 55 years, were seen with signs and symptoms of acute myelitis. Patients 2 and 3 were previously diagnosed with Sjögren's syndrome, and all had more than 4 criteria for the syndrome when acute myelitis appeared. At MRI, a swollen spinal cord with diffuse signal change was observed through the thoracic region in all patients and through the cervical region in one. Erythrocyte sedimentation rates were elevated, and levels of C-reactive protein were normal. All patients had a strongly positive test for antinuclear antibodies with high-titer anti-Ro antibodies and all were negative for antineutrophil cytoplasmic antibodies, antiphospholipid antibodies, and anti-human T-lymphocytic virus-1 antibodies. Patient 1 received oral prednisolone and pulsed monthly IV cyclophosphamide, a therapy patients 2 and 3 also received after IV methylprednisolone alone was ineffective. Clinical improvement occurred within 2 to 3 months, and symptoms completely resolved in time. Spinal cord lesions also resolved in the 2 patients with follow-up MRI. All 3 patients now receive low-dose oral prednisolone and azathioprine for maintenance.

Conclusion.—CNS involvement appears to occur in less than 1% of patients with Sjögren's syndrome, and the symptoms described in these 3 patients seemed to be vasculitic in origin. Marked swelling of the spinal cord, as observed in these patients, is unusual in demyelinating disease, and the antibodies detected are often associated with systemic vasculitis.

▶ Previous reports have detailed signs and symptoms "indistinguishable from multiple sclerosis" in patients with primary Sjögren's syndrome.[1] More recent studies have indicated that such symptoms are quite rare in this patient population; if and when they do occur, they are likely of vasculitic origin.

B. H. Thiers, MD

Reference

1. Alexander EL, Malinow K, Lejewski JE, et al: Primary Sjögren's syndrome with central nervous system disease mimicking multiple sclerosis. *Ann Intern Med* 104:323-330, 1986.

Churg-Strauss Syndrome: Clinical Presentation, Antineutrophil Cytoplasmic Antibodies, and Leukotriene Receptor Antagonists

Keogh KA, Specks U (Mayo Clinic, Rochester, Minn)
Am J Med 115:284-290, 2003   9–19

Introduction.—There are 3 main classification schemes for the Churg-Strauss syndrome: Lanham's criteria, which rely on clinical features; the criteria of the American College of Rheumatology; and the Chapel Hill Consensus Conference, which emphasize pathology (Table 1). This syndrome is frequently associated with the presence of perinuclear antineutrophilic cytoplasmic antibodies (P-ANCAs). It is not known whether these antibodies are associated with clinical course or prognosis. The relationship between ANCAs and leukotriene receptor antagonists with disease activity was examined in a large series of patients with Churg-Strauss syndrome.

Methods.—Potential research subjects were identified by a computerized search of the Mayo Clinic Rochester database for the 1990 to 2000 period. Patients who met 1 of the 3 classification schemes for Churg-Strauss syndrome were included.

Results.—The clinical manifestations of Churg-Strauss syndrome in the 91 patients who met the inclusion criteria (Fig 1) were similar to those in earlier reports. Mortality in this cohort was similar to that of the general population. Seventy-four patients underwent ANCA testing. Twenty-two of the 30 patients (73%) tested before therapy were ANCA positive, as were 12 of the 16 patients (75%) tested during a disease flare. Eight of the 49 patients (16%) tested during disease remission were ANCA-positive.

TABLE 1.—Criteria and Definitions for Churg-Strauss Syndrome

Lanham's criteria (2)
Fulfillment of all of the following:
    Asthma
    Peak peripheral eosinophilia $>1.5 \times 10^9/L$
    Systemic vasculitis involving two or more extrapulmonary organs
American College of Rheumatology (3)
Fulfillment of at least four of the following in the setting of vasculitis:
    Asthma
    Peak peripheral eosinophilia >10% of total white blood cell count
    Peripheral neuropathy attributable to a systemic vasculitis
    Transient pulmonary infiltrates on chest roentgenogram
    Paranasal sinus abnormality
    Biopsy specimen of a blood vessel with extravascular eosinophils
Chapel Hill Consensus Conference (4)
Fulfillment of the following:
    Asthma
    Eosinophilia
    Eosinophil-rich granulomatous inflammation involving the respiratory tract
    Necrotizing vasculitis affecting small to medium vessels

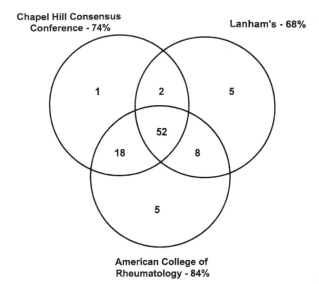

Chapel Hill Consensus
Conference - 74%

Lanham's - 68%

American College of
Rheumatology - 84%

FIGURE 1.—Proportion of patients fulfilling the criteria for Churg-Strauss syndrome of the 3 classification schemes (99 patients). Eight patients were thought to have Churg-Strauss syndrome but did not meet any of the criteria. (Reprinted from Keogh KA, Specks U: Churg-Strauss syndrome: Clinical presentation, antineutrophil cytoplasmic antibodies, and leukotriene receptor antagonists. *Am J Med* 115:284-290, 2003. Copyright 2003, with permission from Excerpta Medica Inc.)

Serial measurements suggested a correlation of ANCA levels with disease activity. CNS involvement was the only clinical manifestation associated with ANCA status ($P = .05$). Of 23 patients who received leukotriene receptor antagonists, 16 (70%) started treatment before diagnosis and 6 (27%) started during remission. Two patients who were treated after diagnosis experienced relapse. The association between disease and leukotriene receptor antagonist use could not be ascertained in 1 patient.

The use of leukotriene receptor antagonists did not influence the time between asthma onset and manifestations of vasculitis. It was not associated with organ manifestations, except for sinus disease.

Conclusion.—No 1 set of criteria described all patients, but the combination of the 3 classification schemes made it possible to identify 92% of patients with Churg-Strauss syndrome. The incidence of ANCA positivity in active disease is higher than previously estimated and justifies inclusion of the Churg-Strauss syndrome as an ANCA-related vasculitis. Leukotriene receptor antagonists do not have a pathogenetic role in Churg-Strauss syndrome.

▶ Keogh and Specks report that Churg-Strauss syndrome has a better prognosis than other ANCA-associated vasculitides. However, their data do not support the hypothesis that leukotriene receptor antagonists may play a role in the pathogenesis of this condition.[1]

B. H. Thiers, MD

Reference

1. Jamaleddine G, Diab K, Tabbarah Z, et al: Leukotriene antagonists and the Churg-Strauss syndrome. *Semin Arthritis Rheum* 31:218-227, 2002.

A Randomized Trial of Maintenance Therapy for Vasculitis Associated With Antineutrophil Cytoplasmic Autoantibodies

Jayne D, for the European Vasculitis Study Group (Addenbrooke's Hosp, Cambridge, England; et al)

N Engl J Med 349:36-44, 2003   9–20

Background.—Wegener's granulomatosis and microscopic polyangiitis are 2 of the primary systemic vasculitides typically associated with autoantibodies to neutrophil cytoplasmic antigens. Whether exposure to cyclophosphamide in patients with generalized vasculitis could be decreased by substituting azathioprine at remission was determined.

Methods.—One hundred fifty-five patients newly diagnosed as having generalized vasculitis and with a serum creatinine level of 5.7 mg/dL or less were studied. All had had at least 3 months of treatment with oral cyclophosphamide and prednisolone. After remission, patients were randomly assigned to continued cyclophosphamide treatment, 1.5 mg/kg of body weight per day, or to a substitute regimen of azathioprine, 2 mg/kg/d. All patients continued to take prednisolone. Follow-up was for 18 months from study entry.

Findings.—Ninety-three percent of the patients entered remission and were randomly assigned to azathioprine or cyclophosphamide. Eight patients died, 7 in the first 3 months, for a mortality rate of 5%. Relapse occurred in 15.5% of the azathioprine group and in 13.7% of the cyclophosphamide group. Ten percent of patients had severe adverse events during the induction phase, 11% in the azathioprine group in the remission phase, and 10% in the cyclophosphamide group in the remission phase. Patients with microscopic polyangiitis had a lower relapse rate than those with Wegener's granulomatosis.

Conclusions.—After remission of generalized vasculitis, cyclophosphamide withdrawal and substitution with azathioprine does not appear to increase relapse rates. This substitution allowed cyclophosphamide exposure duration to be safely reduced.

▶ The authors show that azathioprine can be substituted for the more toxic cyclophosphamide to maintain remission in patients with generalized antineutrophil cytoplasmic antibody-associated vasculitis. Other agents suggested as possible alternatives to cyclophosphamide in the remission phase include methotrexate and mycophenolate mofetil.[1]

B. H. Thiers, MD

Reference

1. Langford CA: Treatment of ANCA-associated vasculitis. *N Engl J Med* 349:3-4, 2003.

Use of a Cyclophosphamide-Induction Methotrexate-Maintenance Regimen for the Treatment of Wegener's Granulomatosis: Extended Follow-up and Rate of Relapse

Langford CA, Talar-Williams C, Barron KS, et al (NIH, Bethesda, Md)
Am J Med 114:463-469, 2003   9–21

Background.—Wegener's granulomatosis can be treated effectively with daily cyclophosphamide and glucocorticoids. However, disease relapse is common, and the prolonged use of cyclophosphamide can result in substantial toxicity. In 1994, a prospective standardized study was launched in which patients with active Wegener's granulomatosis were treated initially with daily cyclophosphamide and glucocorticoids until remission, at which time methotrexate was substituted for cyclophosphamide for remission maintenance. The long-term outcomes and rate of relapse in the patients enrolled in this study were examined.

Methods.—An open-label prospective study enrolled 42 patients with active Wegener's granulomatosis. All the patients underwent treatment with a standardized regimen. Outcomes were assessed by predetermined definitions based on clinical characteristics and pathologic, laboratory, and radiographic findings.

Results.—Remission occurred in all patients in a median of 3 months. The median time to discontinuation of glucocorticoids was 8 months. In a median of 32 months of follow-up, there was 1 death (from myocardial infarction unrelated to vasculitis). Two patients (5%) withdrew from the study because of medication toxicity. Relapse occurred in 22 patients (52%), with glomerulonephritis occurring in 16 patients. Of these 16 patients, 4 had an increase of more than 0.2 mg/dL in serum creatinine level. All 4 patients returned to their previous level of renal function with treatment. Of the 22 patients who had disease relapse, none met the criteria for severe disease.

Conclusions.—This study of patients with active Wegener's granulomatosis found that a protocol of cyclophosphamide and glucocorticoids for induction and methotrexate for maintenance of remission is effective and well tolerated.

▶ The authors describe an effective and well-tolerated therapeutic approach for patients with Wegener's granulomatosis. Nevertheless, relapses do occur, but apparently not more frequently than in historic controls treated with the standard cyclophosphamide regimen.

B. H. Thiers, MD

Association of Mannose-Binding Lectin Genotype with Cardiovascular Abnormalities in Kawasaki Disease

Biezeveld MH, Kuipers IM, Geissler J, et al (Univ of Amsterdam)
Lancet 361:1268-1270, 2003   9–22

Background.—Kawasaki disease, an acute vasculitis of possible infectious cause, typically affects the coronary arteries. In young children, the innate immune system is essential for protection against invading microorganisms. Mannose-binding lectin (*MBL*) is a major component of this system. The role of the gene for this molecule, *MBL*, was investigated in white Dutch patients with Kawasaki disease.

Methods.—Between 1997 and 2001, 90 patients with Kawasaki disease in the Amsterdam area were recruited for the study. A control group consisting of 88 healthy white children comprised a comparison group. Structural mutations in the *MBL* gene were defined with an oligonucleotide ligand assay. Functional promoter variants of this gene were assessed by DNA sequencing.

Findings.—Forty-nine percent of the patients with Kawasaki disease, compared with 32% of the control group, had a mutation in at least 1 of the 3 structural codons. Forty-seven percent of those with Kawasaki disease were in the high-expression group, 36% in the medium-expression group, and 17% in the low-expression group. In the control group, this same distribution was 65%, 20%, and 15%, respectively. Children younger than 1 year with mutations were at greater risk for coronary artery lesions than children without these mutations.

Conclusions.—The frequency of *MBL* gene mutations is higher in children with Kawasaki disease than in healthy children. The innate immune system appears to contribute differently to the functional characteristics of Kawasaki disease at various ages.

▶ Mannose-binding lectin (*MBL*) is part of the innate immune system. This study showed that children with Kawasaki disease who were less than 1 year old and had a deficit in *MBL* gene coding were at increased risk for development of coronary artery disease. Older children, even those with defects in *MBL* gene coding, may not be at increased risk for development of coronary artery abnormalities. Such children have a more mature acquired immune system and therefore rely less than do the very young on *MBL* to eliminate invading pathogens in the acute phase of the disease.

S. Raimer, MD

S100A12 (EN-RAGE) in Monitoring Kawasaki Disease

Foell D, Ichida F, Vogl T, et al (Univ Hosp Münster, Germany)
Lancet 361:1270-1272, 2003   9–23

Background.—The calcium-binding protein S100A12 produces inflammation by interacting with the multiligand receptor for advanced glycation end products (RAGE). In a murine model, blocking S100A12 yielded promising therapeutic effects. The serum concentration of S100A12 in persons with active Kawasaki disease, along with their response to IV gamma globulin therapy, were reported.

Methods and Findings.—Serum levels of S100A12 were measured in 31 patients with Kawasaki disease and in 33 healthy persons. The expression of S100A12 was found to correlate with Kawasaki disease activity. Gamma globulin treatment resulted in a reduction in serum levels of S100A12 in 28 patients who responded to treatment. The mean concentration declined from 463 to 184 µg/L within 24 hours.

Conclusions.—The interaction of S100A12 with multiligand receptors plays a key role in inflammatory responses. Thus, this protein may serve as a novel target for future therapeutic interventions in patients with inflammatory disorders.

▶ The results of this study suggest that S100A12 could be used as an additional serum marker for Kawasaki disease. This protein might also serve as a prognostic indicator as levels tend to be very high in patients with coronary artery disease and appear to decrease in those responding to therapy.

S. Raimer, MD

10 Blistering Disorders

Oral Cyclophosphamide for Treatment of Pemphigus Vulgaris and Foliaceus
Cummins DL, Mimouni D, Anhalt GJ, et al (Johns Hopkins Univ, Baltimore, Md)
J Am Acad Dermatol 49:276-280, 2003   10–1

Introduction.—Some patients with pemphigus vulgaris (PV) and foliaceus (PF) cannot tolerate or fail to respond to the usually effective immunosuppressive antimetabolite agents such as mycophenolate mofetil and azathioprine. Adjuvant cyclophosphamide was evaluated for its efficacy in treating refractory cases of pemphigus.

Methods.—Study participants were 20 patients with PV and 3 with PF, all of whom had failed to achieve clinical remissions with prednisone and antimetabolites. Oral cyclophosphamide was given at a dosage of 2 to 2.5 mg/kg/d each morning and followed by aggressive oral hydration (at least 2-3 L of fluids). Prednisone (1 mg/kg/d) was administered as well but tapered after 2 to 3 months. Patients having more than 40% body surface involvement underwent 4 to 6 plasma exchanges during the first 2 weeks of cyclophosphamide therapy. To produce durable results, patients who achieved a clinical remission were maintained on cyclophosphamide for an additional 9 to 12 months.

Results.—Nineteen patients, 17 with PV and 2 with PF, achieved a complete remission with oral cyclophosphamide; 1 patient with PF had a partial remission. The median time to complete remission was 8.5 months, and the median duration of therapy was 17 months. Nine patients underwent plasma exchange. Fourteen of 23 patients had at least 1 adverse reaction. There were 6 cases of infection, 5 of microscopic or gross hematuria, 3 of gastrointestinal symptoms, and 2 of nonmelanoma skin cancer. One patient had transitional cell cancer of the bladder 15 years after initiation of cyclophosphamide treatment.

Conclusion.—Aggressive or refractory PV or PF often requires adjuvant immunosuppressive therapy, with or without plasma exchange. Oral cyclophosphamide is a potent and effective treatment when first-line agents fail, but close monitoring is required and significant immediate and long-term risks need to be considered, especially in young patients.

▶ It must be recognized that the patients reported by Cummins et al represent a particularly difficult subset of patients who had failed prednisone and adjuvant immunosuppressive therapy. For most patients, azathioprine and mycophenolate mofetil remain satisfactory first-line adjuvant agents because of their favorable safety profile compared with cyclophosphamide. Nevertheless, cyclophosphamide remains an appropriate choice in refractory patients who do not respond to alternative therapies. We have occasionally used monthly IV dosing of cyclophosphamide rather than oral daily dosing to decrease cyclophosphamide exposure.

B. H. Thiers, MD

Protein A Immunoadsorption: A Novel and Effective Adjuvant Treatment of Severe Pemphigus

Schmidt E, Klinker E, Opitz A, et al (Univ of Würzburg, Germany; Inselspital, Berne, Switzerland)

Br J Dermatol 148:1222-1229, 2003   10–2

Background.—Pemphigus foliaceus (PF) and pemphigus vulgaris (PV) are chronic autoimmune blistering diseases associated with antibodies to desmoglein (Dsg) 1 and Dsg 3. PF and PV are usually treated with high-dose systemic corticosteroids and other immunosuppressants that may cause severe side effects. To reduce the often devastating side effects of these regimens, a number of adjuvant therapies have been tried successfully, including IV immunoglobulin and plasmapheresis. In contrast to plasmapheresis, staphylococcal protein A immunoadsorption (PA-IA) specifically removes immunoglobulin from the circulation. PA-IA also allows treatment of larger plasma volumes and does not require substitution of plasma components. The effectiveness and side effects of PA-IA in patients with severe pemphigus were determined.

Methods.—The study group comprised 5 patients with severe pemphigus, including 4 with PV and 1 with PF. Three of these patients had been refractory to various treatment regimens. In addition to treatment with PA-IA, the patients received methylprednisolone, 0.5 mg/kg/d initially, with subsequent tapering.

Results.—Dramatic clinical improvement was manifest in all patients within 2 weeks after initiation of therapy. The patients were free of lesions after 3, 4, 4, 10, and 21 weeks of treatment, respectively. The clinical improvement was accompanied by a rapid decline in autoantibody levels.

Conclusions.—PA-IA is a safe and effective adjuvant therapy for severe pemphigus and should be used more often for this indication. A controlled study should be conducted to compare side effects and effectiveness of PA-IA with other treatment options.

▶ Levels of circulating autoantibodies appear to parallel disease activity in pemphigus, and most available treatments aim to lower the concentration of these antibodies. The staphylococcal PA-IA technique has been available for many years, but its usefulness for the treatment of autoimmune blistering disorders has not been fully explored. This study represents movement in that direction. A larger controlled study using sham immunoadsorption along with systemic immunosuppression will be necessary to convince physicians that this technique can be an important adjunct in the treatment of this debilitating condition.

B. H. Thiers, MD

Paraneoplastic Pemphigus in Children and Adolescents
Mimouni D, Anhalt GJ, Lazarova Z, et al (Johns Hopkins Univ, Baltimore, Md; Thomas Jefferson Univ, Philadelphia; Hosp Clinic, Barcelona)
Br J Dermatol 147:725-732, 2002   10–3

Introduction.—Paraneoplastic pemphigus (PNP), an autoimmune disorder first described in 1990, primarily affects adults. An increasing number of individual reports of PNP among children and adolescents prompted an analysis of the clinical and immunopathologic features of the disease in the pediatric population.

Methods.—A review of PNP cases identified over an 8-year period yielded 14 pediatric patients, 7 boys and 7 girls aged 8 to 18 years. Sera from all patients were analyzed by indirect immunofluorescence and immunoprecipitation for plakin autoantibodies. Immunoblotting was used to detect plectin autoantibodies, and an enzyme-linked immunosorbent assay was used for the detection of desmoglein (Dsg)1 and Dsg3 autoantibodies. Frozen sections of skin biopsy specimens were probed with fluoresceinated antibodies specific for immunoglobulin (Ig) G, IgA, IgM, complement, and fibrin.

Results.—All but 2 patients had Castleman disease. Oral erosions were present in all cases, and genital erosions, conjunctival erosions, and lichenoid lesions were common. Three patients had cutaneous involvement and 10 had pulmonary disease. Indirect immunofluorescence detected IgG autoantibodies in all cases. Histologic patterns identified were a lichenoid/interface infiltrate with variable degrees of cell necrosis and intraepithelial acantholysis. Seven of 14 patients had both of these patterns. Anti-Dsg3 antibodies were found in 10 patients, 3 of whom had anti-Dsg1 antibodies and cutaneous disease. Surgery was performed in 10 patients; 2 also received chemotherapy and 1 radiotherapy. Despite treatment, outcome was fatal in 10 of 14 cases.

Conclusion.—In children and adolescents, PNP most often occurs as a presenting sign of occult Castleman disease. A constant feature is extensive and refractory mucositis, especially in the labial mucosa. In contrast to adult cases of PNP, mucocutaneous lesions were most often lichenoid and not blistering. Respiratory involvement was a major factor in the high mortality rate. Detection of serum antiplakin antibodies is the most reliable serologic diagnostic tool.

▶ While PNP in adults is commonly associated with non-Hodgkin lymphoma, in children and adolescents it is frequently associated with Castleman disease. The diagnosis of PNP in children should therefore prompt a thorough search for this rare lymphoproliferative disorder. Unfortunately, the prognosis for affected children remains dismal even when both the autoimmune and underlying lymphoproliferative conditions are treated.

S. Raimer, MD

Anti-Epiligrin Cicatricial Pemphigoid: Clinical Findings, Immunopathogenesis, and Significant Associations
Egan CA, Lazarova Z, Darling TN, et al (NIH, Bethesda, Md)
Medicine 82:177-186, 2003   10–4

Introduction.—Cicatricial pemphigoid, a rare disorder that typically affects the elderly, is characterized by erosive and/or vesiculobullous lesions that appear on the mucous membranes, particularly in the mouth. The unifying immunopathologic feature is the finding of immunoreactants consisting of IgG, IgA, or both and complement components in perilesional epidermal basement membrane. The 35 patients reported here had anti-epiligrin cicatricial pemphigoid (AECP), a mucosal-predominant subepithelial blis-

FIGURE 2

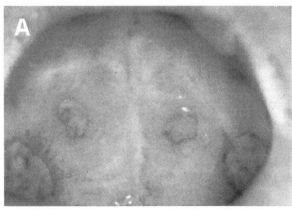
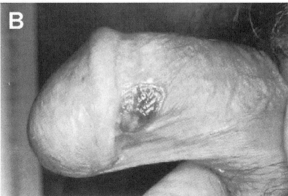

(Continued)

tering disease clinically indistinguishable from other forms of cicatricial pemphigoid. Data on these patients were summarized in a longitudinal study.

Methods.—Patients were recruited over a 12-year period. Anti-laminin 5 autoantibodies, a disease-specific marker for AECP, were present in all cases. Indirect immunofluorescence microscopy revealed binding of circulating IgG autoantibodies to the dermal side of 1M NaCl split skin. The patients' physicians completed questionnaires that sought demographic information, clinical and laboratory findings, disease activity status, and the course of any associated cancers.

Results.—Patients in the cohort (16 men and 19 women; median age, 65 years) had many different racial and ethnic origins. All patients had oral mucosal involvement, and 66% had ocular involvement; other areas were af-

FIGURE 2 (cont.)

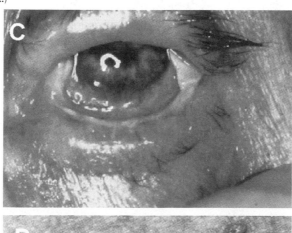

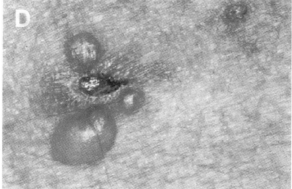

FIGURE 2.—Clinical features of anti-epiligrin cicatricial pemphigoid demonstrating erosions on the hard palate (**A**), an erosion on the shaft of the penis (**B**), ocular involvement with symblephara (**C**), and tense blisters on skin as well as crusted sites corresponding to prior blisters (**D**). (Courtesy of Egan CA, Lazarova Z, Darling TN, et al: Anti-epiligrin cicatricial pemphigoid: Clinical findings, immunopathogenesis, and significant associations. *Medicine* 82(3):177-186, 2003.)

fected at lesser frequencies (Fig 2; see color plate XI). A solid cancer developed in 10 patients (29%) and followed the onset of blistering in 8 patients (within 14 months in 7 patients). Cancers involved the lungs in 3 patients, the stomach in 3, the colon in 2, and the uterus in 2. Most of these cancers were adenocarcinomas and were detected at an advanced stage. Only 4 patients experienced remission of their blistering disease, and 14 (40%) died during follow-up. Eight deaths were cancer related, and 5 were attributed to complications related to therapy of AECP.

Conclusion.—Findings in this series of patients indicate that autoimmune responses in AECP are directed against an autoantigen within or below the lowest portion of the lamina lucida. The high rate of mortality in AECP results from associated cancers and intensive treatment with immunosuppressive agents.

▶ An association between bullous pemphigoid and malignancy has been postulated for years but has never been proven. Many studies suggesting such an association were performed before the development of the elegant immunofluorescent techniques used by Egan et al. It is possible that at least some of those patients presumed to have bullous pemphigoid with an associated neoplasm actually had AECP. Future studies might determine whether laminin 5, the target antigen in AECP, is likewise present in the underlying malignancy.

B. H. Thiers, MD

Hemochromatosis (*HFE*) Gene Mutations and Response to Chloroquine in Porphyria Cutanea Tarda
Stölzel U, Köstler E, Schuppan D, et al (Klinikum Chemnitz, Germany; Hosp Dresden-Friedrichstadt, Germany; Univ of Erlangen-Nürnberg, Germany; et al)
Arch Dermatol 139:309-313, 2003   10–5

Background.—To date, no studies have been published on the clinical implications of hemochromatosis (*HFE*) mutations in patients with porphyria cutanea tarda (PCT) treated with chloroquine. A longitudinal study was conducted to address this question.

Methods.—A database of chloroquine-treated patients with PCT was analyzed to determine whether *HFE* mutations *C282Y* and *H63D* affected clinical response, urinary porphyrin excretion, liver enzyme activities, and serum iron markers. Serum samples and complete sets of data before and after treatment were available for 62 of the 207 patients treated solely with chloroquine. Treatment consisted of low-dose chloroquine diphosphate for a median of 16 months.

Findings.—Sixty percent of the 62 patients carried *HFE* mutations. Chloroquine treatment was associated with clinical remission and decreased urinary porphyrin excretion in 39% of the patients with *HFE* wild type and in 56% of the *HFE* heterozygous patients. Reductions in serum iron markers after chloroquine treatment occurred only in PCT patients with *HFE* wild type. All 3 patients homozygous for the *C282Y* mutation had high serum iron, ferritin, and transferrin saturation. None of these 3 patients responded to chloroquine therapy.

Conclusions.—These data suggest that *C282Y* heterozygosity and compound heterozygosity of *HFE* mutations do not compromise response to chloroquine in PCT patients. However, *HFE C282Y* homozygotes did not respond to such treatment, and reduced serum iron concentrations occurred only in PCT patients with *HFE* wild type. Thus, phlebotomy should be the first-line therapy for PCT patients with *HFE* mutations.

▶ Phlebotomy and chloroquine therapy are both effective treatments for PCT, although the latter is certainly more invasive and time consuming. Few criteria exist to guide the clinician as to which modality would be the best approach for the individual patient. The data presented by Stölzel et al should help in that regard.

B. H. Thiers, MD

The Sensitivity and Specificity of "Caterpillar Bodies" in the Differential Diagnosis of Subepidermal Blistering Disorders
Fung MA, Murphy MJ, Hoss DM, et al (Univ of Connecticut, Farmington)
Am J Dermatopathol 25:287-290, 2003   10–6

Background.—Caterpillar bodies (CBs), eosinophilic, elongated, segmented globules arranged linearly within the roofs of blisters (Fig 1), are said to be a specific histopathologic feature of porphyria, including porphyria cutanea tarda (PCT). This belief is based on a small number of cases. Thus, 76 cases of subepidermal vesiculobullous disorders were reviewed to determine the specificity of CBs in diagnosing PCT.

Methods.—The medical records of 76 patients with subepidermal blistering conditions were reviewed. Hematoxylin and eosin–stained specimens

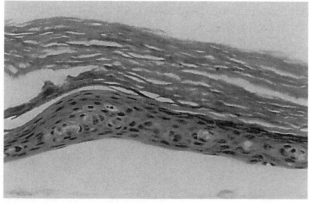

FIGURE 1.—Classic caterpillar body in porphyria cutanea tarda. (Courtesy of Fung MA, Murphy MJ, Hoss DM, et al: The sensitivity and specificity of "caterpillar bodies" in the differential diagnosis of subepidermal blistering disorders. *Am J Dermatopathol* 25:287-290, 2003.)

were examined to identify CBs, CB-like clusters (ie, discrete clustered or linear collections of cells in the blister roof containing pale or eosinophilic cytoplasm), and festooning (ie, preservation of papillary dermal tips along the blister floor).

Results.—PCT was diagnosed in 14 of the 76 cases (18.4%) (Table 1). However, CBs were seen in only 6 of these cases (sensitivity, 43%). In addition, CBs were noted in 1 blister associated with venous stasis (specificity, 98%). CB-like clusters were seen in 36% of cases of PCT, but they were also seen in 100% of bullous impetigo cases, in 100% of pseudoporphyria cases, in 60% of epidermolysis bullosa cases, in 33% of erythropoietic protoporphyria cases, and in 29% of bullous pemphigoid cases. Thus, the sensitivity and specificity of CB-like clusters in the diagnosis of PCT were 35% and 77%, respectively. Some cases had both CB and CB-like clusters in the blister roof. Festooning was present in 86% of PCT cases, in 100% of linear IgA bullous dermatosis/chronic bullous disease of childhood cases, in 100% of pseudoporphyria cases, in 66% of erythropoietic protoporphyria cases, in 50% of epidermolysis bullosa acquisita cases, in 50% of bullous impetigo cases, in 29% of wound-healing reactions, and in 13% of bullous pemphigoid cases.

Conclusion.—CBs are a highly specific feature of PCT, but they are not very sensitive. CBs appear to contain degenerating keratinocytes and basement membrane material. Positive staining of CBs with periodic acid-Schiff, as has been reported in other studies, may reflect a specific reactivity with the basement membrane materials. Thus, one reason for the low sensitivity found in this study may be because CBs might not be distinguishable from the cytoplasm of degenerating keratinocytes whose nuclei have been removed by sectioning. The fact that none of the periodic acid-Schiff staining results in this article (when available) were positive for CB-like clusters supports this hypothesis.

TABLE 1.—Histologic Features of Subepidermal Blistering Disorders

Diagnosis	#	CB	CB-Like Clusters	Festooning
PCT	14	6	5	12
Pseudoporphyria	1	0	1	1
EPP	3	0	1	2
Epidermolysis bullosa, junctional or dystrophic	5	0	3	0
EBA	4	0	0	2
BP	24	0	7	3
Linear IgA bullous dermatosis/chronic bullous disease of childhood	3	0	0	3
Bullous impetigo	2	0	2	1
Scar/wound-healing	7	0	0	2
Stasis/edema	1	1	0	0

Abbreviations: PCT, Porphyria cutanea tarda; *EPP*, erythropoietic protoporphyria; *EBA*, epidermolysis bullosa acquisita; *BP*, bullous pemphigoid; *CB*, caterpillar bodies.

(Courtesy of Fung MA, Murphy MJ, Hoss DM, et al: The sensitivity and specificity of "caterpillar bodies" in the differential diagnosis of subepidermal blistering disorders. *Am J Dermatopathol* 25:287-290, 2003.)

▶ This study is one of several recent publications that attempts to discern the significance of various histopathologic criteria for the diagnosis of inflammatory blistering diseases. Fung et al demonstrate that CBs are highly specific, although not highly sensitive, for the diagnosis of PCT. It is always welcome to have specific criteria on which to hang one's hat. This clue should be useful in distinguishing PCT from other subepidermal blistering diseases that have little or no inflammatory infiltrate and, therefore, may mimic PCT.

J. C. Maize, MD

Treatment of Toxic Epidermal Necrolysis With Intravenous Immunoglobulin in Children
Tristani-Firouzi P, Petersen MJ, Saffle JR, et al (Univ of Utah, Salt Lake City)
J Am Acad Dermatol 47:548-552, 2002   10–7

Introduction.—Mortality rates remain quite high among patients with toxic epidermal necrolysis (TEN), even when optimal wound care, fluid management, and control of infection are provided in a burn unit setting. IV immunoglobulin (IVIg) has had some success in both adult and pediatric patients with TEN. The charts of 8 pediatric patients who were safely and effectively treated with IVIg were retrospectively reviewed.

Methods.—Patients were 4 girls and 4 boys aged 22 months to 21 years. A drug etiology was confirmed in 7 cases. Diagnosis of TEN was based on the finding of acute, widespread epidermal sloughing that involved more than 10% of body surface area and biopsy results. Treatment at 1 center included mechanical debridement of necrotic tissue and coverage of denuded areas with Biobrane, discontinuation of corticosteroids and all unnecessary medications, and aggressive fluid resuscitation and nutritional support. Debridement and Biobrane placement were omitted at the second study center. The IVIg protocol consisted of 0.5 to 0.75 g/kg per day for 4 consecutive days. Three pediatric patients in a historic control group were treated similarly, but with plasmapheresis instead of IVIg.

Results.—The mean BSA involvement in the 8 patients was 67%. The average length of time between the onset of signs and symptoms of TEN and the onset of treatment was 3.2 days. Arrest of progression of TEN occurred after an average of 2.1 days; the average time to complete re-epithelialization was 8.1 days. No deaths occurred, and most complications were infectious in nature. The average length of hospital stay was 13.6 days. In the historic control group, which had an average body surface area involvement of 38%, survival was 100%, the mean time to arrest in the progression of lesions was 4.5 days, and the mean time to complete re-epithelialization was 11.7 days.

Conclusion.—The pathophysiology of TEN is unknown, but this severe drug reaction may be mediated by apoptosis. Keratinocytes from patients with TEN show upregulation of lytically active Fas ligand expression, and the therapeutic effect of IVIg may be mediated by binding of naturally occurring Fas-blocking antibodies present in IVIg. The potential adverse side effects of IVIg did not develop in these patients with TEN.

▶ In the 8 children with TEN reported by Tristani-Firouzi et al, cessation of epidermal detachment and time to epithelialization appeared to have been hastened by a 4-day course of IVIg. IVIg is not without risk, and serious complications such as renal failure and anaphylaxis may accompany its use. In addition, when biologic substances such as immunoglobulin preparations are derived from plasma pools, there may be differences in the product depending on the purification procedures used by different manufacturers, and there may be batch-to-batch variation. Moreover, IVIg is quite expensive and is not always readily available. For maximum efficacy, it appears advisable to administer IVIg as early as possible in the course of the disease. Cyclosporine, which has less potential for serious side effects with short-term use, appears to be beneficial in the treatment of TEN in adults. A comparative study of these 2 agents would be of interest.

S. Raimer, MD

Treatment of Toxic Epidermal Necrolysis With High-Dose Intravenous Immunoglobulins: Multicenter Retrospective Analysis of 48 Consecutive Cases

Prins C, for the TEN-IVIG Study Group (Geneva Univ, Switzerland; et al)
Arch Dermatol 139:26-32, 2003   10–8

Background.—Toxic epidermal necrolysis (TEN) is an acute and life-threatening mucocutaneous disease that is usually related to sulfonamide, anticonvulsant, or nonsteroidal anti-inflammatory drug use. TEN is associated with a high mortality rate, which increases with the extent of skin detachment. These authors have previously demonstrated that the keratinocyte apoptosis that occurs in TEN is due to increased FasL (CD95L) expression. Commercially available IV immunoglobulins (IVIGs) have been reported to inhibit the progression of TEN. The effect of high-dose IVIG treatment of patients with TEN was examined in a retrospective study.

Study Design.—This multicenter study examined the response to treatment with high-dose (0.2-2.9 g/kg/d for 1-5 days) IVIG of 48 patients with TEN who had epidermal detachment involving at least 10% of total body surface area. Patients with Stevens-Johnson syndrome were excluded. The main outcome measures were response to IVIG treatment, final outcome by day 45, parameters that affected response to treatment, and tolerance of treatment. Variability in inhibition of Fas-mediated cell death among different IVIG batches was assessed.

Findings.—High-dose infusion of IVIG was associated with a rapid cessation of skin and mucosal detachment in 90% of patients and survival of 88%. Patients who responded to IVIG received treatment early in the course of their disease with high doses of IVIG. Analysis of 35 IVIG batches revealed significant variability in inhibition of Fas-mediated cell death in vitro.

Conclusion.—This retrospective multicenter study found that early infusion of high-dose, commercially available IVIG is safe, well tolerated, and effective in the treatment of patients with TEN. Early treatment of patients with TEN with IVIG at a total dose of 3 g/kg over 3 consecutive days (1 g/kg/d) is recommended. This study also found significant variability among batches of commercially available IVIG. The anti-Fas activity of batches of IVIG used to treat nonresponding patients should be assessed. These data are presented to pave the way for a controlled clinical trial of the efficacy of IVIG for patients with TEN.

Intravenous Immunoglobulin Treatment for Stevens-Johnson Syndrome and Toxic Epidermal Necrolysis: A Prospective Noncomparative Study Showing No Benefit on Mortality or Progression
Bachot N, Revuz J, Roujeau J-C (Hôpital Henri Mondor, Crèteil, France)
Arch Dermatol 139:33-36, 2003   10–9

Background.—Toxic epidermal necrolysis (TEN) and Stevens-Johnson syndrome (SJS) are severe skin reactions to medications. SJS is a more limited form. These diseases are rare but are associated with high mortality rates. There is no accepted treatment. It has been suggested that a Fas-Fas ligand (FasL) interaction is responsible for the apoptosis of epidermal cells that characterizes these diseases and that high-dose IV immunoglobulin (IVIG) could be used to treat these patients. The efficacy of high-dose IVIG in the treatment of patients with SJS and TEN was prospectively examined at a single institution.

Study Design.—The study group consisted of 34 consecutive patients hospitalized with SJS or TEN between 1999 and 2000. Patients with normal renal function received IVIG for a total dose of 2 g/kg within 2 days of admission. Three different brands of IVIG were used. A prognosis score (SCORTEN) was calculated at admission and compared to actual mortality. The extent of epidermal detachment was measured at admission and on days 3 and 11 to assess the efficacy of the therapy.

Findings.—At admission, epidermal detachment involved an average of almost 20% of the total body surface area. After IVIG treatment, epidermal detachment involved over 30% of the total body surface area. The SCORTEN predicted 8.2 deaths; there were 11 actual deaths in the patient group. Most deaths occurred in elderly patients with impaired renal function.

Conclusion.—This open trial of patients with SJS and TEN treated at a single institution with high-dose IVIG found that the treatment was not associated with reduced mortality. This suggests that high-dose IVIG cannot be recommended as a treatment for patients with SJS and TEN and should not be used in elderly patients with impaired renal function.

Analysis of Intravenous Immunoglobulin for the Treatment of Toxic Epidermal Necrolysis Using SCORTEN: The University of Miami Experience

Trent JT, Kirsner RS, Romanelli P, et al (Univ of Miami, Fla)
Arch Dermatol 139:39-43, 2003   10–10

Background.—Toxic epidermal necrolysis (TEN) is a rare, severe skin disorder that results from drug-hypersensitivity. In patients with TEN, keratinocytes undergo apoptosis due to upregulation of FasL. IV immunoglobulin (IVIG) inhibits Fas-mediated keratinocyte apoptosis and may be a useful treatment. IVIG was used to treat 16 patients with TEN in a single-institution study. The efficacy of IVIG was assessed with the use of the SCORTEN, a TEN-specific severity of illness scale, which has been developed to predict mortality in affected patients.

Study Design.—The study group consisted of 16 consecutive patients with TEN who were treated with IVIG. Patients with Stevens-Johnson syndrome were excluded. The patients were managed with a standard TEN protocol plus IVIG 1 g/kg/d for 4 days (one patient received 0.4 g/kg/d). SCORTEN risk factors were recorded for each patient at admission. Standardized mortality ratio analysis was performed to determine whether IVIG treatment reduced mortality for these patients.

Findings.—One of the 16 patients died. This patient showed improvement in TEN symptoms but died due to preexisting medical conditions. Based on the SCORTEN, more than 5 patients were expected to die. Standardized mortality ratio analysis indicated that patients treated with IVIG were 83% less likely to die than if they had not been treated with IVIG.

Conclusion.—Until a randomized, placebo-controlled clinical trial of treatment of TEN patients can be performed, this study lends support to the use of high-dose IVIG for this condition.

▶ A thoughtful editorial by Wolff and Tappeiner appeared in the same issue of the journal.[1] In their article, these authors underscored some reasons for the ongoing problems in defining an appropriate treatment for TEN. These include the uncertain pathogenetic mechanisms involved in the disease, the ethical problems in conducting comparative controlled studies for this often fatal condition, and the variable biological activity of the various immunoglobulin preparations. In the studies abstracted above, 2 were retrospective (Abstracts 10–8 and 10–10), 1 was prospective (Abstract 10–9), and all 3 were nonrandomized and uncontrolled.

B. H. Thiers, MD

Reference

1. Wolff K, Tappeiner G: Treatment of toxic epidermal necrolysis: The uncertainty persists but the fog is dispersing. *Arch Dermatol* 139:85-86, 2003.

11 Genodermatoses

Spectrum of PTCH1 Mutations in French Patients With Gorlin Syndrome
Boutet N, Bignon Y-J, Drouin-Garraud V, et al (Institut Bergonié, Bordeaux, France; Ctr Jean Perrin, Clermont-Ferrand, France; CHU Charles Nicolle, Rouen, France; et al)
J Invest Dermatol 121:478-481, 2003   11–1

Background.—Gorlin syndrome or nevoid basal cell carcinoma syndrome (NBCCS) is an autosomal dominant genetic disease characterized by developmental abnormalities and tumor predisposition. Three major criteria are used in the diagnosis of Gorlin syndrome: the presence of basal cell carcinomas, palmar and plantar epidermal pits, and jaw keratocysts. Genetic linkage studies have localized the NBCCS gene to 9q22-31. The responsible gene *PTCH* was identified by positional cloning as the human homolog of the *Drosophila patched* gene. Two initial reports (1996) described germline mutations of *PTCH* gene in patients with Gorlin syndrome, and since then many PTCH germline mutations have been described. The spectrum of PTCH germline mutation was assessed in the French population.

Methods.—Sixty-five families were identified, 23 familial cases and 42 sporadic cases. Included in the familial cases were 46 patients and 33 nonaffected siblings. A control population consisted of nonaffected unrelated individuals from the same area. A geneticist evaluated patients for the presence of at least 1 of the 3 main features of NBCCS.

Results.—With the use of polymerase chain reaction single-strand conformation polymorphism or heteroduplex analysis to screen the *PTCH* gene for mutations, 19 new mutations and 5 new polymorphisms were found in 65 family or sporadic cases of NBCCS. Twenty patients bearing a PTCH mutation were identified. There were 2 nonsense mutations: Y224X, localized after the first transmembrane domain, and Y873X, after the first group of transmembrane domains. Seven frameshift mutations gave rise to various truncated Ptc proteins. A 2-nucleotide microdeletion at 1208-1209 in exon 8 was identified in 1 sporadic and 2 familial cases of NBCCS. These cases came from different parts of France and had no apparent familial links. In a sporadic case, a 3-nucleotide microdeletion was identified in exon 3 deleting a conserved glutamine among vertebrate species. None of the 100 controls had this microdeletion. Six missense mutations in familial cases exhibited sequence variations not found in a population of 200 control chromosomes.

The 11 polymorphisms identified appear in the general population in frequencies ranging from less than 1% to 14.5%.

Discussion.—Nineteen new mutations with 11 polymorphisms were identified in French patients with NBCCS. Frameshift mutations were the most common, and half of the typical familial cases showed no PTCH mutations. The high frequency of PTCH spontaneous mutation is illustrated by the high prevalence of sporadic cases. Mutations in PTCH may activate the hedgehog protein pathway and play a role in the development of the basal cell carcinomas that characterize NBCCS.

▶ Germline mutations of the *Ptch-1* gene have been identified in several studies of patients with NBCCS (Gorlin syndrome). These investigators screened a large number of both familial and sporadic cases of this syndrome and determined that although frameshift mutations were most commonly detected, as had been previously reported, several novel polymorphisms were identified. Importantly, no mutations were found in half of the patients with familial disease; the authors note the need for investigation of other genetic and environmental factors in the cause of this syndrome.

G. M. P. Galbraith, MD

Dilemmas in Distinguishing Between Dominant and Recessive Forms of Dystrophic Epidermolysis Bullosa
Mallipeddi R, Bleck O, Mellerio JE, et al (St Thomas' Hosp, London)
Br J Dermatol 149:810-818, 2003   11–2

Background.—The blistering skin disorder dystrophic epidermolysis bullosa (DEB) is caused by mutations in the type VII collagen gene (*COL7A1*), which is the major protein of the anchoring fibrils at the dermal–epidermal junction. DEB may be inherited by autosomal dominant or autosomal recessive transmission. Differentiating between dominant and recessive inheritance is important for genetic counseling, but it is difficult to do based on clinical features. Different mutations in *COL7A1* appear to be involved in the dominant and recessive forms of DEB. For example, autosomal dominant DEB usually involves glycine substitutions within the triple helix of *COL7A1*, whereas severe autosomal recessive DEB usually involves nonsense, frameshift, or splice-site mutations in *COL7A1* on both alleles, most commonly compound heterozygous changes. Whether *COL7A1* mutation analysis would be useful in determining the mode of inheritance in patients with mild to moderate DEB was examined.

Methods.—The subjects were 4 girls 2 to 16 years of age with mild to moderate DEB and clinically unaffected parents. Genomic DNA from the patients and their parents was extracted from peripheral blood lymphocytes and analyzed by polymerase chain reaction amplification and heteroduplex analysis.

Results.—Each patient had a heterozygous glycine substitution within the type VII collagen triple helix. In patient 1 (Table 1), 1 mutation from exon 13

TABLE 1.—Results of COL7A1 Screening

Patient No.	Exons Which Revealed Heteroduplex Bands With Conformation-Sensitive Gel Electrophoresis			Automated Nucleotide Sequencing of PCR Products From Patient	
	Patient	Mother	Father	cDNA Sequence Change	Nucleotide Change
1	13 and 86	13	86	Exon 13 1732 C → T	Arg 578 → Stop (R578X)
				Exon 86 6788 G → T	Gly 2263 → Val (G2263V)
2	13 and 108	N/A	N/A	Exon 13 1732 C → T	Arg 578 → Stop (R578X)
				Exon 108 8021 G → A	Gly 2674 → Asp (G2674D)
3	73	None	None	Exon 73 6016 G → A	Gly 2006 → Ser (G2006S)
4	73	None	None	Exon 73 6127 G → A	Gly 2043 → Arg (G2043R)

Abbreviations: PCR, Polymerase chain reaction; N/A, not available.
(Courtesy of Mallipeddi R, Bleck O, Mellerio JE, et al: Dilemmas in distinguishing between dominant and recessive forms of dystrophic epidermolysis bullosa. *Br J Dermatol* 149:810-818, 2003. Reprinted by permission of Blackwell Publishing.)

was also present in her mother, and 1 mutation from exon 86 was also present in her father, which confirmed autosomal recessive transmission. Samples were not available from the parents of patient 2, but her sample showed compound heterozygous changes characteristic of severe autosomal recessive DEB. Both patients 3 and 4 had only 1 heteroduplex band, and neither of their parents had this mutation, which suggested de novo dominant DEB.

Conclusion.—DNA sequencing can be useful in distinguishing dominant from recessive DEB. A thorough clinical examination may be helpful in this regard but is often noncontributory. Because both dominant and recessive DEB involve glycine substitution mutations, comprehensive screening for additional mutations in both the patient and the parents is necessary to make the diagnosis with confidence.

▶ When patients present with DEB and no family history of the disease, it may be important for reasons of genetic counseling to differentiate between mild recessive and de novo dominantly inherited disease. *COL7A1* mutation screening appears to be a useful tool to aid in distinguishing between the 2 conditions.

S. Raimer, MD

Clinical Study of 40 Cases of Incontinentia Pigmenti
Hadj-Rabia S, Froidevaux D, Bodak N, et al (Hôpital Necker–Enfants-Malades, Paris)
Arch Dermatol 139:1163-1170, 2003   11–3

Background.—Incontinentia pigmenti (IP) is a rare X-linked dominant genodermatosis. The typical phenotype results from a functional mosaicism, which results from lyonization, or the random inactivation 1 of the 2 X chromosomes in women. The distribution of manifestations of IP were investigated in a cohort of children, and guidelines were presented for follow-up of patients with this disorder.

Methods and Findings.—Forty-seven children referred to 1 center with a diagnosis of IP between 1986 and 1999 were included in the retrospective analysis. Seven children were found to be misdiagnosed. Most children with IP had erythema, vesicles, and hyperkeratotic lesions in the neonatal period. Ocular and neurologic abnormalities were documented in 20% and 30% of the children, respectively. However, these abnormalities were severe in only 8% and 7.5%, respectively.

Conclusions.—Correct phenotype-genotype correlation in patients with IP, which relies on clinical diagnosis, is essential to better understand the pathologic mechanisms of and to develop new treatments for IP. Molecular analysis is helpful in some uncertain cases. Characteristic histologic features must be included as major criteria for diagnosing IP. Multidisciplinary follow-up is mandatory to identify ophthalmologic and neurologic complications, especially in the first year of life. When neurologic findings are abnormal or vascular retinopathy is found, neuroimaging is indicated.

▶ This retrospective study of 40 children with IP carefully documents the clinical, histologic, and laboratory findings in this uncommon condition.

S. Raimer, MD

Medical Management of Neurofibromatosis 1: A Cross-sectional Study of 383 Patients

Drappier JC, Khosrotehrani K, Zeller J, et al (Paris XII Univ, Créteil, France)
J Am Acad Dermatol 49:440-444, 2003   11–4

Introduction.—The morbidity and mortality caused by neurofibromatosis 1 (NF1) are due to complications that could involve any of the body systems. Two management models have been proposed in specialized neurofibromatosis clinics: investigation protocols focused on identifying the various complications (including extensive imaging and analysis of 24-hour urinary catecholamine levels) or clinical follow-up (including history and physical examination) with no further assessment unless symptoms occur.

Ideal care for patients with NF1 may lie between these 2 models. The strategy of clinical follow-up (without routine imaging and 24-hour urinary catecholamine levels) was examined by comparing 2 successive periods: 1 period of screening investigations and 1 of clinical follow-up.

Methods.—The numbers of treated complications during the 2 successive periods were retrospectively compared from the database. Screening investigations were monitored between November 1988 and June 1995 and clinical examination results were tabulated between July 1995 and June 2000.

Results.—There was no statistically significant difference in the number of complications treated during the 2 evaluation periods ($P = .39$).

Conclusion.—Systematic screening investigations add little to clinical follow-up of patients with NF1, particularly in adults. The nonscreening approach is now recommended in most guidelines for management of patients with NF1.

▶ The results echo the recommendations of the National Institutes of Health, whose consensus statement on NF1 concluded, "Tests should be dictated by findings on clinical examination. Laboratory tests when aimed at asymptomatic patients are unlikely to be of value, particularly cranial computed tomography, MRI, electroencephalograms, and evoked potentials."

B. H. Thiers, MD

Bone Mineral Density and Fractures in Turner Syndrome

Bakalov VK, Chen ML, Baron J, et al (IH, Bethesda, Md)
Am J Med 115:259-264, 2003   11–5

Introduction.—Osteopenia and osteoporosis have been reported in two thirds of women with Turner syndrome and appear to be linked to deficient estrogen treatment. An increased incidence of fractures has been reported in some trials. Bone density and fracture history were compared in women with Turner syndrome and age-matched healthy women to ascertain whether women with Turner syndrome who receive standard hormone replacement therapy from the mid teens or the time of ovarian failure have normal or near-normal bone mineralization as well as more fractures.

Methods.—Dual-energy x-ray absorptiometry was used to determine areal bone density for the lumbar spine and femoral neck in 40 adult females with Turner syndrome and 43 age-matched healthy women. Personal interviews were performed to obtain histories of estrogen treatment and fractures.

Results.—The mean areal bone density was significantly lower at the lumbar spine (0.87 g/cm^2 vs 0.98 g/cm^2; $P < .001$) in women with Turner syndrome compared with control subjects. The diagnostic criteria for osteoporosis (T-score below -2.5) was met by 8 women with Turner syndrome (20%) with scores at the lumbar spine and by 3 (8%) with scores at the femoral neck. All women diagnosed with osteoporosis were shorter than 150 cm in height. Areal bone density was significantly correlated with height (lumbar spine: $R^2 = 0.4$; $P < .001$). Adjustments for skeletal size diminished the differences between groups, along with the number of women diagnosed with osteoporosis (eg, from 8 to 2 women, based on lumbar spine score). There were no significant between-group differences in the prevalence and type of fractures.

Conclusion.—The prevalence of osteoporosis and bone fractures is not significantly increased in women with Turner syndrome who are treated with standard estrogen replacement therapy. Women shorter than 150 cm in height are likely to be misdiagnosed as having osteoporosis when areal bone density is measured, unless adjustments for body size are considered.

▶ The data support the use of standard estrogen therapy to protect against osteoporosis and bone fractures in women with Turner syndrome. However, questions still remain whether increased bone fragility develops more often in women with Turner syndrome despite hormone replacement. The optimal time to initiate sex steroid therapy and the most effective dose and route of administration require further investigation.[1]

B. H. Thiers, MD

Reference

1. Bachrach LK, Neely EK: Pitfalls in the hunt for osteoporosis. *Am J Med* 115:322-323, 2003.

A Progeroid Syndrome in Mice Is Caused by Defects in A-Type Lamins
Mounkes LC, Kozlov S, Hernandez L, et al (Natl Cancer Inst, Frederick, Md)
Nature 423:298-301, 2003   11–6

Introduction.—Hutchinson-Gilford progeria syndrome (HGPS) is a rare genetic disorder that results in premature aging and early death. In addition to the findings of shortened stature, craniofacial disproportion, thin skin, alopecia, and osteoporosis, recent reports suggest that developmental abnormalities may be important in HGPS. The derivation of mice carrying an autosomal recessive mutation in the lamin A gene (*Lmna*) encoding A-type lamins, major components of the nuclear lamina is described.

Observations.—The varied role of lamins in diverse developmental processes may explain their growing association with certain human diseases. Two overall categories of laminopathies are identified: those affecting striated muscle and those with phenotypes affecting adipose tissue and bone. Because phenotypic overlap continues to be discovered in these disease categories, they may represent a spectrum of disorders rather than separate diseases. One of the most severe extremes in such a spectrum is found in a progeroid syndrome associated with $Lmna^{L530P/L530P}$ mutant mice. Homozygous mice exhibit defects consistent with HGPS, including a marked reduction in growth rate and death by 4 weeks of age. Disease of the heart, skin, skeletal muscle, and bone in these 4-week-old mice suggest developmental defects consistent with progeria. Nuclear morphology defects and decreased lifespan of homozygous fibroblasts suggest premature cell death. Tissues most affected in both patients with progeria and the mutant mice arise from

TABLE 1.—Comparison of HGPS Phenotypes in Human and $Lmna^{L530/L530P}$ Mouse

Human	Mouse
Severe growth retardation	Severe growth retardation
Short stature; failure to thrive	Short stature; failure to thrive
Mean death at 12-15 years	Death at 4-5 weeks
Craniofacial disproportion; micrognathy	Micrognathy
Abnormal dentition	Abnormal dentition
Very thin skin; loss subcutaneous fat	Loss of subcutaneous fat
Decreased eccrine, sebaceous glands	Decreased eccrine, sebaceous glands
Scleroderma	Increased collagen deposition in skin
Alopecia, onset at about 1 year	Decreased hair follicle density
Hyperkeratosis in some patients	Hyperkeratosis
Bone hypoplasia and resorption; osteoporosis	Decreased bone density; thin trabeculae
Hypoplasia/resorption of clavicles	Malformation of scapulae
Resorption of hip-girdle joints; shuffling gait	Waddling gait
Congestive heart failure; descrease in vascular smooth muscle	Heart pathology; subtle changes consistent with pulmonary hypertension
Incomplete sexual maturation	Hypogonadism
No consistent dyslipidaemia	Normal TTG and FFA; low cholesterol
Hypoplastic facial bones	Not determined
Thin diaphyses	Thinner femur; other diaphyses not studied
Osteolysis of terminal digits	None observed
Protruding ears; prominent eyes	Protruding ears
Myocardial fibrosis	Increased cardiac collagen and fibrocyte number
Atherosclerosis	No obvious defects in aorta, small vessels
Poor muscle development; atrophy	Poor muscle development and/or atrophy

Abbreviations: HGPS, Hutchinson-Gilford progeria syndrome; *TTG*, total triglycerides; *FFA*, free fatty acids.

Note: Online Mendelian inheritance in Man (OMIN) cites HGPS cases from 2 families in which consanguineous siblings were affected with progeroid syndrome, suggesting possible autosomal recessive inheritance. However, many HGPS patients arise from a nonconsanguineous union, suggesting an autosomal dominant mode of inheritance. Both modes of inheritance may be possible. $Lmna^{L530/L530P}$ mice are consistent with the autosomal recessive inheritance pattern.

(Reprinted with permission of *Nature* from Mounkes LC, Kozlov S, Hernandez L, et al: A progeroid syndrome in mice is caused by defects in A-type lamins. *Nature* 423:298-301, 2003. Copyright 2003 Macmillian Magazines Limited.)

the mesenchymal cell lineage. Clear parallels exist (Table 1) between HGPS phenotypes in humans and the $Lmna^{L530/L530P}$ mouse.

Lamin A Truncation in Hutchinson-Gilford Progeria
De Sandre-Giovannoli A, Bernard R, Cau P, et al (Inserm U491, Marseille, France; Hôpital la Timone, Marseille, France; Hôpital Conception, Marseille, France; et al)
Science 300:2055, 2003   11–7

Introduction.—Hutchinson-Gilford progeria syndrome (HGPS) is a rare disorder characterized by postnatal growth retardation, premature athero-sclerosis, and generalized osteodysplasia with osteolysis and pathologic fractures. The median age at death is 13.4 years; coronary artery disease is the usual cause. Many human disorders are ascribed to mutations at the *LMNA* locus, and *LMNA* is a strong candidate gene for HGPS.

Observations.—A genomic and transcriptional analysis of *LMNA* in chil-dren affected with HGPS revealed that 2 patients had a heterozygous C to T transition at nucleotide 1824 (C1824 to T1824) in exon 11 of the coding sequence. Because this substitution was not found in the parents or on 300 control chromosomes, an attempt was made to determine whether it af-fected transcript splicing. Two fragments were found on 1 patient's lympho-cytes, the larger corresponding to the expected transcript size, as in controls. The shorter transcript had a 150-base pair deletion starting at G1819. Fifty amino acids were predicted to be removed from lamin A tail, leaving lamin C unmodified. The other transcript, although it carried a T at position 1824, had a normal coding sequence length. Further analysis indicated that in pa-tients lamin A may not be transcribed from the normal allele (C at position 1824). The mutation would thus result in truncated and normal messenger RNAs (mRNAs) in cis; in trans, it would inhibit transcriptional processing of the normal allele, acting as a dominant negative mutation. Immunocyto-chemical analyses with specific antibodies to lamins A/C, A, and B1 showed most cells to have strikingly altered nuclear sizes and shapes. Lamin A was detected in only 10% to 20% of HGPS lymphocytes and lamin B1 was delo-calized to the nucleoplasm. These and other alterations were significant compared with control cells.

Conclusion.—Hutchinson-Gilford progeria syndrome appears to repre-sent a novel laminopathy that results from a single heterozygous splicing mutation in the *LMNA* gene. This mutation leads to a major loss of lamin A expression and associated nuclear alterations.

▶ One approach to elucidating the underlying causes of aging has been to study diseases associated with premature aging, such as Werner syndrome and Hutchinson-Gilford progeria syndrome (Abstracts 11–6 to 11–8). The latter is a rare genetic disorder with a phenotype suggestive of accelerated aging. The lamin A gene encodes a protein that is a critical component of the inner nuclear membrane. Mutations of this gene in mice result in nuclear morphologic defects and decreased life span of homozygous fibroblasts, suggesting premature cell death. Mice homozygous for this gene mutation display clinical defects consistent with HGPS, including a marked reduction in growth rate, premature death, and abnormalities of bone, muscle, and skin, and thus may serve as an animal model for this disorder. In this context, Eriksson et al (Abstract 11–8) and De Sandre-Giovannoli et al (Abstract 11–7) observed lamin A mutations in their patients with HGPS.

B. H. Thiers, MD

Recurrent De Novo Point Mutations in Lamin A Cause Hutchinson–Gilford Progeria Syndrome

Eriksson M, Brown WT, Gordon LB, et al (NIH, Bethesda, Md; New York State Inst for Basic Research in Development Disabilities, Staten Island, NY; Tufts Univ, Boston; et al)
Nature 423:293-298, 2003   11–8

Introduction.—Children affected with Hutchinson–Gilford progeria syndrome (HGPS) age rapidly and die on average at 13 years, most from progressive atherosclerosis of the coronary and cerebrovascular arteries. This rare genetic disorder is thought to be of sporadic autosomal dominant inheritance, but some studies suggest the possibility of autosomal recessive inheritance. To search for evidence of homozygosity, DNA samples from 12 individuals considered to represent classical HGPS and from 16 unaffected first-degree relatives underwent a whole-genome scan, including 403 polymorphic microsatellite markers with an average spacing of 9.2 cM.

Findings.—No evidence of homozygosity was found in the overall sample set, but 2 HGPS samples did have uniparental isodisomy of chromosome 1q. It was determined that the HGPS gene must lie in an interval of 4.82 Mb on proximal chromosome 1q, which contains roughly 80 known genes. One of them, the *LMNA* gene, encodes 2 protein products (lamin A and lamin C), and mutations in *LMNA* are known to cause 6 different recessive and dominant disorders. Polymerase chain reaction amplification of all of the exons of the *LMNA* gene, followed by direct sequencing, identified a heterozygous base substitution, G608G(GGC/GGT), within exon 11 of the *LMNA* gene in 18 of 20 samples from patients with classical HGPS. This single-base substitution was de novo and identical in all 18 cases. An additional case was identified with a different substitution within the same codon. Both mutations result in activation of a cryptic splice site within exon 11, leading to production of a protein product that deletes 50 amino acids near the carboxy terminus.

Discussion.—HGPS is one of many human genetic disorders resulting from mutations in the *LMNA* gene. Because most cases of the disorder appear to have a de novo mutation in the same codon, molecular diagnostics should be feasible for both diagnostic confirmation and prenatal counseling.

Discovery of the molecular basis for HGPS also suggests that *LMNA* may play a role in normal aging.

▶ This important article reports evidence of the genetic basis for HGPS, a syndrome characterized by dramatically premature aging and early death. These investigators determined that a single base substitution (C to G) was present within exon 11 of the lamin A gene in 18 of 20 patients with this syndrome. A different base change at the same position was observed in another patient. This mutation results in the creation of a splice site and abnormal protein product. Although the role of the lamin A gene mutation in this disease is not known, the authors suggest that the abnormal splicing may result in incomplete processing of the precursor protein, prelamin A. It is noteworthy that other mutations within this gene have been associated with human diseases, including certain forms of muscular dystrophy, and a mouse knockout of the gene is characterized by growth retardation and nuclear abnormalities. Studies of the role of lamin A in the normal aging process are awaited with interest.

G. M. P. Galbraith, MD

Permanent Correction of an Inherited Ectodermal Dysplasia With Recombinant EDA
Gaide O, Schneider P (Univ of Lausanne, Switzerland)
Nat Med 9:614-618, 2003   11–9

Background.—X-linked hypohidrotic dysplasia (XLHED) is a genetic disorder characterized by absence or deficient function of the hair, teeth, and sweat glands. It is caused by mutations of the ectodysplasin A gene (*Eda*) on the X chromosome. Mutations in this gene are responsible for the Tabby phenotype in mice. There are 2 major splice variants of *Eda*, which encode EDA1 and EDA2. This study examined rescue of prenatal Tabby mice with recombinant EDA1.

Methods and Results.—Recombinant proteins containing the receptor-binding domain of EDA fused to the C terminus of an IgG Fc domain (Fc:EDA1 and Fc:EDA2) were generated. The Fc component allowed the protein to pass through the placental barrier. These proteins were administered to pregnant Tabby mice on gestational days 11, 13, and 15. The pregnant mice appeared unaffected by these injections, but administration of Fc:EDA1, although not Fc:EDA2, rescued the mutant phenotype of their offspring. Hair, sebaceous glands, jaws, teeth, eyes, meibomian glands, and sweat glands appeared to be rescued by prenatal administration of recombinant EDA1. These changes persisted into adulthood. When Fc:EDA1 was administered at different prenatal and ante-natal time points, it was apparent that different aspects of the phenotype could be rescued at different times.

Conclusions.—Prenatal administration of recombinant EDA1 can permanently rescue the phenotype of the murine Tabby syndrome (human

XLHED). Similar approaches might be taken in humans and with other developmental disorders caused by deficient prenatal ligand expression.

▶ This report is of particular interest in that it describes the correction of a genetic defect by the antenatal administration of a recombinant protein. The investigators used a murine model (Tabby mice) of the human disease XLHED. Both murine and human diseases are characterized by mutations of the ectodysplasin A gene located on the X chromosome, which codes for the EDA1 protein that is required for normal formation of hair, teeth, and sweat glands. In this study, recombinant fusion proteins comprised of EDA protein and the C-terminus of a murine IgG1 Fc molecule were administered to pregnant Tabby mice at various times of gestation. The Fc moiety was included to ensure transplacental delivery of the EDA protein to the fetuses. The results showed that this treatment rescued the offspring of the Tabby mice from many of the features of the deficient phenotype, including formation of sweat glands, and these effects were maintained into adult life. This study may hold important implications for development of novel therapies for human genetic disorders.

G. M. P. Galbraith, MD

Late Presentation of Dyskeratosis Congenita as Apparently Acquired Aplastic Anaemia Due to Mutations in Telomerase RNA
Fogarty PF, Yamaguchi H, Wiestner A, et al (Natl Heart, Lung, and Blood Inst, Bethesda, Md; NIH, Bethesda, Md; Univ of British Columbia, Vancouver)
Lancet 362:1628-1630, 2003   11–10

Introduction.—Aplastic anemia is typically an acquired disorder in adults and can be treated with immunosuppressive therapy. Constitutional bone marrow failure, in contrast, is usually diagnosed in children with a strong family history of blood diseases, and typical physical anomalies are often present. The 2 families described here each had an adult diagnosed with acquired aplastic anemia. Two novel point mutations in the telomerase RNA gene (*TERC*) were detected in each family.

Observations.—The index patient of family A, a man, 30 years, with severe pancytopenia, had bone marrow findings consistent with acquired aplastic anemia. The proband died of sepsis 188 days after receiving a hemopoietic stem cell transplantation from his healthy 48-year-old sister whose bone marrow harvest yielded suboptimal numbers of CD34$^+$ cells. The proband of family B showed moderate pancytopenia at age 21. Five years later, immunosuppressive therapy was started because of worsening anemia. An attempt at hemopoietic stem cell transplantation from a healthy brother was unsuccessful. Treatment of the proband with androgens yielded clinical improvement. Assessment of family members of the index patients found individuals with mutated *TERC*. None had physical signs of dyskeratosis congenita, and blood counts were nearly normal, but these affected individuals had extremely short telomeres in all cell types analyzed. Additional abnormalities were reduced hemopoietic function and elevated serum erythropoietin and thrombopoietin.

Discussion.—Low stem cell numbers in a family member considered a potential donor for a patient with aplastic anemia, or a family history of even mild blood count abnormalities, should suggest that an underlying hereditary syndrome may be present. Bone marrow failure linked to dyskeratosis congenita may occur in otherwise phenotypically normal adults. Such findings suggest that a trial of androgens may be beneficial and that the conditioning program before stem cell transplantation be modified.

▶ The telomerase enzyme maintains the protective structures, called telomeres, at the end of chromosomes. When telomerase expression is suppressed, telomeres shorten progressively with each cell division, eventually leading to cell death. An article reviewed in the 2000 YEAR BOOK OF DERMATOLOGY AND DERMATOLOGIC SURGERY suggested that compromised telomerase function in dyskeratosis congenita might limit the normal proliferative capacity of human somatic cells in the epithelium and blood. This would explain the skin defects that characterize that disorder, as well as the increased mortality rate from bone marrow failure associated with the reduced regenerative capacity of hematopoietic stem cells.[1] Fogarty et al observed the same gene defect associated with some cases of dyskeratosis congenita in 2 families with adult onset pancytopenia, suggesting that occult dyskeratosis congenita in otherwise phenotypically normal adults can masquerade as acquired aplastic anemia.

B. H. Thiers, MD

Reference

1. Mitchell JR, Wood E, Collins K: A telomerase component is defective in the human disease dyskeratosis congenita. *Nature* 402;551-555, 1999. (2000 YEAR BOOK OF DERMATOLOGY AND DERMATOLOGIC SURGERY, p 272.)

Loss of Kindlin-1, a Human Homolog of the *Caenorhabditis elegans* Actin–Extracellular-Matrix Linker Protein UNC-112, Causes Kindler Syndrome
Siegel DH, Ashton GH, Penagos HG, et al (Univ of California, San Francisco; Hosp of Sick Children, London; Social Security Bureau of Panama, David; et al)
Am J Hum Genet 73:174-187, 2003   11–11

Introduction.—Kindler syndrome is an autosomal recessive disorder involving neonatal blistering, sun sensitivity, atrophy, abnormal pigmentation, and fragility of the skin. Evidence that it may be caused by an actin–extracellular-matrix (ECM) linkage protein deficiency is discussed.

Methods.—Blood samples were drawn from members of 24 families from Panama, the United States, Britain, Italy, Oman, Jordan, Turkey, Saudi Arabia, Afghanistan, Pakistan, and Japan. Specimens of blood or biopsy or both underwent several analyses including genome-wide screen and genetic linkage analysis, cell culture and RNA extraction, cDNA synthesis, multiple-tissue Northern blot, multiple-tissue cDNA panels, mutation identification, anti-kindlin-1 antibody generation, immunohistochemistry, and kindlin-1 transfections.

Results.—Linkage and homozygosity testing in an isolated Panamanian cohort and in additional inbred families mapped the gene to 20p12.3. Loss-of-function mutations were observed in the *FLJ20116* gene (renamed "*KIND1*"[encoding kindlin-1]). Kindlin-1 is a human homolog of the *Caenorhabditis elegans* protein UNC-112, a membrane-related structural/signaling protein involved in linking the actin cytoskeleton to the ECM.

Conclusion.—Kindler syndrome is the first known skin fragility disorder caused by a defect in actin–ECM linkage and not in the keratin–ECM linkage.

▶ The authors show that the features observed in Kindler syndrome are associated with mutations in the *KIND1* gene. Its gene product, kindlin-1, is thought to anchor the actin-myosin cytoskeleton in muscle to the ECM and thus appears to play an important role in muscle-matrix stability. However, the absence of significant muscle symptomatology in affected patients suggests that other proteins may compensate for the *KIND1* deficit or that the gene has other unknown functions responsible for the typical manifestations of the condition, which include photosensitivity, blistering, pigmentation, atrophy, and skin fragility. An alternative explanation might be that other genes are responsible for these characteristic symptoms. For example, Rothmund-Thomson syndrome and Bloom syndrome exhibit phenotypic similarities to Kindler syndrome but display a distinctly different genetic defect, that is, a dysfunction of DNA helicase.

B. H. Thiers, MD

Griscelli Syndrome Restricted to Hypopigmentation Results From a Melanophilin Defect (GS3) or a *MYO5A* F-exon Deletion (GS1)

Ménasche G, Hsuan Ho C, Sanal O, et al (Hôpital Necker-Enfants Malades, Paris)
J Clin Invest 112:450-456, 2003   11–12

Background.—Griscelli syndrome (GS) is a rare autosomal recessive disorder characterized by pigmentary dilution of skin and hair, clumps of pigment in hair shafts, and accumulation of end-stage melanosomes in the center of melanocytes. Type 1 GS (GS1), caused by mutations in the myosin 5A gene (*MYO5A*), is also characterized by severe primary neurologic impairment. Type 2 GS (GS2) is characterized by an immune defect and mutations in the RAB27A gene. Murine models exist of GS1 (*dilute*) and GS2 (*ashen*). Identical pigment defects have been described in *leaden* mice, which have a mutation in melanophilin (*Mlph*). This report describes the molecular characterization of 2 patients who presented with a novel form of GS characterized exclusively by pigment defects.

Methods and Results.—Both patients presented with silver-gray hair and large clumps of pigment in the hair shaft, characteristic of GS. Longitudinal follow-up of 6 and 8 years, respectively, revealed that phenotypic presentation was restricted to pigment defects. Genomic DNA was extracted and mutational analyses performed. In the case of patient A (PA), mutational analysis excluded the known GS mutations, so based on findings in *leaden* mice, mutations were assayed in *Mlph*. A mutation was detected in both copies of PA's *Mlph* gene. In the case of patient B, *Mlph* was excluded by mutational analysis and a homozygous deletion was identified in the F-exon of the MYO5A gene, which is expressed in melanocytes.

Conclusions.—This report describes a third form of Griscelli syndrome (GS3) restricted to pigmentation defects. This hypopigmentation defect can occur as the result of either of 2 mutations, 1 in the melanophilin gene and the other a deletion of the F-exon of the MYO5A gene. The spectrum of GS types helps to define the pathways used by melanocytes, neurons, and immune cells for secretory granule exocytosis.

▶ GS is a fascinating inherited genetic disorder with 2 previously characterized clinical phenotypes. Type 1 GS presents with hypopigmentation of the skin and hair with associated neurologic deficits, whereas in type 2 GS patients, the pigmentary loss is associated with an unusual defect of immune regulation that results in uncontrolled activation of T cells and macrophages (hemophagocytic syndrome). These syndrome variants result from mutations in the myosin 5A gene (type 1) and the Rab27a gene (type 2), respectively. These investigators describe evidence for a third phenotype of GS, characterized by hypopigmentation alone, which appears to result from mutations of the melanophilin gene. This study highlights the complexity of the genetic factors responsible for the diverse phenotypes of inherited disorders such as Griscelli syndrome.

G. M. P. Galbraith, MD

Identification of *PEX7* as the Second Gene Involved in Refsum Disease
van den Brink DM, Brites P, Haasjes J, et al (Univ of Amsterdam; King's College London; Imperial College Med School, London)
Am J Hum Genet 72:471-477, 2003   11–13

Background.—Refsum disease (RD) is characterized by increased levels of phytanic acid resulting from a deficiency of the peroxisomal enzyme phytanoyl-CoA hydroxylase (PhyH). Disease-causing mutations in the *PHYH* gene have been identified in most patients with RD. However, in a subgroup, no mutations are found, which indicates that the condition is genetically heterogeneous. Biochemical investigations of fibroblasts from 2 probands with clinically diagnosed RD but no mutations in the *PHYH* gene were performed.

Methods and Findings.—Linkage analysis of these patients suggested a second locus on chromosome 6q22-24, including the *PEX7* gene, which codes for the peroxin 7 receptor protein needed for peroxisomal import of proteins containing a peroxisomal targeting signal type 2. Typically, *PEX7* mutations cause rhizomelic chondrodysplasia punctata type 1, a severe peroxisomal disease. Biochemical analyses in the patients with RD demonstrated defects in phytanic acid α-oxidation and in plasmalogen synthesis and peroxisomal thiolase. Mutations in the *PEX7* gene were also identified.

Conclusions.—Mutations in the *PEX7* gene may result in a broad clinical spectrum, ranging from severe rhizomelic chondrodysplasia punctata to relatively mild RD. A full screen of peroxisomal functions may be needed to clinically diagnose conditions that involve retinitis pigmentosa, ataxia, and polyneuropathy.

▶ RD is caused by a deficiency of a peroxisomal enzyme, resulting in disturbed branched-chained lipid metabolism and elevated levels of phytanic acid. Clinical findings include ichthyosis, cataracts, skeletal abnormalities, cardiac arrhythmias, peripheral neuropathy, ataxia, and progressive adult retinitis pigmentosa. Previous studies have identified disease-causing mutations in the *PHYH* gene; however, in some affected patients no such mutations are found, which suggests that the condition is genetically heterogeneous. van den Brink et al identify the *PEX7* gene as an important underlying factor in some patients with this disorder. This gene has also been associated with another peroxisomal disorder, rhizomelic chondrodysplasia punctata, which emphasizes the broad clinical spectrum of disorders that may be associated with its mutation. It is likely that other as yet unidentified modifier genes affect the clinical phenotype associated with these gene mutations.

B. H. Thiers, MD

Role of *TBX1* in Human Del22q11.2 Syndrome
Yagi H, Furutani Y, Hamada H, et al (Tokyo Women's Med Univ; Chiba Univ, Japan; Kelo Univ, Tokyo; et al)
Lancet 362:1366-1373, 2003   11–14

Introduction.—Del22q11.2 syndrome is a contiguous gene syndrome characterized by a variety of abnormalities, including T-cell deficits, facial anomalies, velopharyngeal insufficiency, and cardiac abnormalities. DiGeorge syndrome and conotruncal anomaly face syndrome are included in the clinical spectrum. The syndrome has an incidence of 1 in 4000 to 5000 live births, making it the most frequent known chromosomal microdeletion syndrome. At least 30 genes have been mapped to the deleted region, but the association of these genes with the cause of the del22q11.2 syndrome remains uncertain. An attempt was made to localize the *TBX1* mutation, which has been suggested as a candidate gene for the syndrome.

Methods.—The study included 235 unrelated patients with a diagnosis of the del22q11.2 syndrome who underwent assessment by history and physical examination. Fluorescence in situ hybridization analysis with 10 probes on 22q11.2 was used to test for the chromosomal deletion. Genetic analysis in 13 patients from 10 families with the syndrome phenotype but no detectable deletion of 22q11.2 was designed to investigate mutations in the coding sequence of *TBX1*.

Results.—All but 10 of the 235 patients had a defined 1.5 to 3Mb deletion at 22q11.2, and all patients had features of the conotruncal anomaly face syndrome. Dysmorphism of the nose was observed consistently. Three mutations of *TBX1* were identified in 2 unrelated patients without the deletion (1 with sporadic conotruncal anomaly face syndrome and velocardiofacial syndrome and 1 with sporadic DiGeorge syndrome) and in 3 patients from a family with conotruncal anomaly face syndrome and velocardiofacial syndrome. A study of 555 healthy control subjects showed no evidence of these 3 mutations.

Conclusion.—Mutation in *TBX1*, a recently described member of the T-box gene family, appears to be responsible for 5 major phenotypes (but not typical mental retardation) in del22q11.2 syndrome. Thus, *TBX1* is considered a major determinant of the del22q11.2 syndrome.

▶ The authors have identified a mutation in the *TBX1* gene that yields a variable phenotype. They suggest that environmental factors, as well as altered interaction with downstream genes that are regulated by T-box transcription factors, may play an essential role in embryogenesis. Other phenotypic expressions may represent carriers of *TBX1*-inactivating mutations.[1]

B. H. Thiers, MD

Reference

1. Baldini A: DiGeorge's syndrome: A gene at last. *Lancet* 362:1342-1343, 2003.

Immune Tolerance After Long-term Enzyme-Replacement Therapy Among Patients Who Have Mucopolysaccharidosis I
Kakavanos R, Turner CT, Hopwood JJ, et al (Women's and Children's Hosp, North Adelaide, South Australia; Univ of Adelaide, South Australia; Harbor-Univ of California, Torrance)
Lancet 361:1608-1613, 2003   11–15

Introduction.—One trial in patients with mucopolysaccharidosis I, an autosomal recessive inherited lysosomal storage disorder, reported positive responses to enzyme-replacement therapy. Both animal and human studies, however, suggest that an immune response to the replacement protein develops in some subjects. Ten patients who had taken part in a clinical trial of enzyme-replacement therapy were investigated for a humoral immune response to recombinant human α-L-iduronidase replacement protein.

Methods.—Titers and specific linear sequence epitope reactivity of serum antibodies to α-L-iduronidase were characterized in the patients at the start of treatment and after 6, 12, 26, 52, and 104 weeks. IV infusions of 125,000 U per kilogram of body weight were administered over 3-hour periods, once weekly. The values for the patients' serum samples were compared with the values for serum samples from normal control subjects.

Results.—Patients ranged in age from 5 to 22 years; 8 had Hurler-Scheie intermediate phenotypes, 1 had Hurler's syndrome, and 1 had Scheie's syndrome. Before enzyme-replacement therapy, all 10 patients had serum antibodies to recombinant human α-L-iduronidase within the control range (512 to 32,000 for control subjects and 1000 to 20,000 for patients). Early during the course of treatment, 5 of 10 patients had elevated titers of antibody to the replacement protein (serum antibody titers 130,000 to 500,000 and high-affinity epitope reactivity). Antibody reactivity was reduced, however, by week 26 of therapy, and all patients had low antibody titers (100 to 100,000) and only low-affinity epitope activity by week 104. All patients with antibody titers in the normal range at 6 to 12 weeks remained in the normal range throughout treatment.

Conclusion.—Long-term enzyme replacement therapy did not produce lasting immune responses in these patients with mucopolysaccharidosis I. After 2 years of treatment with recombinant human α-L-iduronidase replacement protein, patients who initially had an immune reaction developed immune tolerance.

▶ The finding of immune tolerance after a long-term enzyme-replacement therapy is reassuring and has positive implications for the safety and effectiveness of such treatment. Moreover, this so-called natural induction of immune tolerance may have significant advantages over the costly and aggressive immune-tolerance programs currently recommended for some immune-responsive enzyme-replacement therapies that have been used for conditions such as Gaucher disease.[1] For mucopolysaccharidosis I, it will be important to confirm when immune tolerance to α-L-iduronidase develops and whether it is maintained throughout the course of treatment.

B. H. Thiers, MD

Reference

1. Rosenberg M, Kingma W, Fitzpatrick MA, et al: Immunosurveillance of alglucerase enzyme therapy for Gaucher patients: Induction of humoral tolerance in seroconverted patients after repeated administration. *Blood* 93:2081-2088, 1999.

12 Drug Development and Promotion

The Effect of Incentive-Based Formularies on Prescription-Drug Utilization and Spending
Huskamp HA, Deverka PA, Epstein AM, et al (Harvard School of Public Health, Boston; Brigham and Women's Hosp, Boston)
N Engl J Med 349:2224-2232, 2003   12–1

Background.—In an attempt to control the cost of prescription drugs, many employers and health plans have adopted incentive-based formularies. This study investigated the utilization of and spending on drugs in 2 employer-sponsored health plans that implemented changes in formulary administration.

Methods.—One plan changed from a 1-tier to a 3-tier formulary, increasing all enrollee co-payments. The second plan changed from a 2-tier to a 3-tier system, raising the co-payments only for tier-3 drugs (Table 1). The utilization of angiotensin-converting enzyme (ACE) inhibitors, proton-pump inhibitors, and statins was analyzed.

Findings.—The probability of the use of a drug showed a slower growth in the plan implementing the more substantial changes. In this plan, a major shift in spending from the plan to enrollees occurred. Among those initially taking tier-3 statins, more enrollees in this plan switched to tier-1 or tier-2 drugs than did persons in a comparison group, at 49% and 17%, respectively. Twenty-one percent of the former group quit taking statins completely, compared with 11% in the comparison group. Similar patterns were seen for ACE inhibitors and proton-pump inhibitors. Enrollees in the plan that made more moderate changes were more likely than the comparison group to switch to tier-1 or tier-2 drugs but not to quit taking a certain class of medications entirely.

Conclusions.—Different changes in employer-sponsored health plan formulary administration schemes can have markedly different effects on utilization and spending. In many instances, enrollees discontinue treatment altogether. Quality of care may be affected by dramatic changes in formulary administration.

TABLE 1.—Summary of Changes in Pharmaceutical Benefits*

Employer No.	Characteristics of the Company†	Old Design of Pharmaceutical Benefit	New Design of Pharmaceutical Benefit
1	Large firm with mostly hourly workers	One-tier benefit: Retail—$7 generic or brand-name Mail order—$15 generic or brand-name	Three-tier benefit: Retail—$8 generic, $15 preferred brand-name, $30 nonpreferred brand-name Mail order—$16 generic, $30 preferred brand-name, $60 nonpreferred brand-name Three-tier formulary structure plus across-the-board increase in copayments
2	Large firm with mostly salaried workers	Two-tier benefit: Retail—$6 generic, $12 brand-name Mail order—same as for retail	Three-tier benefit: Retail—$6 generic, $12 preferred brand-name, $24 nonpreferred brand-name Mail order—same as for retail Three-tier formulary structure only

*Typically, an enrollee receives a 90-day supply of a drug when purchasing it through a mail-order program, as compared with a 30-day supply when purchasing it in a retail setting.
†We do not provide additional details about the characteristics of the employers in order to protect their anonymity.
(Reprinted by permission of *The New England Journal of Medicine* from Huskamp HA, Deverka PA, Epstein AM, et al. The effect of incentive-based formularies on prescription-drug utilization and spending. *N Engl J Med* 349:2224-2232, 2003. Copyright 2003 Massachusetts Medical Society. All rights reserved.)

▶ As noted by Thomas[1] in an accompanying editorial, incentive-based formularies cannot solve the underlying problem, which is the high cost of drugs in the United States. Nevertheless, the shifting of costs and responsibility for health care decisions to consumers is a growing trend, and incentive-based formularies have an important role in this strategy. What remains to be determined is the effect of these formularies on patients' health outcomes.

B. H. Thiers, MD

Reference

1. Thomas CP: Incentive-based formularies. *N Engl J Med* 349:2186-2188, 2003.

Disclosure of Financial Competing Interests in Randomised Controlled Trials: Cross Sectional Review
Gross CP, Gupta AR, Krumholz HM (Yale Univ, New Haven, Conn)
BMJ 326:526-527, 2003   12–2

Background.—The 1997 uniform requirements require authors to acknowledge in the manuscript all financial support for their work. When industry provides support for specific projects, authors are to describe the sponsor's role in the design, analysis, and reporting of the study. Previous research has revealed that many published papers do not contain statements of financial competing interests. Less is known about journals' compliance with other parts of the disclosure guidelines and about the nature of interests disclosed.

Methods.—Published randomized controlled studies in 5 major medical journals were reviewed to determine adherence to the 1997 disclosure requirements. The trials appeared in the *Annals of Internal Medicine, British Medical Journal, Journal of the American Medical Association, Lancet,* and *New England Journal of Medicine* between April 1, 1999, and March 31, 2000.

Findings.—Sixty-nine of the 100 industry-sponsored studies included statements about the nature of the relationship between the authors and the study sponsor. In the papers providing this information, the most commonly cited relationships were employment (43%), consultant/honorarium (32%), grants (26%), stock ownership (10%), and participation in a speaker's bureau (10%). The 30 papers coauthored by industry sponsor employees represented 30% of all published industry-sponsored trials and 11% of all randomized controlled trials in the sample. Only 8 of the 100 industry-sponsored studies stated the role of the sponsor in the methods section. Two of these 8 studies explicitly stated that the sponsor had no role, and 6 described the sponsor's role. The degree of sponsor involvement varied greatly and was typically described vaguely.

Conclusions.—Industry involvement in published randomized controlled studies appears to be substantial, but the extent and nature of that involvement are difficult to assess critically because adherence to disclosure guidelines varies. Currently, the editors of major journals are moving toward the more stringent measure of asking authors to document that they had access to the data and were allowed to make publication decisions independently.

▶ Gross et al demonstrate that the complex financial relationships between investigators and industry are difficult to assess because of variable adherence to disclosure guidelines. Some prominent medical journals now require that authors document that they had access to the data and were able to make publication decisions independently.[1] Nevertheless, given the poor adherence to existing uniform requirements, it is uncertain whether journals will adhere to these more stringent guidelines.

B. H. Thiers, MD

Reference

1. Davidoff F, DeAngelis C, Drazen JM, et al: Sponsorship, authorization, and accountability. *Lancet* 358:854-856, 2001.

Association of Funding and Conclusions in Randomized Drug Trials: A Reflection of Treatment Effect or Adverse Events?
Als-Nielsen B, Chen W, Gluud C, et al (Copenhagen Univ)
JAMA 290:921-928, 2003   12–3

Introduction.—Conclusions in randomized trials have been shown to be more positive toward experimental interventions when funded by for-profit organizations. A meta-analysis was performed in an observational investigation to determine whether there is an association between funding and conclusions in randomized drug trials that reflects the magnitude of treatment effect or occurrence of side effects.

Methods.—A total of 370 randomized drug trials were included in meta-analyses from Cochrane reviews selected from the Cochrane Library, May 2001. From a random sample of 167 Cochrane reviews, 25 randomized drug trials contained eligible meta-analyses (evaluated a binary outcome; pooled a minimum of 5 full-paper trials of which at least 1 reported adequate and 1 reported inadequate allocation concealment). The main binary outcome from each meta-analysis was considered the primary outcome for all investigations included in each meta-analysis.

The relationship between funding and conclusions was examined by logistic regression with adjustment for treatment effect, adverse events, and additional confounding factors (methodological quality, control intervention, sample size, publication year, and place of publication). The primary outcome measure was conclusions in trials, classified into whether or not the experimental drug was recommended as the treatment of choice.

Results.—The experimental drug was recommended as the treatment of choice in 16%, 30%, 35%, and 51% of trials funded by nonprofit organizations, trials not reporting funding, trials funded by both nonprofit and for-profit organizations, and trials funded by for-profit organizations, respectively ($P < .001$). Logistic regression analyses showed that funding, treatment effect, and double-blinding were the only significant predictors of conclusions.

Adjustment analyses revealed that trials funded by for-profit organizations were significantly more likely to recommend the experimental drug as the treatment of choice (odds ratio, 5.3; 95% confidence interval, 2.0-14.4) than were trials funded by nonprofit organizations. This relationship did not seem to reflect treatment effect or adverse events.

Conclusion.—Conclusions in trials funded by for-profit organizations may be more positive as a result of biased interpretation of trial findings. Readers need to carefully determine whether conclusions in randomized trials are adequately supported by data.

▶ The authors provide yet additional evidence to emphasize the need for critical interpretation of the results of industry-sponsored clinical trials. Readers must determine independently whether the conclusions offered by the authors are supported by the data presented.

B. H. Thiers, MD

Pharmaceutical Industry Sponsorship and Research Outcome and Quality: Systematic Review
Lexchin J, Bero LA, Djulbegovic B, et al (York Univ, Toronto; Univ of California, San Francisco; Univ of South Florida, Tampa, et al)
BMJ 326:1167-1170, 2003   12–4

Background.—Clinical research sponsored by pharmaceutical companies influences medical practice. The relationship between the source of research funding and reported outcomes was investigated, and the methodologic quality of industry-sponsored research was compared with that of other research.

Methods.—A MEDLINE search of the literature published between 1966 and 2002 and an Embase search of literature between 1980 and 2002 were conducted. Additional material was identified by a review of the references in these studies. The authors' files were also analyzed. Three authors independently abstracted data from the 30 studies included.

Findings.—Analysis indicated that studies funded by drug companies were less likely to be published than studies with other sources of funding. Research sponsored by the pharmaceutical industry was more likely to yield outcomes favoring the sponsor than was research with other sponsors, the odds ratio being 4.05. The methods of industry-sponsored research did not appear to be of lower quality than that of other research.

Conclusions.—Published research funded by pharmaceutical companies has a systematic bias favoring products made by the funding companies. The reasons for this include selection of an inappropriate comparator and publication bias.

Evidence B(i)ased Medicine—Selective Reporting From Studies Sponsored by Pharmaceutical Industry: Review of Studies in New Drug Applications

Melander H, Ahlqvist-Rastad J, Meijer G, et al (Med Products Agency, Uppsala, Sweden)

BMJ 326:1171-1173, 2003   12–5

Background.—The standard basis for treatment guidelines is systematic literature reviews or meta-analyses of all randomized controlled studies. The relative effect on bias caused by multiple publication, selective publication, and selective reporting in research sponsored by the pharmaceutical industry was investigated.

Methods.—The studies analyzed were 42 placebo-controlled trials of 5 selective serotonin reuptake inhibitors for the treatment of major depression that were submitted to the Swedish drug regulatory authority to support marketing approval. Also analyzed were published versions of the same studies that appeared between 1983 and 1999. The degree of selection bias in the published studies compared with those submitted to the regulatory authority (which are obliged to be inclusive of all data gathered during clinical trials) was determined.

Findings.—Instances of multiple publication were noted. Twenty-one studies yielded at least 2 publications each. Five publications were based on 3 studies. Selective publication was also identified. Studies demonstrating significant drug effects were stand-alone publications more often than studies yielding nonsignificant findings. In addition, there was evidence of selective reporting, with many publications ignoring the findings of intention-to-treat analyses and reporting only the more favorable per protocol analyses.

Conclusions.—Publicly available data on specific selective serotonin reuptake inhibitors for the treatment of depression are likely to be biased. For clinicians who rely on published data alone to choose a specific drug, these findings are cause for concern.

▶ Physicians are aware that when a pharmaceutical company funds drug research, the published results are likely to be favorable to the sponsoring company's product. Lexchin et al (Abstract 12–4) confirm that drug company–funded research more often has an outcome that favors the sponsor's product than research funded by other sources. This likely is not due to methodologic deficiencies, but probably represents the use of inappropriate comparators or publication bias. One example of inappropriate comparators was illustrated in an article reviewed in the 2002 YEAR BOOK OF DERMATOLOGY AND DERMATOLOGIC SURGERY. In this article, an inappropriately low dose of griseofulvin was compared with 1 of the newer systemic antifungal drugs for the treatment of tinea capitis.[1] Publication bias is also demonstrated by the occasional attempt by drug manufacturers to prevent publication of studies that cast their product in an unfavorable light.[2,3] Melander et al (Abstract 12–5) investigated duplicate publication, selective publication, and selective reporting. They found these factors to be a major source of bias in published research and argue that, without access to unpublished, perhaps negative data, physicians may be unable to draw sound conclusions regarding the benefits and risks of new drugs. The uneasy relationship between medical journals and pharmaceutical companies was addressed in articles appearing in the same issue of the *British Medical Journal*[4,5]

Another source of concern is the relationship between drug companies and regulatory agencies. Drug companies need positive research data to petition regulatory agencies for permission to market their drugs. Over the past several years, the pharmaceutical industry has become quite vocal in pressuring regulatory agencies for rapid drug approvals. In many countries, these same regulatory agencies have become heavily dependent on industry fees for their survival and often find themselves competing with each other for industry fees for regulatory work.[6]

B. H. Thiers, MD

References

1. Fuller LC, Smith CH, Cerio R, et al: A randomized comparison of 4 weeks of terbinafine vs. 8 weeks of griseofulvin for the treatment of tinea capitis. *Br J Dermatol* 144:321-327, 2001.
2. Nathan DG, Weatherall DJ: Academia and industry: Lessons from the unfortunate events in Toronto. *Lancet* 327:771-772, 1999.
3. McCarthy M: Company sought to block paper's publication. *Lancet* 356:1659, 2000.
4. Smith R: Medical journals and pharmaceutical companies: Uneasy bedfellows. *BMJ* 326:1202-1205, 2003.
5. Burton B, Rowell A: Unhealthy spin. *BMJ* 326:1205-1207, 2003.
6. Abraham J: Making regulation responsive to commercial interests: Streamlining drug industry watchdogs. *BMJ* 325:1164-1169, 2002.

Role of a Research Ethics Committee in Follow-up and Publication of Results

Pich J, Carné X, Arnaiz J-A, et al (Hosp Clínic, Barcelona; Institut d'Investigacions Biomèdiques August Pi i Sunyer [IDIBAPS], Barcelona)
Lancet 361:1015-1016, 2003   12–6

Background.—Research ethics committees assess the scientific and ethical aspects of submitted protocols. These committees approve protocols and are responsible for following and monitoring the trial until it is completed. However, lack of time and resources makes it difficult to meet this last responsibility. The outcomes of protocols submitted to the Hospital Clinic Ethics Committee (HCEC), to which most clinical trial protocols in Spain are submitted for approval, were assessed in the current study.

Methods.—The ouctomes of all protocols submitted to the HCEC in 1997 were reviewed. Of 166 clinical trials submitted during that year, 158 were approved. Principal investigators, sponsors, contract research organizations, or a combination of these were interviewed.

Findings.—The recruitment rate was lower than expected in 45% of all clinical trials initiated. Sixty-four percent of the trials were completed in accordance with their protocol. After 3 years, only 21% of the completed clinical trials had their findings published in peer-reviewed journals. When articles in press were included, this percentage increased to 31%. Only 27% were presented at scientific meetings.

Conclusions.—A relatively low percentage of the clinical trials approved by the HCEC in the year studied resulted in the publication or presentation of their findings. Research ethics committees should devote more effort and resources to promote the public dissemination of clinical trial findings.

▶ Clearly, clinical trials with positive results are more likely to be published than those with negative findings. The authors argue that the research ethics committee should ensure public dissemination of results of clinical trials, whether favorable or unfavorable.

B. H. Thiers, MD

Synergy Between Publication and Promotion: Comparing Adoption of New Evidence in Canada and the United States
Majumdar SR, McAlister FA, Soumerai SB (Univ of Alberta, Edmonton, Canada; Harvard Med School, Boston)
Am J Med 115:467-472, 2003   12–7

Background.—How new evidence from clinical studies affects physician practice is not well documented. Whether publication of new evidence changes practice and how such changes are influenced by differences in promotional activity in Canada and the United States was investigated for the Heart Outcomes Prevention and Evaluation (HOPE) study and the Randomized Aldactone Evaluation Study (RALES).

Methods.—Longitudinal dispensing data were obtained between 1998 and 2001 to assess changes in prescribing patterns for ramipril and other angiotensin-converting enzyme inhibitors before and after the HOPE trial. Estimates for promotional expenditures were also obtained. Analyses were stratified by country in an attempt to isolate the effect of promotion. Interrupted time series methods were used to adjust for pre-existing prescribing trends. In similar analyses, spironolactone use before and after RALES was investigated.

Findings.—Publication of the findings from the HOPE study correlated with rapid increases in ramipril use. These increases were associated with an increase in detailing expenditures in both countries. After adjustment for previous trends in prescribing, after study publication, ramipril prescription increased by 12% per month in Canada compared with 5% per month in the United States. One year after publication, ramipril prescriptions comprised 30% of the ACE inhibitor market in Canada and 6% in the United States. Publication of the RALES findings was associated with more modest increases of 2% per month in spironolactone prescription in Canada and the United States. No promotional activity for RALES occurred in either country.

Conclusions.—The publication of new evidence from clinical trials correlated with modest changes in practice. Promotional activity seemed to increase such changes. More active promotion appears to be needed to accelerate the adoption of new evidence.

▶ Being a bit cynical, this reviewer was hardly surprised by the findings reported by Majumdar et al. They concluded that publication of new evidence in peer-reviewed journals is associated with only modest changes in clinical practice. Active promotion, whether carried out by the pharmaceutical industry or by the study investigators themselves, plays a major role in accelerating adoption of such evidence. The bottom line is that "educational" programs supported by pharmaceutical companies are highly effective in changing physicians' prescribing habits.

B. H. Thiers, MD

Characteristics of General Practitioners Who Frequently See Drug Industry Representatives: National Cross Sectional Study
Watkins C, Moore L, Harvey I, et al (Blackwell and Nailsea Med Group, Bristol, England; Cardiff Univ, Wales; Univ of East Anglia, Norwich, England; et al)
BMJ 326:1178-1179, 2003   12–8

Background.—Prescribing costs among general practitioners are known to vary. Previous research has shown that frequent contact between general practitioners and drug industry representatives correlates strongly and independently with higher prescribing costs. The attitudes and behaviors of general practitioners who reported frequent contacts with drug company representatives were investigated.

Methods.—A questionnaire was mailed to all 1714 general practitioners in 200 UK practices selected randomly from 3 groups classified as the bottom, middle, and top fifths of prescribing costs. Personal and practice characteristics were elicited. The clinicians were then asked whether they agreed with a series of statements about prescribing attitudes and behaviors. The response rate was 64%.

Findings.—In a multivariate logistic regression analysis, frequent contact with a drug company representative correlated significantly with a greater willingness to prescribe new drugs. Physicians with frequent contact were also significantly more willing to agree to prescribe a drug not clinically indicated because the patient requested it. These physicians also had greater dissatisfaction with specialists whose consultations offered advice only, and receptiveness to drug advertising and promotional materials from drug companies.

Conclusions.—Compared with general practitioners who report less frequent contacts with drug company representatives, those reporting weekly contacts were more likely to develop habits that lead to unnecessary prescribing. Further research on the nature of the relationship between general practitioners and drug company representatives is needed to help define policies that encourage more cost-effective prescribing.

▶ Watkins et al confirm what most pharmaceutical companies already know: that physicians who interact with sales representatives tend, either consciously or unconsciously, to be quite accommodative in prescribing their products. The thin line between medical education and medical marketing was discussed in several articles in the same issue of the *British Medical Journal* and may involve drug company interaction with patient support groups as well.[1-4]

B. H. Thiers, MD

References

1. Moynihan R: Who pays for the pizza? Redefining the relationships between doctors and drug companies. 1: Entanglement. *BMJ* 326:1189-1192, 2003.
2. Moynihan R: Who pays for the pizza? Redefining the relationships between doctors and drug companies. 2: Disentanglement. *BMJ* 326:1193-1196, 2003.
3. Wager E: How to dance with porcupines: Rules and guidelines on doctors' relations with drug companies. *BMJ* 326:1196-1198, 2003.
4. Herxheimer A: Relationships between the pharmaceutical industry and patients' organizations. *BMJ* 326:1208-1210, 2003.

Validity of Indirect Comparison for Estimating Efficacy of Competing Interventions: Empirical Evidence From Published Meta-analyses
Song F, Altman DG, Glenny A-M, et al (Univ of Birmingham, England; Inst of Health Sciences, Oxford, England; Univ Dental Hosp of Manchester, England)
BMJ 326:472-476, 2003   12–9

Background.—The most valid evidence for the relative efficacies of different interventions comes from well-designed, randomized, controlled trials. However, not all competing interventions have been compared directly in randomized studies. The validity of adjusted indirect comparisons was determined by using data from published meta-analyses of randomized studies.

Methods.—Forty-four published meta-analyses were identified and data extracted. The analysis included direct comparisons of different interventions in randomized studies and adjusted indirect comparisons in which 2 interventions were compared through their relative effect versus a common comparator. Discrepancies between the direct and adjusted indirect comparison were determined by the difference between the 2 estimates.

Findings.—In general, the results of adjusted indirect comparisons did not differ significantly from those of direct comparisons. In 3 of the 44 comparisons, there was a significant discrepancy between the direct and adjusted indirect estimates. The statistical conclusions from direct and adjusted indirect comparisons showed moderate agreement. The discrepancy direction between the 2 estimates was not consistent.

Conclusions.—Adjusted indirect comparisons usually, though not always, agree with the findings of direct comparisons in randomized trials. In the absence of adequate direct evidence from randomized studies, adjusted indirect comparisons may provide useful or supplementary information on the relative efficacies of different interventions. The validity of the adjusted indirect comparisons relies on the internal validity and similarities of the studies included.

▶ This article addresses the difficulty in assessing the relative efficacy of competing interventions when they have not been subjected to head-to-head comparison in randomized trials. Song et al demonstrate that results of adjusted indirect comparisons usually, but not always, agree with those of head-to-head randomized trials. As expected, the internal validity and similarity of the trials under consideration have an impact on the validity of these adjusted indirect comparisons.

B. H. Thiers, MD

Survey of Claims of No Effect in Abstracts of Cochrane Reviews

Alderson P, Chalmers I (UK Cochrane Centre, Oxford, England)
BMJ 326:475, 2003   12–10

Introduction.—Because it is impossible to prove a negative or that 2 treatments have the same effects, the possibility of a small difference between 2 treatments can never be excluded. Claims of no effect or no difference may cause patients to be exposed to harmful interventions or to be denied potentially beneficial ones, and promising research avenues may be overlooked. To determine the prevalence of claims of no effect or difference, the first 2 issues of the *Cochrane Database of Systematic Reviews* were examined.

Methods.—A total of 989 complete reviews appeared in issue 1, 2001, and 80 reviews were published for the first time in issue 2, 2002. Sections headed "Main Results" and "Reviewers' Conclusions" were extracted and assessed.

Results.—Claims of no effect or difference were made in 240 (22.5%) Cochrane abstracts published in 2001 and in 19 (13.3%) first published in 2002, a −9.2% difference in proportions. Thus, inappropriate claims of no effect or no difference occurred in about one fifth of the abstracts of Cochrane reviews.

Discussion.—The claims of no effect or no difference in abstracts of reviews published in the *Cochrane Database of Systematic Reviews* may have resulted from careless wording. Such errors, which have been reported to the relevant editorial teams, appear to be decreasing. Phrases such as "no significant differences were detected" or "there is insufficient evidence either to support or to refute" are recommended alternatives.

▶ Stating that "it is impossible to prove a negative or that two treatments have the same effect," the authors argue that it is never correct to claim that treatments have no effect or that there is no difference in the effects of treatments. They stress the importance of qualifying terms such as *clinical* or *statistical significance* in describing the results of clinical trials.

B. H. Thiers, MD

13 Drug Actions, Reactions, and Interactions

Absence of Cross-Reactivity Between Sulfonamide Antibiotics and Sulfonamide Nonantibiotics

Strom BL, Schinnar R, Apter AJ, et al (Univ of Pennsylvania, Philadelphia; Pfizer, New York)

N Engl J Med 349:1628-1635, 2003   13–1

Background.—The safety of sulfonamide nonantibiotic agents in patients with previous allergic reactions to sulfonamide antibiotics has not been established (Table 1). The risk of allergic reactions within 30 days after receiving a sulfonamide nonantibiotic was investigated in a retrospective cohort study.

Methods.—Data were obtained from the General Practice Research Database in the United Kingdom. Patients with previous hypersensitivity after receiving a sulfonamide antibiotic and patients with no such response were compared.

Findings.—Ten percent of 969 patients who had had allergic reactions after previously receiving a sulfonamide antibiotic had an allergic reaction af-

---

TABLE 1.—Sulfonamide Nonantibiotic Drugs

Acetazolamide	Cyclopenthiazide	Glyburide	Probenecid
Acetohexamide	Dapsone	Glymidine	Quinethazone
Bendroflumethiazide	Diazoxide	Hydrochlorothiazide	Sulfasalazine
Benzthiazide	Dichlorphenamide	Hydroflumethiazide	Sulthiame
Bumetanide	Furosemide	Indapamide	Tolazamide
Chlorothiazide	Glibornutide	Mefruside	Tolbutamide
Chlorpropamide	Gliclazide	Methyclothiazide	Torsemide
Chlorthalidone	Glimepiride	Metolazone	Xipamide
Clopamide	Glipizide	Piretanide	
Clorexolone	Gliquidone	Polythiazide	

ter subsequent sulfonamide nonantibiotic use compared with 1.6% of 19,257 patients who had had no allergic reaction after previous sulfonamide antibiotic use. The former group had an adjusted odds ratio of 2.8 (95% CI, 2.1-3.7). The risk of allergic reactions was even higher after penicillin use in patients with a previous hypersensitivity reaction to a sulfonamide antibiotic compared with patients without this history: the odds ratio was 3.9 (95% CI, 3.5-4.3). The risk of an allergic reaction after receiving a sulfonamide nonantibiotic was lower among patients with previous hypersensitivity to sulfonamide antibiotics than among patients with a history of hypersensitivity to penicillins: the odds ratio was 0.6 (95% CI, 0.5-0.8).

Conclusions.—Hypersensitivity after sulfonamide antibiotic use is associated with a subsequent reaction to such agents. This relationship seems to be the result of a predisposition to allergic reactions rather than the result of cross-reactivity with sulfonamide-based agents.

▶ The cross-reactivity between sulfonamide antibiotics and sulfonamide nonantibiotics is of importance to dermatologists. The findings of this article suggest that, for example, patients with dermatitis herpetiformis may attempt treatment with dapsone even with a history of a documented reaction to a sulfonamide antibiotic. If dapsone does, however, cause a reaction, it may simply reflect that individual's predisposition to allergic drug reactions in general, rather than any specific cross-reactivity with sulfonamide-based drugs.

B. H. Thiers, MD

Inhaled or Systemic Corticosteroids and the Risk of Hospitalization for Hip Fracture Among Elderly Women

Lau E, Mamdani M, Tu K (Univ of Toronto; Inst for Clinical Evaluative Sciences, Toronto; Toronto Western Hosp)
Am J Med 114:142-145, 2003   13–2

Introduction.—High-dose, long-term systemic corticosteroid therapy leads to bone loss and increased fracture risk in postmenopausal women, but the risks of inhaled corticosteroid use are uncertain. A retrospective cohort study examined the effects of inhaled and systemic corticosteroids on the incidence of hospitalization for hip fracture in women aged 66 years or older.

Methods.—Women included in the analysis were identified using the Ontario (Canada) Registered Persons Database. The Canadian Institute for Health Information provided data on hip fractures and comorbid conditions; medications prescribed were obtained from the Ontario Drug Benefit database. Excluded were women who had been hospitalized within 5 years for hip fracture, epilepsy, trauma, pathologic fracture, or certain cancers. Four drug groups were studied: inhaled corticosteroids, systemic corticosteroids, proton pump inhibitors (not known to be associated with hip fractures), and estrogen replacement (a potentially protective therapy). The observation period extended from January 1, 1993, to March 31, 2000.

Results.—Each of the 4 drug groups included more than 24,000 women; mean ages of the groups ranged from 71.4 to 75.6 years. Medical conditions and the use of other medications varied among the drug groups. During follow-up, 931 hip fractures occurred. The incidence was highest in women who used systemic corticosteroids (12.1 per 1000 person-years) and lowest in those who used estrogen (3.1 per 1000 person-years). The risk of hip fractures did not differ significantly between users of proton pump inhibitors and users of inhaled corticosteroids (10.7 vs 9.6 per 1000 person-years).

Conclusion.—Systemic but not inhaled corticosteroids were associated with an increased risk of hip fractures in elderly women. In contrast to a previous report linking inhaled corticosteroid use with hip fracture, this study included a large sample and controlled for comorbid conditions and medications that might affect the risk of hip fracture.

▶ Dermatologists have some concern over the systemic effects of topical corticosteroids when they are applied to large areas of the skin over an extended time duration. Unfortunately, the findings of this study, while reassuring, are not directly comparable to therapy with topical corticosteroids. It would be quite helpful if such a study was done with dermatology patients to assess the effects of topically applied corticosteroids on bone mineral density and the risk of fractures.

B. H. Thiers, MD

Effect of Non-steroidal Anti-inflammatory Drugs on Risk of Alzheimer's Disease: Systematic Review and Meta-analysis of Observational Studies
Etminan M, Gill S, Samii A (Royal Victoria Hosp, Montreal)
BMJ 327:128-131, 2003   13–3

Background.—There are limited pharmacologic treatments available for Alzheimer's disease. However, recent observational studies have shown that the use of nonsteroidal anti-inflammatory drugs (NSAIDs) may protect against the development of the disease. It is not known whether this benefit is a class effect or whether it is restricted to specific agents. The role of aspirin in particular has been examined. The risk of Alzheimer's disease in users of all NSAIDs and users of aspirin was quantified, and whether duration of use has any influence on the protective effect against Alzheimer's disease in these subjects was investigated.

Methods.—This systematic review and meta-analysis examined observational studies published from 1996 to October 2002 that investigated the role of NSAID use in the prevention of Alzheimer's disease. The studies were identified through searches of MEDLINE, EMBASE, International Pharmaceutical Abstracts, and the Cochrane Library.

Results.—Nine studies examined the use of all NSAIDs in adults older than 55 years. Six of these were cohort studies with a total of 13,211 participants, and 3 were case-control studies with 1443 participants. The pooled relative risk of Alzheimer's disease among NSAID users was 0.72 (95% confidence interval [CI], 0.56-0.94), with a risk of 0.95 (95% CI, 0.70-1.29) among short-term users (less than 1 month) and a risk of 0.83 (95% CI, 0.65-1.06) and 0.27 (95% CI, 0.13-0.58) among intermediate-term (less than 24 months) and long-term (more than 24 months) users, respectively. The pooled relative risk in the 8 studies that examined aspirin users was 0.87 (95% CI, 0.70-1.07).

Conclusion.—NSAIDs may provide some protection against the development of Alzheimer's disease. However, the appropriate dosage and duration of drug use and the risk-to-benefit ratios have not been determined.

▶ NSAIDs are commonly used in dermatology, and the findings reported by Etminan et al suggest a possible additional benefit in preventing Alzheimer's disease. These investigators found that the use of NSAIDs seemed to lower the risk of developing Alzheimer's disease in patients more than 55 years of age. The benefits appeared to be greater the longer the drugs were used. The appropriate dose, duration, and risk-benefit ratio of the use of NSAIDs in this clinical setting remain to be determined. Also needing further study is whether the various classes of NSAIDs differ in their purported ability to prevent Alzheimer's disease and whether aspirin differs from other NSAIDs in terms of effectiveness.[1,2]

B. H. Thiers, MD

References

1. Ho L, Purohit D, Haroutunian V, et al: Neuronal cyclooxygenase 2 expression in the hippocampal formation as a function of the clinical progression of Alzheimer disease. *Arch Neurol* 58:487-492, 2001.
2. Cryer B, Feldman M: Cyclooxygenase-1 and cyclooxygenase-2 selectivity of widely used nonsteroidal anti-inflammatory drugs. *Am J Med* 104:413-421, 1998.

Nonsteroidal Anti-inflammatory Drugs and the Risk of Parkinson Disease
Chen H, Zhang SM, Hernán MA, et al (Harvard Med School, Boston; Massachusetts Gen Hosp, Boston)
Arch Neurol 60:1059-1064, 2003   13–4

Background.—In animal models of Parkinson disease (PD), nonsteroidal anti-inflammatory drugs (NSAIDs) have been found to decrease dopaminergic neuron degeneration. However, there have been no epidemiologic studies on the relationship between NSAID use and PD risk. Possible associations between nonaspirin NSAID or aspirin use and the risk of PD were investigated.

Methods.—Data were obtained on cohorts of 44,057 men and 98,945 women enrolled in the Health Professionals Follow-up Study, 1986 to 2000, and the Nurses' Health Study, 1980 to 1998. The cohorts were free of PD, stroke, and cancer on study enrollment.

Findings.—Four hundred fifteen incident cases of PD were documented during follow-up. Participants reporting regular nonaspirin NSAID use at study enrollment had a lower PD risk than those without regular use. The pooled multivariate relative risk was 0.55. Compared with nonusers, men and women taking 2 or more aspirin tablets per day had a nonsignificantly lower risk of PD, the relative risk being 0.56.

Conclusions.—Regular users of nonaspirin NSAIDs have a 45% lower risk of PD than do nonusers. A similar risk reduction was documented among persons taking 2 or more aspirin tablets per day compared with non-users.

▶ The results are similar to previous observations that NSAIDs may reduce the risk of Alzheimer disease (Abstract 13–3).[1] This suggests a possible neuroprotective effect of this class of drugs.

B. H. Thiers, MD

Reference

1. in t'Veld BA, Ruitenberg A, Hofman A, et al: Nonsteroidal antiinflammatory drugs and the risk of Alzheimer's disease. *N Engl J Med* 345:1515-1521, 2001.

Exposure to Non-steroidal Anti-inflammatory Drugs During Pregnancy and Risk of Miscarriage: Population Based Cohort Study

Li D-K, Liu L, Odouli R (Kaiser Permanente, Oakland, Calif)
BMJ 327:368-371, 2003

13–5

Introduction.—A recent case-control trial reported a link between the use of prescribed nonsteroidal anti-inflammatory drugs (NSAIDs) and miscarriage. The effect of NSAIDs on the risk of miscarriage was examined by analyzing data from the Kaiser Permanente Medical Care Program, a large health care delivery system in the San Francisco area.

Methods.—A total of 1055 pregnant women were recruited and interviewed immediately after a positive pregnancy test regarding their prenatal use of NSAIDs, aspirin, and paracetamol (acetaminophen) in a population-based cohort investigation. The median gestational age at trial entry was 40 days. The primary outcome measure was pregnancy outcomes up to 20 weeks' gestation.

Results.—Fifty-three women (5%) reported prenatal NSAID use around the time of conception or during pregnancy. After adjusting for potential confounders, prenatal NSAID use was linked with an 80% increased risk of miscarriage (adjusted hazard ratio, 1.9; 95% confidence interval, 1.0-3.2). The correlation was stronger if the initial NSAID use was around the time of conception or if NSAID use lasted for over a week. Prenatal aspirin use was similarly linked with increased risk of miscarriage, regardless of timing and duration of use.

Conclusion.—There was a link between the prenatal use of NSAIDs and aspirin and increased risk of miscarriage. These findings need to be verified in trials designed specifically to examine the apparent correlation; nevertheless, it may be prudent for physicians and women who are planning to become pregnant to be aware of this potential risk and avoid using NSAIDs around the time of conception.

▶ A previous study that reported an increased risk of miscarriage with NSAID use during pregnancy was compromised by its reliance on linkage of data from registers. This population-based cohort study provides stronger evidence for an association between NSAID and aspirin use and miscarriage. The highest risk of miscarriage was with NSAID use around the time of conception, a finding that supports the hypothesis that normal implantation is altered by these drugs. Acetaminophen did not appear to have an effect on the risk of miscarriage.

B. H. Thiers, MD

Gastrointestinal Safety of NO-Aspirin (NCX-4016) in Healthy Human Volunteers: A Proof of Concept Endoscopic Study
Fiorucci S, Santucci L, Gresele P, et al (Università di Perugia, Italy; Università degli Studi di Milano, Italy; Nicox SA, Sophia Antipolis, France)
Gastroenterology 124:600-607, 2003   13–6

Background.—A major disadvantage of aspirin use is its potential for severe adverse gastrointestinal effects. Nitro-aspirin (NCX-4016) is a derivative of aspirin that releases nitric oxide (NO) and has antiplatelet activity. The effects of NCX-4016 on gastrointestinal mucosa and platelet functions in healthy individuals were investigated in a parallel-group, double-blind, placebo-controlled study.

Methods.—Forty healthy volunteers were assigned randomly to 7 days of treatment with NCX-4016, equimolar doses of aspirin, or placebo. Upper endoscopies were conducted before and at the end of treatment. Gastroduodenal lesions were graded using a predefined scoring system.

Findings.—The mean mucosal endoscopic injury scores were 0.63 on day 7 in the placebo group, 11 in individuals given 200 mg aspirin twice daily, and 16.1 in those given 420 mg aspirin twice daily. By contrast, NCX-4016 was nearly free of gastric and duodenal toxicity and had total gastric and duodenal endoscopic scores of 1.38 and 1.25, respectively. NCX-4016 inhibited arachidonic acid–induced platelet aggregation and serum thromboxane B_2 and platelet thromboxane B_2 production induced by arachidonic acid to a degree similar to aspirin.

Conclusions.—These data show that adding an NO-donating moiety to aspirin produces a new chemical entity that almost completely avoids gastrointestinal damage while maintaining cyclo-oxygenase (COX)-1 and platelet inhibitory activity.

▶ Although the COX-2 inhibitors are associated with a significant reduction in major gastrointestinal adverse events, they do not affect platelet aggregation; thus, they do not confer cardioprotective benefits.[1,2] The observations of Fiorucci et al suggest that the addition of NO-releasing activity to aspirin results in a new chemical entity that maintains COX-1 and platelet inhibitory activity with little gastrointestinal toxicity. To determine whether long-term administration of this drug is truly as effective and safer than aspirin while maintaining its cardioprotective qualities will require long-term clinical trials.[3] It should be emphasized that this was only a 1-week study; thus, any conclusions based on its results should be considered preliminary at best.

B. H. Thiers, MD

References

1. FitzGerald GA, Patrono C: The coxibs, selective inhibitors of cyclooxygenase-2. *N Engl J Med* 345:433-442, 2001.
2. Bombardier C, for the VIGOR Study Group: Comparison of upper gastrointestinal toxicity of rofecoxib and naproxen in patients with rheumatoid arthritis. *N Engl J Med* 343:1520-1528, 2000.
3. Peura DA: Mandate to modify a medicinal mantra: Maybe not yet? *Gastroenterology* 124:842-844, 2003.

Cervical Cancer and Use of Hormonal Contraceptives: A Systematic Review

Smith JS, Green J, Berrington de Gonzalez A, et al (Internatl Agency for Research on Cancer, Lyon, France; Cancer Research UK Epidemiology Unit, Oxford, England; Inst of Cancer Research, Sutton, Surrey, England; et al)
Lancet 361:1159-1167, 2003   13–7

Introduction.—The most important cause of cervical cancer appears to be persistent infection with certain sexually transmitted, high-risk types of human papillomavirus (HPV). Recent studies suggest that the risk of cervical cancer is increased in HPV-DNA–positive women who use oral contraceptives for more than 5 years. This relationship was examined in a review of published studies.

Methods.—A MEDLINE search (January 1966 to July 2002) and references cited in identified studies were used to retrieve peer-reviewed articles that reported on the duration of use of hormonal contraceptives. Results were combined to assess the relationship between invasive and in situ cervical cancer and the duration and recency of use of these contraceptives, with particular attention to HPV infection.

Results.—Twenty-eight eligible studies (24 case-control and 4 cohort) included a total of 12,531 women with invasive or in situ cervical cancer. Two of the studies were restricted to women who were positive for HPV. When all findings were combined, the relative risk of cervical cancer increased with increasing duration of hormonal contraceptive use. Relative risks were 1.1 for durations of less than 5 years, 1.6 for 5 to 9 years, and 2.2 for 10 or more years. When analysis was limited to HPV-positive women, relative risks were 0.9, 1.3, and 2.5, respectively. Findings were generally similar for invasive and in situ cervical cancers, for squamous cell and adenocarcinoma and, when adjustment was made for HPV status, for number of sexual partners, cervical screening, smoking, or use of barrier contraceptives.

Discussion.—The use of hormonal contraceptives for periods longer than 5 years was found to be associated with an increased risk of cervical cancer. Because study designs varied and there was evidence of statistical heterogeneity between studies, the magnitude of the summary relative risks should be interpreted with caution. Available data could not determine whether risk is reduced after women discontinue the use of hormonal contraceptives.

▶ Prolonged intake of hormonal contraceptives has been associated with an increased risk of cervical cancer. However, how long this increased risk remains after their use has been discontinued is unknown. Limited published data suggest that the risk might decline after cessation of oral contraceptive administration, although the analysis of the data is hampered by the different methods employed in various studies and the lack of published information cross-classifying women by duration of use and time since last use.

B. H. Thiers, MD

Angioedema and Oral Contraception
Bouillet L, Ponard D, Drouet C, et al (CHU de Grenoble, France; Hôpital Edouard-Herriot, Lyon, France)
Dermatology 206:106-109, 2003   13–8

Background.—The use of oral contraceptives (OCs) can induce attacks of both hereditary and acquired forms of angioedema (ANE). A group of patients with ANE beginning during OC use and disappearing after OC discontinuation was reported.

Methods and Findings.—The 5 patients were seen between 1996 and 2001. Symptoms appeared 6 to 18 months after OC initiation. The mean age at symptom onset was 24.6 years. The patients reported relapsing swelling of the lips, hands, neck, and feet. Two patients had larygneal edema that necessitated hospitalization. Another patient reported attacks of abdominal pain. The diagnoses were made 2 months to 10 years after symptom onset. Serum values were normal for C4, C1q, carboxypeptidase N, and C1Inh antigen. In none of the patients was C1Inh antibody detected. However, C1Inh activity was reduced to 23% to 89% of normal values. The C1Inh serpin function, assessed by immunoblot, failed with a substantially cleaved C1Inh protein and an impaired association with C1s. When the OC was discontinued, C1Inh activity and serpin function returned to normal.

Conclusions.—These 5 patients had ANE beginning after OC initiation and disappearing after OC discontinuation. The mechanism underlying this phenomenon is not understood, but it may result from negative modulation of C1Inh expression by androgens or an imbalance between coagulation proteins favoring C1Inh cleavage by its target proteases.

Recurrent Episodes of Skin Angioedema and Severe Attacks of Abdominal Pain Induced by Oral Contraceptives or Hormone Replacement Therapy

Bork K, Fischer B, Dewald G (Johannes-Gutenberg Univ, Mainz, Germany; Univ of Bonn, Germany)

Am J Med 114:294-298, 2003   13–9

Background.—Recurrent angioedema is characterized by skin swelling, colicky attacks of abdominal pain, and life-threatening laryngeal edema. It is either hereditary or acquired. Anecdotal reports suggest that it may be associated with the use of oral contraceptives (OC) and hormone replacement therapy (HRT). Interactions between these medications and different types of recurrent angioedema were investigated in a large cohort of women.

Methods and Findings.—Five hundred sixteen women with recurrent angioedema underwent a medical examination and were classified by angioedema type, using standard criteria (Table 1). Two hundred twenty-eight (44%) of the women had used OC or HRT. This subgroup included 45% of women with urticaria-related angioedema, 22% with idiopathic angioedema, 17% with hereditary angioedema type III, 14% with hereditary angioedema type I, and 2% with angioedema induced by angiotensin-converting enzyme inhibitors. In 46 women (20%), OC or HRT led to angioedema attacks. This subgroup included 63% of the women with hereditary angioedema type I, 62% with hereditary angioedema type III, and 4% with idiopathic angioedema. Twenty-six of these 46 women had symptoms occurring for the first time after the use of these medications. In the remaining 20, preexisting recurrent angioedema markedly worsened.

Conclusions.—These data show that OC and HRT can induce or exacerbate symptoms of hereditary angioedema type I or III or idiopathic an-

---

TABLE 1.—Classification of Recurrent Angioedema

---

1. Hereditary angioedema due to deficiency of C1 inhibitor protein and activity (hereditary angioedema type I)
2. Hereditary angioedema due to deficiency of C1 inhibitor activity (hereditary angioedema type II)
3. Hereditary angioedema with normal C1 inhibitor activity in women (hereditary angioedema type III)
4. Acquired angioedema due to increased consumption of C1 inhibitor or autoantibody formation (acquired angioedema types I and II)
5. Recurrent angioedema due to angiotensin-converting enzyme inhibitors or angiotensin II-receptor antagonists
6. Urticaria-related angioedema
7. Idiopathic angioedema

gioedema. However, many women with recurrent angioedema can tolerate these medications without adverse effects.

▶ Although OC or HRT can induce or exacerbate symptoms of type I or type III hereditary angioedema, estrogen administration does not always result in the appearance or worsening of symptoms. Such disparate responses may be explained by genetic polymorphisms in the kinin system, and information about such polymorphisms might help identify women whose angioedema might be aggravated by administration of estrogen-containing medications.

B. H. Thiers, MD

Dose-Dependent Severe Cutaneous Reactions to Imatinib
Ugurel S, Hildenbrand R, Dippel E, et al (German Cancer Research Ctr, Heidelberg; Univ Hosp of Mannheim, Germany)
Br J Cancer 88:1157-1159, 2003   13–10

Background.—Imatinib is a protein kinase inhibitor used to treat chronic myelogenous leukemia and gastrointestinal stromal tumors. It is generally well tolerated, but imatinib can cause severe cutaneous reactions that may require drug discontinuation. Four patients with advanced melanoma who experienced severe cutaneous adverse events during imatinib therapy are described.

 Case Reports.—Four patients (1 man and 3 women, 41-71 years old) with advanced melanoma began receiving imatinib, 400 mg twice daily, as part of a phase II trial. Within the first 2 weeks of therapy, 3 patients had a moderate to strong cutaneous reaction with a macular or urticarial pattern. The eruptions began on the face and trunk and spread to the extremities, and were so severe in 2 patients that that imatinib dosage had to be reduced by 50%. The cutaneous eruptions regressed in all 3 patients within 2 to 3 weeks. Thereafter, the dosage was escalated to 600 mg/d in the 2 patients whose dose had been reduced to 400 mg/d. However, dose escalation to 600 mg/d resulted in a resurgence of the skin eruptions, and the dosage was again reduced to 400 mg/d.

 Histologic analysis showed a cutaneous reactivity pattern different from that of allergic hypersensitivity, with loose mononuclear cells infiltrating the dermis in a perivascular pattern. There was marked edema of the upper dermis and, surprisingly, an increased number of mast cells.

Conclusion.—In these 4 patients with advanced melanoma, imatinib triggered dose-dependent adverse cutaneous reactions that were severe enough to require dosage reduction in 2 patients. These data and other reports suggest that, to minimize the risk of cutaneous reactions, imatinib should be administered at low to intermediate doses (200-600 mg/d) whenever possible.

Gynaecomastia in Men With Chronic Myeloid Leukaemia After Imatinib

Gambacorti-Passerini C, Tornaghi L, Cavagnini F, et al (Natl Cancer Inst, Milan, Italy; San Gerardo Hosp, Monza, Italy; Univ of Milano Bicocca, Monza, Italy; et al)

Lancet 361:1954-1956, 2003   13–11

Background.—Imatinib inhibits cKit and platelet-derived growth factor receptor (PDGFR) expression in the testes. A possible association between gynecomastia and imatinib therapy in men with chronic myeloid leukemia was investigated.

Methods.—Sex hormone concentrations were measured in 38 men (median age, 50 years) with chronic myeloid leukemia, both before (n = 21) and during (n = 38) a median 25.5 months of imatinib therapy (400-800 mg/d). Hormones assayed included follicle-stimulating hormone, luteinizing hormone, β human chorionic gonadotropin, 17-β-estradiol, progesterone, dehydroepiandrosterone, 17-hydroxyprogesterone, testosterone, free testosterone, androstenedione, and prolactin. Subjects were evaluated at each clinic visit for the development of gynecomastia.

Results.—During imatinib treatment, 92% of the subjects had abnormally low testosterone levels, 73% had low free testosterone levels, 49% had high progesterone levels, and 42% had high 17-hydroxyprogesterone levels. Seven of the subjects (18%) developed gynecomastia after 5 to 13 months of imatinib therapy. Multivariate analyses showed a significant correlation between hormonal abnormalities (ie, low testosterone plus high progesterone) and the presence of gynecomastia. The effect was dose-dependent and was stronger at dosages of more than 600 mg/d than at dosages of 400 mg/d.

Conclusion.—Imatinib has a dose-dependent association with the development of gynecomastia in men with chronic myeloid leukemia. This effect is likely due to imanitib's inhibition of cKit and PDGFR in the testes and the resultant reduction in testosterone production.

▶ Imatinib is commonly prescribed for the treatment of chronic myeloid leukemia, and its utility in the treatment of other forms of neoplasia is the subject of intense investigation. As use of imatinib will likely increase significantly in future years, dermatologists need to be aware of its associated cutaneous side effects. Moreover, the ability of imatinib to reduce testosterone production may lead to new avenues of research into the treatment of disorders of the pilosebaceous apparatus.

B. H. Thiers, MD

Adverse Drug Events in Ambulatory Care

Gandhi TK, Weingart SN, Borus J, et al (Brigham and Women's Hosp, Boston; Beth Israel Deaconess Med Ctr, Boston; Harvard Risk Management Found, Boston; et al)

N Engl J Med 348:1556-1564, 2003   13–12

Introduction.—Adverse drug-related events are known to occur frequently among inpatients, but few data are available on adverse drug events in the outpatient setting in which most prescribing occurs. The frequency, type, severity, and consequences of adverse drug events among outpatients were examined.

Methods.—Data were collected between September 1999 and March 2000 from 4 adult primary care practices in Boston, all of which were affiliated with academic medical centers. Two practices were hospital based and 2 were community based; 1 of each practice type used a basic computerized system for prescribing drugs, and 1 of each used a manual system. A total of 1202 outpatients received at least 1 prescription during 4-week study periods. Possible adverse events reported by patients were reviewed independently by 2 physicians.

Results.—Surveys were completed by 661 patients (55%) at 2 weeks and by 600 of these responding patients (91%) at 3 months. A total of 181 adverse drug events were experienced by 162 patients. Twenty-four events (13%) were serious but not fatal or life-threatening; 51 (28%) were ameliorable; and 20 (11%) were preventable. Thirty-two ameliorable events (63%) were attributed to physician failure to respond to medication-related symptoms and 19 (37%) were attributed to patient failure to report symptoms to the physician. Drugs often involved in adverse events were selective serotonin-reuptake inhibitors (10%), β-blockers (9%), angiotensin-converting-enzyme inhibitors (8%), and nonsteroidal anti-inflammatory agents (8%). Adverse events occurred at similar rates in computerized and manual prescription systems. Only the number of drugs taken was significantly associated with adverse events.

Conclusion.—Over a 3-month period, 25% of the outpatients at 4 primary care practices had adverse drug events. An important cause was failure of communication between physician and patient. Preventable adverse events resulted from prescribing errors, many of which could be avoided by the use of advanced computerized systems.

▶ Typically, adverse drug reactions occur in elderly patients who take multiple medications from several physicians who do not communicate well with one another. Although various computer programs have been designed to identify potential harmful interactions, such strategies often fail when prescriptions are filled at multiple pharmacies.[1] As demonstrated by Gandhi et al, many adverse events are preventable and may involve either errors of commission or errors of omission (eg, missed opportunities to prescribe appropriate medications, such as failure to recommend β-blockers or aspirin to patients discharged after a myocardial infarction). Better physician-physician and physician-patient communication is essential to reduce the frequency of adverse drug reactions.

B. H. Thiers, MD

Reference

1. Tierney WM: Adverse outpatient drug events—A problem and an opportunity. *N Engl J Med* 348:1587-1589, 2003.

Excess Length of Stay, Charges, and Mortality Attributable to Medical Injuries During Hospitalization
Zhan C, Miller MR (Ctr for Quality Improvement and Patient Safety, Rockville, Md; Johns Hopkins Univ, Baltimore, Md)
JAMA 290:1868-1874, 2003   13–13

Introduction.—Medical injuries are a known and important hazard within the health care system, yet little is understood about their prevalence, adverse outcomes, or effective prevention. What is considered preventable is debatable. Medical injures may occur during all stages of care, vary widely in nature, and are relatively infrequent. Patient Safety Indicators (PSIs) were used to evaluate length of stay, charges, and deaths attributable to medical injuries during hospitalization.

Methods.—The Agency for Healthcare Research and Quality (AHRQ) PSIs were used to identify medical injuries in 7.45 million hospital discharge abstracts from 994 acute care hospitals across 28 states in 2000 in the AHRQ Healthcare Cost and Utilization Project Nationwide Inpatient Sample database. The primary outcome measures were length of stay, charges, and mortality that were documented in hospital discharge abstracts and were attributable to medical injuries according to 18 PSIs.

Results.—Excess length of stay due to medical injuries ranged from 0 days for injury to a neonate to 10.89 days for postoperative sepsis. Excess charges ranged from $0 for obstetric trauma (without vaginal instrumentation) to $57,727 for postoperative sepsis. The rate of excess mortality ranged from 0% for obstetric trauma to 21.96% for postoperative sepsis ($P < .001$). After postoperative sepsis, the second most serious event was postoperative wound dehiscence (9.42 extra days in the hospital, $40,323 in excess charges, and 9.63% in attributable mortality). Infection resulting from medical care was linked with 9.58 extra days, $38,656 in excess charges, and 4.31% in attributable mortality.

Conclusion.—Medical injuries in hospitals pose a substantial risk to patients and are associated with significant costs to society.

▶ As discussed in an accompanying editorial,[1] to be maximally useful, tools to measure patient safety should focus on preventable injuries. Such injuries—in contrast to complications secondary to appropriately administered, clearly risky therapies—offer viable targets for quality improvement. Unfortunately, such preventable injuries are technically difficult to identify.

B. H. Thiers, MD

Reference

1. Weingart SN, Iezzoni LI: Looking for medical injuries where the light is bright. *JAMA* 290:1917-1919, 2003.

14 Miscellaneous Topics in Clinical Dermatology

Influence of Controllable Lifestyle on Recent Trends in Specialty Choice by US Medical Students

Dorsey ER, Jarjoura D, Rutecki GW (Evanston Northwestern Healthcare, Chicago; Northwestern Univ, Chicago; Northeastern Ohio Univ, Rootstown)

JAMA 290:1173-1178, 2003   14–1

Background.—Lifestyle concerns may be an increasingly important variable in medical students' choice of specialty. The role of lifestyle characteristics in recent changes in the specialty preferences of senior medical students in the United States was investigated.

Methods.—Data were obtained from the National Resident Matching Program, the San Francisco Matching Program, and the American Urological Association Matching Program from 1996 to 2002. Previous research was used to define specialty lifestyles and controllable versus uncontrollable characteristics. Log-linear models were developed to investigate specialty preferences along with the controllability of the specialty, its income and work hours, and the number of years of graduate medical education needed to attain it.

Findings.—Senior medical students' specialty preferences, determined by the distribution of applicants in certain specialties, showed significant changes between 1996 and 2002. The log-linear model showed that a controllable lifestyle explained 55% of the variability in specialty preferences between 1996 and 2002, after adjustment was made for income, work hours, and years of graduate education needed.

Conclusions.—A controllable lifestyle was strongly associated with the recent specialty preferences of US senior medical students. This may result in a significant change in the composition of the physician workforce over time.

Trends in Career Choice by US Medical School Graduates

Newton DA, Grayson MS (East Carolina Univ, Greenville, NC; New York Med College, Valhalla, NY)

JAMA 290:1179-1182, 2003   14–2

Background.—The percentage of US medical student graduates seeking a career in primary care has declined recently. Trends in the career choices of graduates of allopathic US medical schools were investigated.

Methods.—Data were obtained from the Association of American Medical Colleges Graduation Questionnaire (AAMC GQ), the National Resident Matching Program, and the National Graduate Medical Education census. The numbers of US medical doctors entering residencies in primary care, general or subspecialty surgical, and nonprimary care and nonsurgical specialties between 1987 and 2002 were analyzed.

Findings.—In 1987, 49.2% of graduates matched to internal medicine, pediatrics, or family medicine. In the early 1990s, the percentage of students matching to primary care specialties declined. In 1998, it peaked at 53.2%, then decreased to 44.2% in 2002. Concurrent with this decrease, AAMC GQ data revealed a reduction in graduates' interest in primary care careers, from 35.6% in 1999 to 21.5% in 2002. Between 1987 and 2002, the total percentage matching to general or subspecialty surgical residences remained stable, from 11% to 12%, respectively. During this time, those graduates matching to emergency medicine and plastic surgery increased. Anesthesiology, pathology, and psychiatry were more variable.

Conclusions.—Career choice distribution among specialties between 1987 and 2002 has varied widely. Health care professionals will continue to debate the appropriate specialty mix within the workforce.

▶ What are the implications of the preference of medical students for specialties characterized by a controllable lifestyle? The most obvious of these would be an alteration in the distribution of physicians by specialty. This has become clearly apparent by the trend in recent years for significantly lower fill rates in primary care residency programs (Abstracts 14–1 and 14–2). Factors such as the increasing number of women in medicine, the rising level of debt among medical students, and the changing reward structure in medicine (reflected, at least in part, by decreased professional autonomy) suggest that income and lifestyle will remain important variables in the career choices of medical students well into the future.

B. H. Thiers, MD

Virtual Outreach: Economic Evaluation of Joint Teleconsultations for Patients Referred by Their General Practitioner for a Specialist Opinion
Jacklin PB, for the Virtual Outreach Project Group (London School of Hygiene and Tropical Medicine; et al)
BMJ 327:84-88, 2003   14–3

Background.—From 6% to 10% of patient visits to primary care physicians result in referral to a specialist. Studies in The Netherlands have found that the involvement of general practitioners in joint consultation with specialists can provide better patient management, reductions in hospital follow-up appointments, fewer tests and investigations, improved health status 1 year after referral, and fewer subsequent referrals to the hospital. The use of videoconferencing for such joint consultation would eliminate the need for all participants to be in the same location. It would also potentially provide the same benefits in communication without increasing costs. The use of videoconferencing in the United Kingdom was examined to test the hypothesis that videoconferencing, compared with conventional outpatient consultation, would incur no additional costs to the National Health Service (NHS), would reduce costs to patients, and would reduce absences from work by patients and their caregivers.

Methods.—A cost consequences study was conducted in parallel with a randomized controlled trial in 2 hospitals and in 29 general practices in rural and urban areas. A total of 2094 patients were included, with 1051 assigned to videoconferencing (virtual outreach) and 1043 to standard outpatient appointments. The main outcome measures were NHS costs, patient costs, health status, time spent attending the index consultation, and patient satisfaction.

Results.—The overall 6-month costs were greater for the virtual outreach consultations than for conventional outpatient appointments (£724 vs £625 per patient). Virtual outreach costs remained greater than those of conventional outpatient consultation costs even when analysis was restricted to resource items deemed attributable to the index consultation. In both analyses, the index consultation was the source of the excess cost. Savings to patients in terms of cost and time occurred in both analyses, with a difference in mean total patient cost of £8. There was also a reduction in the time lost from work in the virtual outreach group, with a difference in mean cost of £11.

Conclusion.—These findings do not support the main hypothesis that videoconferencing for consultations between general practitioners and specialists would be cost neutral for the NHS. However, the findings support the contention that such virtual outreach would reduce costs to patients and losses in productivity.

▶ This study from England investigated the cost-effectiveness of joint teleconsultations between the patient, the general practitioner, and hospital specialists. Surprisingly, the investigators found that virtual outreach consultations actually incurred greater costs to the payer (in this case, the NHS) than standard outpatient appointments. However, such consultations did result in cost and time savings to patients. Nevertheless, the authors concluded that adoption of virtual outreach could not be justified on economic grounds alone.

B. H. Thiers, MD

A Double-blind Randomized Trial of 0.1% Tacrolimus vs 0.05% Clobetasol for the Treatment of Childhood Vitiligo
Lepe V, Moncada B, Castanedo-Cazares JP, et al (Universidad Autónoma de San Luis Potosi, Mexico)
Arch Dermatol 139:581-585, 2003   14–4

Background.—Vitiligo is a common idiopathic, acquired, depigmenting disease of the skin and hair. An estimated 0.5% of the world's population is affected. Tacrolimus is an immunosuppressor macrolide lactone that can inhibit activation and maturation of T cells by blocking the action of calcineurin and interleukin (IL)-2, IL-4, and IL-5 transcription. The efficacy and safety of topical 0.1% tacrolimus was compared with those of 0.05% clobetasol propionate in children with vitiligo.

Methods.—This randomized double-blind trial included 20 children who had received no topical or systemic therapy for 2 months before enrollment. Two symmetric lesions of comparable size and evolution were selected on each patient and treated with topical tacrolimus and clobetasol, respectively, for 2 months.

Findings.—Some repigmentation occurred in 90% of the patients. The mean percentages for tacrolimus and clobetasol were 41.3% and 49.3%, respectively. Clobetasol treatment in 3 patients was associated with atrophy and in 2 patients with telangiectasias. Tacrolimus treatment caused a burning sensation in 2 patients.

Conclusions.—Tacrolimus appears to be almost as effective as clobetasol in restoring skin color in children with vitiligo. Because tacrolimus is not associated with atrophy or other adverse effects, this agent may be very useful for younger patients and for sensitive areas of the skin. Tacrolimus should also be considered for treatments of other skin disorders that are currently treated with topical steroids for prolonged periods.

▶ The authors demonstrate in a small group of patients that 0.1% tacrolimus ointment appears to have efficacy similar to 0.05% clobetasol cream for the treatment of vitiligo. From personal experience, I would agree that tacrolimus works well for vitiligo on the face, where it is likely that the thin stratum corneum allows penetration of the rather large tacrolimus molecule. Tacrolimus obviously has the advantage of causing no atrophy, and it appears to be safe to use on the eyelids. Class II or III topical corticosteroids are likely to be more efficacious for the treatment of lesions on the trunk or extremities. Long-term use of class I corticosteroids, such as clobetasol, should generally be avoided in children, particularly on the face and eyelids.

S. Raimer, MD

Epidermal Grafting in Vitiligo: Influence of Age, Site of Lesion, and Type of Disease on Outcome

Gupta S, Kumar B (Postgraduate Inst of Med Education and Research, Chandigarh, India)
J Am Acad Dermatol 49:99-104, 2003   14–5

Background.—Various factors influence the success of suction blister epidermal grafting. The effects of patient age, vitiligo patch site, and disease type on the outcome of suction blister epidermal grafting were determined in a series of patients.

Methods.—In addition to a retrospective analysis of the case series, the literature on suction blister epidermal grafting was reviewed. Published studies of this procedure in 10 or more patients were included. All patients had stable, recalcitrant vitiligo.

Findings.—In the authors' series, 117 of 143 patients undergoing the procedure had a follow-up time of 6 months or longer. In previous publications, information on various factors was limited. In the current case series, the success rate for patients with generalized disease was 53%, and for those with segmental or focal disease, it was 91%. In the literature, these rates were 61% and 88%, respectively.

In the current case series, the success rate in patients younger than 20 years was 82%, and for those aged 20 years or older, it was 58%. In the literature, these rates were 100% and 66%, respectively. Success rates did not differ significantly by body site in the current case series or in the literature. Adverse reactions included hyperpigmentation in 32% of the current case series and 17% of the previously reported patients. Infection occurred in 6% and 0%, respectively, and contact dermatitis in 1% and 1% (Table 2).

Conclusion.—The results of suction blister epidermal grafting appear to be better in segmental/focal vitiligo than in the generalized type of disease and in persons younger than 20 years compared with those aged 20 or older.

TABLE 2.—Adverse Effects of Epidermal Grafting in the Current Study and in Reported Literature

	Adverse Effect	Current Study N = 117 No. (% [95% CI])	Literature N = 462 No. (% [95% CI])
Recipient area	Hyperpigmentation	38 (32.4 [24-41])	76 (16.5 [13-20])
	Infection	7 (6 [2-10])	0 (0 [0-0])
	Contact dermatitis	1 (1 [0-2])	5 (1 [0-2])
	Scarring/keloid formation	0 (0 [0-0])	3 (0.6 [0-1.2])
Donor area	Hyperpigmentation	117 (100 [100-100])	111 (24 [20-28])
	Koebner phenomenon	0 (0 [0-0])	8 (1.7 [0.5-3])

Abbreviation: CI, Confidence interval.

However, the location of the vitiligo patch did not significantly affect treatment outcomes.

▶ Epidermal grafting has been shown to be effective in treating recalcitrant vitiligo. In this report, the authors summarize their experience and that of others with this technique. Successful repigmentation was observed in 64% to 87% of patients. Young patients and those with localized vitiligo appeared to achieve better results. The location of the vitiligo did not appear to affect the outcome. Patients with disease that had been stable for at least a year had better results and were less likely to koebnerize. The most common side effect of the procedure was hyperpigmentation of the donor and recipient sites.

P. G. Lang, Jr, MD

Cutaneous Involvement in Sarcoidosis: Analysis of the Features in 170 Patients
Yanardağ H, Pamuk ÖN, Karayel T (Univ of Istanbul, Turkey; Univ of Trakya, Edirne, Turkey)
Respir Med 97:978-982, 2003   14–6

Introduction.—Nearly 25% of patients with sarcoidosis are reported to have skin involvement. A group of patients with sarcoidosis and skin involvement was retrospectively evaluated for clinical and demographic features and compared with a group of patients with sarcoidosis but no skin involvement.

Methods.—During a 36-year period, 516 patients (341 females and 175 males) seen at the study institution fulfilled clinical features, radiologic features, or both, of sarcoidosis. Skin involvement was present in 170 (32.9%) of these patients (136 females and 34 males); the remaining 346 patients served as controls. Chest radiographs were classified as stage I (bilateral hilar lymphadenopathy [BHL]), stage II (BHL plus pulmonary parenchymal infiltration), or stage III (parenchymal involvement infiltration without BHL).

Results.—Erythema nodosum, the most common skin lesion, was found in 20.5% of patients. Also present were skin plaques and subcutaneous nodules (4.3% of cases), maculopapular eruptions (3.7% of cases), and scar lesions (2.9% of cases). All types of skin lesions were more frequent in female patients than in male patients. Pulmonary parenchymal involvement was most common in patients with lupus pernio (64.3% of the 14 cases) and in those with scar lesions (40% of the 15 cases); only 10.4% of patients with erythema nodosum had parenchymal involvement.

Discussion.—In this series of patients with sarcoidosis, approximately one third had skin involvement. Women were more likely than men to have skin involvement, and among patients with skin lesions, parenchymal involvement was more frequent in those with lupus pernio and scar lesions, and less frequent in those with erythema nodosum, maculopapular eruptions, and plaque lesions.

▶ Most interesting was the authors' observation in patients with sarcoidosis of a positive association between lupus pernio, scar lesions, and parenchymal lung disease. In contrast, patients with erythema nodosum were less likely to have parenchymal lung involvement.

B. H. Thiers, MD

Nephrogenic Fibrosing Dermopathy: A Novel Cutaneous Fibrosing Disorder in Patients With Renal Failure
Swartz RD, Crofford LJ, Phan SH, et al (Univ of Michigan, Ann Arbor)
Am J Med 114:563-572, 2003   14–7

Background.—Nephrogenic fibrosing dermopathy, a newly identified cutaneous fibrosing disorder, is characterized by acute onset of induration involving the upper and lower limbs of patients with renal failure. Typically, affected patients develop painful, acute, lumpy, plaque-like induration on the legs and occasionally also on the arms or torso (Fig 1). Some degree of functional disability results. The etiology, pathogenesis, associated clinical conditions, and ultimate course of 1 series of patients were reported.

Methods and Findings.—Thirteen patients diagnosed as having nephrogenic fibrosing dermopathy at 1 center were included in the review. Renal failure predated nephrogenic fibrosing dermopathy in all patients. Eight

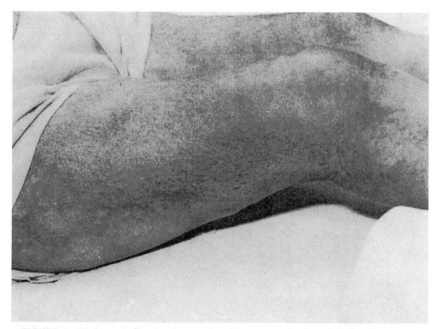

FIGURE 1.—Nephrogenic fibrosing dermopathy with pronounced induration and a "lumpy" appearance in some areas. The lesions were painful and impeded mobility. (Reprinted from Swartz RD, Crofford LJ, Phan SH, et al: Nephrogenic fibrosing dermopathy: A novel cutaneous fibrosing disorder in patients with renal failure. *Am J Med* 114:563-572, 2003. Copyright 2003, with permission from Excerpta Medica Inc.)

TABLE 5.—Differential Diagnosis for Nephrogenic Fibrosing Dermopathy

Disease	Appearance of Skin Lesions	Affected Sites	Laboratory Findings	Associated Diseases or Disorders	Histologic Findings
Nephrogenic fibrosing dermopathy	Nodular/lumpy induration, may coalesce to form plaques	Lower limbs, occasionally upper limbs, hands, and trunk	Elevated serum creatinine level	Acute or chronic renal failure	Diffuse fibroblastic proliferation in dermis, usually with subcutaneous extension; minimal to slight increase in dermal mucin; minimal inflammation
Scleromyxedema	Papulonodules coalescing to form plaques	Hands, elbows, upper trunk, frequently neck and face	Serum paraprotein	Occasional multiple myeloma, or involvement of viscera, muscle, or peripheral nerves	Diffuse fibroblastic proliferation in dermis with focal moderate to marked dermal mucinous deposition; often slight perivascular chronic inflammation
Scleredema	Peau d'orange skin thickening and induration	Face, neck, and upper trunk; infiltration of viscera and tongue; effusions	Sometimes serum paraprotein detected	Upper respiratory tract infection, diabetes, multiple myeloma (rarely)	Fibroblasts in normal numbers; scant chronic inflammation sometimes present in superficial dermis; dermis markedly thickened by abundant mucin and abnormally thickened collagen
Pretibial myxedema	Pink or yellow waxy plaques or nodules	Anterolateral lower legs; rarely arms, abdomen, neck, and face	Abnormal thyroid function test; positive for long-acting thyroid stimulator antibody	Hyperparathyroidism (Grave's disease)	Fibroblasts in normal numbers; no substantial inflammation; collagen bundles separated by abundant mucin; hyperkeratotic epidermis with follicular plugging
Systemic sclerosis/scleroderma (diffuse and limited types)	Diffuse edema ± telangiectasias; sclerotic and atrophic in late stage	Hands, feet, extremities, trunk and face (diffuse type); hands and face (limited type)	Antinuclear and anticentriole anticentriole antibody; anti-Scl 70 and anti-RNA polymerase III in diffuse type; anticentromere antibodies in limited type	Syndrome of calcinosis, Raynaud's phenomenon, esophageal dysmotility, sclerodactyly, telangiectasia, and pulmonary hypertension (limited type); pulmonary, cardiac, gastrointestinal, and renal involvement in diffuse SS; sometimes overlap syndrome with other connective tissue disease features such as Sjögren's syndrome and myositis (mixed connective tissue disease)	Early changes include an infiltrate of lymphocytes, histiocytes, and plasma cells in dermis, around blood vessels and along dermal-subcutaneous junction with slight fibroblastic proliferation; established lesions show thickened, swollen eosinophilic collagen fibers and atrophy of periadnexal adipocytes; fibroblasts are usually sparse

Eosinophilic fasciitis	Tender peau d'orange swelling and induration, groove sign	Extremities and trunk; spares hands and feet	Elevated erythrocyte sedimentation rate and gamma globulins, peripheral blood eosinophilia	Sometimes, serious hematologic abnormalities	Changes localized to deep dermis and fascia, sometimes extending into muscle; fibrinoid necrosis and myxoid change with eosinophils, lymphoid follicles, and chronic inflammation in early lesions; marked fibrosis and sclerosis in later stage
Spanish toxic oil syndrome	Erythematous rash (initially); edema and diffuse induration (early); firm atrophic plaques (late)	Upper and lower limbs and face	Peripheral eosinophilia; elevated serum major basic protein at all phases of disease	Acute and chronic multisystem dysfunction (pneumonitis, myositis, thromboembolism, contractures, muscle atrophy, neuropathy)	Superficial and deep perivascular chronic inflammation, endothelial swelling and hyperplasia; obliteration of vascular lumina; dermal and subcutaneous fibrosis; atrophy of sweat glands and hair follicles
Eosinophilia-myalgia syndrome	Edema, erythematous rash, peau d'orange swelling and induration	Extremities and trunk; early edema but otherwise sparing of hands and feet	Peripheral eosinophilia	Disabling generalized myalgias, pneumonitis, myocarditis, neuropathy, and encephalopathy	Perivascular and diffuse mixed inflammation with eosinophils in deep dermis, fascia, and perimysium; narrowed or occluded vascular lumina; fibrosis and sclerosis in later stage

(Reprinted from Swartz RD, Crofford LJ, Phan SH, et al: Nephrogenic fibrosing dermopathy: A novel cutaneous fibrosing disorder in patients with renal failure. *Am J Med* 114:563-572, 2003. Copyright 2003, with permission from Excerpta Medica Inc.)

were undergoing chronic hemodialysis and 2 were undergoing chronic peritoneal dialysis. The remaining 3 had acute renal failure and had not had dialysis before dermopathy developed. Other serious underlying medical conditions were present in most patients. Many were taking erythropoietin or cyclosporine before the onset of dermopathy.

In patients who had undergone transplantation, no histocompatibility antigens correlated with the disease. Histopathologic analysis of skin biopsy specimens obtained 7 to 180 days after dermopathy onset indicated possible tissue reaction to injury. The presence of smooth muscle actin-positive myofibroblasts was also noted.

Conclusion.—Nephrogenic fibrosing dermopathy can be distinguished from other sclerosing or fibrosing skin disorders by distinctive clinical and histopathologic findings and its occurrence in patients with renal failure (Table 5). In this series, other than renal failure, the patients had no clinical risk factors or laboratory findings in common. Fibrogenic cytokines may be involved in the development of this condition.

▶ Swartz et al confirm that this "scleromyxedema-like cutaneous disease," initially observed exclusively in hemodialysis patients, can occur in patients with renal failure who have never been dialyzed. They found no consistent laboratory abnormality associated with this condition and suggest that myofibroblasts found in biopsy specimens may have pathogenetic significance.

B. H. Thiers, MD

Clinical and Pathologic Features of Nephrogenic Fibrosing Dermopathy: A Report of Two Cases
Streams BN, Liu V, Liégeois N, et al (Massachusetts Gen Hosp, Boston; Lahey Clinic, Burlington, Mass; Harvard Med School, Boston)
J Am Acad Dermatol 48:42-47, 2003   14–8

Introduction.—Nephrogenic fibrosing dermopathy (NFD) is a recently described skin disorder that occurs in patients with a history of renal disease. Forty-nine cases have been reported in the United States and Europe since 1997. In those affected, large areas of hardened skin with fibrotic plaques develop on the trunk and extremities.

> *Case 1.*—Woman, 40, was on hemodialysis for 9 months when diffuse skin thickening appeared on her lower extremities and rapidly spread to her back, upper chest, and upper extremities. No systemic symptoms were present, but painful flexion contractures of her fingers and knees limited mobility. The patient's medical history included long-standing insulin-dependent diabetes mellitus, chronic renal failure, rejection of a cadaver renal allograft, and renal cell carcinoma. A skin biopsy specimen showed spindle cell proliferation intercalated between compact, clefted collagen bundles.

TABLE 1.—Clinical and Pathologic Features of Various Fibrosing Disorders

Disorder	Clinical Manifestations	Pathologic Features
NFD	Firm, thickened skin; papules and subcutaneous nodules on extremities and trunk, usually spares face	Early lesions–thickened collagen bundles with clefts, CD-34+ spindle cells, mucin; late lesions–less clefting, less mucin, fewer CD-34+ cells, elongated elastic fibers
Scleromyxedema	Waxy, linear distributed papules on face, neck; furrowing of glabella, sclerodactyly, IgG λ paraproteinemia	Thickened collagen bundles, stellate fibroblasts, mucin pools, lymphoplasmacytic infiltrate
Morphea	Ivory-colored plaque with violaceous borders	Thickened, homogenized collagen bundles, lymphoplasmactyic infiltrate, atrophy of adnexae; mucin in early stages
Systemic sclerosis	Diffuse, local, or widespread sclerosis; subcutaneous calcification, telangiectases; facial constriction; pulmonary, cardiac, renal involvement	Thickened, homogenized collagen bundles, vascular fibrosis, calcification, less inflammation than seen in morphea
Porphyria cutanea tarda	Bullae, scarring, and milia in photosensitive areas, hypertrichosis, skin thickening	Noninflammatory subepidermal bulla with festooning base; caterpillar bodies; IgG, C3 deposition at dermoepidermal junction and in vessel walls in linear fashion
Eosinophilic fasciitis	Swelling, induration of extremities, "groove sign"	Hyalinization and thickening of collagen of deep fascia and subcutis; focal collections of eosinophils
Eosinophilia-myalgia syndrome	Diffuse skin thickening, papules, on trunk and face, sparing hands and feet; peripheral eosinophilia, severe myalgias	Thickened collagen bundles, variable inflammatory infiltrate, mucin deposition
β₂-Microglobulin amyloidosis	Variable features including papules, nodules, and hyperpigmentation	Hyaline deposits in dermis, which stain with Congo red, crystal violet, thioflavin T
Fibroblastic rheumatism	Symmetric polyarthritis of distal, extremities, cutaneous nodules, sclerodactyly, Raynaud's phenomenon	Thickened collagen bundles in deep dermis, subcutis; spindle cell proliferation, decreased elastic fibers

(Reprinted by permission of the publisher from Streams BN, Liu V, Liégeois N, et al: Clinical and pathologic features of nephrogenic fibrosing dermopathy: A report of two cases. *J Am Acad Dermatol* 48:42-47, 2003. Copyright 2003 by Elsevier.)

Case 2.—Woman, 37, was seen for a diffuse eruption of firm yellow and tan plaques of 1 year's duration. Lesions had appeared on the palms, elbows, and lower extremities and were accompanied by joint stiffness and pain. The patient had been receiving hemodialysis for chronic renal failure, secondary to glomerulonephritis, for about 18 months. Additional medical problems included pulmonary embolism and seropositive rheumatoid arthritis. Examination of a skin punch-biopsy specimen revealed plump spindle cells interwoven among sclerotic bundles and around adipose tissue.

Discussion.—Initial reports of NFD involved patients undergoing renal dialysis, yet renal insufficiency in general appears to be a unifying feature among known cases. Clinical features of NFD include skin thickening with hyperpigmentation, firm papules and plaques on the extremities and trunk, stiffening of the hands, and flexion contractures. There are similarities, but also clear differences, between scleromyxedema and NFD (Table 1). In both cases reported here, there were no systemic symptoms other than joint stiffness and pain, and laboratory studies were unremarkable. Cutaneous manifestations improved in 2 previously reported patients when renal abnormalities were corrected.

Nephrogenic Fibrosing Dermopathy (Scleromyxedema-like Illness of Renal Disease)
Mackay-Wiggan JM, Cohen DJ, Hardy MA, et al (Columbia Univ, New York)
J Am Acad Dermatol 48:55-60, 2003   14–9

Introduction.—A report published in 2000 described a new disorder that was termed "scleromyxedema-like cutaneous disease." All 14 affected patients had undergone hemodialysis or renal transplantation and had acute-onset thickening and hardening of the skin. Four additional cases are reported here, together with a review of features of the disease and possible causes.

Case Report.—A white woman, 49, had a history of antiphospholipid antibody syndrome and renal insufficiency. After an episode of acute superimposed on chronic renal insufficiency, erythematous indurated plaques developed on her arms, hands, thighs, and back. The disease progressed, causing contractures of the hands, incapacitating pain, and a burning sensation. Hemodialysis was started 9 months after onset of the skin lesions. A skin biopsy specimen revealed a sparse interstitial fibrohistiocytic infiltrate, and mucin deposition was confirmed with alcian-blue stain. Antinuclear antibody testing and anticardiolipin antibody testing produced positive results. No evidence of peripheral eosinophilia or plasmacytosis was found. Treatment with plasmapheresis and photophoresis was yielding slow improvement when the patient died secondary to aspergillus sinusitis, cerebrovascular hemorrhage, and congestive heart failure.

Discussion.—The clinical features of this disease entity are distinctive and consistent. Onset of the skin lesions was acute, and laboratory studies were unrevealing, although all 4 patients had positive anticardiolipin antibodies. No lesions were located on the head and neck, as usually seen in scleromyxedema. Patients with scleromyxedema usually have a detectible paraprotein, but none was found in the 18 patients with this new entity. Scleromyxedema-like illness of renal disease, or nephrogenic fibrosing dermopathy, has no single, universally effective therapy, and the incidence, prevalence, and cause are unknown.

Scleromyxoedema-like Changes in Four Renal Dialysis Patients
Hubbard V, Davenport A, Jarmulowicz M, et al (Royal Free Hosp, London)
Br J Dermatol 148:563-568, 2003   14–10

Introduction.—Four patients undergoing renal dialysis experienced skin changes with both clinical and histologic features of scleromyxedema. All patients were affected during the 6-month period between August 2000 and February 2001, and no additional cases have been seen at the study institution. Findings in these patients are presented together with a comparison of their skin changes and those of classical scleromyxedema.

> *Case Report.*—Man, 36, had end-stage renal failure at age 18, a result of bilateral ureteric obstruction and reflux nephropathy. A cadaveric renal transplant performed in 1985 failed because of recurrent urinary tract infections. Hemodialysis was resumed until the time of a second cadaveric renal transplant, complicated by acute vascular rejection on the ninth postoperative day. An emergency transplant nephrectomy was performed and hemodialysis resumed. Two weeks after the failed transplant and 3 days after returning to hemodialysis, patches of erythematous, indurated skin appeared on the patient's legs, buttocks, and left arm. The dermal plaques were initially firm and well-defined, then became confluent and more widely distributed. Skin changes over the fistula (left) arm were most notable. A flexion contracture of the left elbow and fingers subsequently developed.

Observations.—Biopsy specimens from patients 1 and 2 showed a diffuse proliferation of spindle-shaped cells with ill-defined cytoplasmic membranes throughout the dermis. Immunohistochemical findings suggested that the spindle cells were fibroblasts. In contrast, minimal abnormalities were seen in biopsy specimens from patients 3 and 4. All 4 patients had normal immunoglobulins and were antinuclear antibody negative, and no infectious cause was identified. Plasma exchange, intralesional triamcinolone, and intralesional methotrexate were not effective treatments.

Discussion.—Features of skin lesions in these renal dialysis patients were similar, but not identical, to scleromyxedema. In addition, the systemic signs of scleromyxedema were absent. It is possible that the skin changes were precipitated by an unidentified environmental agent.

▶ There still appear to be more questions than answers regarding the entity that has come to be known as nephrogenic fibrosing dermopathy (Abstracts 14–8 to 14–10). Although many of the early cases were associated with hemodialysis, it has become clear that the condition occurs in patients with compromised renal function in general rather than specifically in patients on dialysis. No unifying etiologic agent has been defined; specifically, there are no specific autoantibodies or paraproteins associated with the condition, and no environmental toxin has been identified. There is no known effective treatment. The association with anticardiolipin antibodies reported by Mackay-Wiggan et al (Abstract 14–9) is a new observation and is of uncertain significance.

B. H. Thiers, MD

Brachioradial Pruritus: A Symptom of Neuropathy
Cohen AD, Masalha R, Medvedovsky E, et al (Ben-Gurion Univ of the Negev, Beer-Sheva, Israel)
J Am Acad Dermatol 48:825-828, 2003   14–11

Background.—Brachioradial pruritus (BRP) is a localized form of pruritus that affects the skin of the dorsolateral aspect of the arms. The pruritus appears during the summer and remits in the winter in some patients, whereas in other patients the disease remains stable throughout the year. Patients with BRP experience disturbing symptoms and present a therapeutic challenge because they do not respond to antipruritic treatments such as topical corticosteroids or antihistamines. The cause of BRP is controversial—some authors consider it to be a photodermatosis, whereas others have attributed BRP to compression of the cervical nerve roots. The results of electrophysiologic studies in a series of patients with BRP were presented.

Methods.—Electrophysiologic studies of the median, ulnar, and radial nerves were performed in 7 consecutive patients with BRP (5 men and 2 women). The patients had an average age of 58.3 years. The electrophysiologic studies included measurement of sensory and motor distal latency, conduction velocity and F responses of the median and ulnar nerves, and sensory distal latency of the radial nerves in both upper arms.

Results.—Four of 7 patients (57%) had abnormal F responses that were diagnostic for cervical radiculopathy, and 3 of these patients had prolonged distal latencies of the tested nerves, which may be interpreted as sensory motor neuropathy secondary to chronic radiculopathy. The fourth patient had polyneuropathy secondary to diabetes mellitus.

Conclusions.—BRP may be attributable to a neuropathy, such as chronic cervical radiculopathy. The possibility of an underlying neuropathy should be considered in the evaluation and treatment of all patients with BRP.

Brachioradial Pruritus: Cervical Spine Disease and Neurogenic/Neurogenic Pruritus

Goodkin R, Wingard E, Bernhard JD (Univ of Massachusetts, Worcester)
J Am Acad Dermatol 48:521-524, 2003   14–12

Introduction.—Patients with brachioradial pruritus (BRP) experience itching with such neuropathic features as burning, stinging, or pain. Many report relief from the application of ice packs or wet towels. These symptoms, and the lack of a recognizable skin condition, suggest an underlying abnormality in the skeletal or nervous system. The medical records of patients with BRP were retrospectively analyzed to determine whether a relationship exists between BRP and cervical spine disease.

Methods.—Patients were seen in the dermatology division of the study institution between 1993 and 2000. Data of interest were patient age and sex, duration of symptoms, history of cervical spine trauma, results of any available cervical spine radiographs, and response to treatment. In addition, MEDLINE was searched from 1966 to 2000 for patients with BRP.

Results.—Eleven of 22 patients in the study center database had cervical spine radiographs. All were found to have abnormalities of the cervical spine, particularly at C3 to C7. None had a history of neck injury. Four of 11 patients without radiographs had reported a history of cervical trauma. Patients ranged in age from 39 to 70; 15 were women and 7 were men. Bilateral BRP was present in 15, and duration of symptoms ranged from 2 months to 11 years. Helpful treatments included capsaicin, pramoxine, gabapentin, topical cooling, and cervical epidural injection. Thirty of 98 patients identified in the MEDLINE search had cervical spine disease detected at radiography.

Conclusion.—Some patients with BRP may have an underlying cervical spine disorder. In the literature review, the location of pruritus correlated with alteration in sensory innervation of the involved skin area in 13 of 30 patients. At the study institution, similar findings were present in all 11 patients with cervical spine radiographs. Patients with BRP may benefit from neurologic investigation and treatment.

▶ Certainly, a controlled study would be needed to confirm that the rate of cervical spine disease in patients with BRP is higher than in a matched group of asymptomatic individuals.

B. H. Thiers, MD

Autoantibodies to Extracellular Matrix Protein 1 in Lichen Sclerosus

Oyama N, Chan I, Neill SM, et al (Guy's, King's, and St Thomas' School of Medicine, London; Churchill Hosp, Oxford, England; St Thomas' Hosp, London)
Lancet 362:118-123, 2003   14–13

Background.—Lichen sclerosus is a common acquired inflammatory disorder of the skin and mucous membranes, with a prevalence that may be as high as 1 in 1000 persons. Women and girls are more commonly affected than men. Symptoms may include intractable itching and soreness, and the chronic inflammation of the skin and mucous membranes may lead to scarring. The etiology of lichen sclerosus is unknown, but HLA-subtype susceptibility and high rates of other autoimmune disorders in affected patients have led to suggestions that autoantibodies to specific mucocutaneous antigens are involved. The clinicopathologic similarities between lichen sclerosus and lipoid proteinosis, which results from loss-of-function mutations in extracellular matrix protein 1 (ECM1), suggest this protein as an autoantigen. Whether lichen sclerosus is associated with the presence of autoantibodies to ECM1 was determined.

Methods.—Serum antibody profiles were analyzed in 171 persons (86 with lichen sclerosus and 85 healthy controls) by immunoblotting of extracts from normal human skin and lipoid proteinosis skin, which lacked ECM1. A full-length glutathione-S-transferase fusion protein for ECM1 was generated to confirm specific immunoreactivity. Serum from patients with lichen sclerosus was affinity purified, and indirect immunofluorescence microscopy was performed on normal skin with or without preabsorption with recombinant ECM1.

Results.—Immunoblotting revealed IgG autoantibodies in 20 (67%) of 30 lichen sclerosus serum samples. The highest titer was 1 in 20. The bands were not detected in ECM1-deficient substrate. These samples and the samples from 56 other patients with lichen sclerosus showed immunoreactivity to the recombinant ECM1 protein (64 of 86 positive, or 74%). Only 6 of 85 samples from controls were positive. Affinity-purified IgG from serum of patients with lichen sclerosus labeled skin in a manner similar to that observed with a polyclonal antibody to ECM1. Positive staining was blocked by preabsorption with excess recombinant ECM1 protein.

Conclusions.—These findings provide insight into the diagnosis, monitoring, and treatment of lichen sclerosus and support the concept that a specific humoral immune response to ECM1 is involved in the etiology of this disease.

▶ The authors found circulating autoantibodies to a specific skin protein, ECM1, in most patients with lichen sclerosus. Importantly, this does not establish that these antibodies cause the disease, but the data do provide further evidence for humoral autoimmunity in the pathogenesis of this chronic inflammatory disorder. A question that still must be answered is whether the synthesis of these autoantibodies is a primary or secondary pathogenetic event or simply an epiphenomenon.

B. H. Thiers, MD

Childhood Vulvar Lichen Sclerosus: The Course After Puberty
Powell J, Wojnarowska F (Radcliffe Hosp, Oxford, England)
J Reprod Med 47:706-709, 2002   14–14

Introduction.—In adults, lichen sclerosus (LS) of the vulva is known to be associated with the development of squamous cell carcinoma (SCC). Recent research suggests that adolescent girls with childhood-onset LS might also be at risk for the development of vulvar SCC. Twenty-one postpubertal girls with LS who had been attending a pediatric vulvar clinic were assessed for current symptoms, treatment requirements, and related problems.

Methods.—All patients were examined for physical signs and had blood samples sent for immunogenetic analysis and autoantibody detection. Vulvar scrapings and urine were collected for herpesvirus DNA detection. A cohort of 251 postmenopausal adults and a group of 12 young adult premenopausal patients with LS who attended an adult vulvar dermatology clinic were asked to recall any childhood symptoms associated with LS.

Results.—Five of the 21 postpubertal girls with childhood-onset LS reported their symptoms were unchanged and 16 reported improvement; 11 of 16, however, did admit to using topical steroid preparations for occasional pruritus. Intermittent dysuria was also reported, but no problems were noted with menarche, coitus, pregnancy, or delivery. Physical examination revealed persistent signs of LS in 16 of 21 girls. Four of 12 young women with premenopausal LS recalled symptoms in childhood. In 1 case, LS appeared to have resolved at puberty, but vulvar SCC was subsequently diagnosed and the patient died at age 32 with widespread metastases. An unexpected finding was that only 5 of the 251 postmenopausal adults with LS could recall symptoms in childhood. Immunogenetic studies on 30 of 75 girls with LS confirmed a 67% association with HLA class DQ7, similar to that reported in adults with LS.

Conclusion.—Vulvar LS in prepubertal girls is common, but the condition often resolves during puberty. In this series of 21 girls, however, the signs of LS were persistent in 16. There is concern that without symptoms, such patients may not continue follow-up and may be at risk for the development of vulvar carcinoma in early adult life.

▶ In this study of girls with LS, it was noted that although symptoms improved with puberty in 75% of individuals, physical signs persisted in an equal number. Because of the potential to develop SCC of the vulva, girls affected by LS and their parents should be advised that regular examinations are important to detect possible early signs of malignancy.

S. Raimer, MD

How Common Is Obsessive-Compulsive Disorder in a Dermatology Outpatient Clinic?

Fineberg NA, O'Doherty C, Rajagopal S, et al (Queen Elizabeth II Hosp, Welwyn Garden City, England; Univ of Hertfordshire, Hatfield, England; Guy's Hosp, London)
J Clin Psychiatry 64:152-155, 2003   14–15

Background.—Only a small proportion of individuals with obsessive-compulsive disorder (OCD) receive appropriate treatment. Many affected individuals are ashamed of their symptoms and do not discuss them with physicians. Because of skin damage from excessive, ritualized washing or picking, a large number of individuals with OCD may seek care from dermatologists. Thus, the dermatology clinic may be a place for screening and identifying persons with OCD.

Methods.—Ninety-two consecutive patients referred to dermatologic practices were screened for *Diagnostic and Statistical Manual of Mental Disorders, Fourth Edition* (DSM-IV)-defined OCD. The Mini-International Neuropsychiatric Interview, the Yale-Brown Obsessive Compulsive Scale (YBOCS), and the 5-item screening questionnaire from the International Council on OCD were administered. Disease severity was rated on the YBOCS. Symptom profiles and dermatologic diagnoses were determined for patients with positive screening results.

Findings.—Twenty percent of the patients met DSM-IV criteria for the diagnosis of OCD. Seventeen of these 20 patients did not have a previous OCD diagnosis. The range and type of symptoms represented the normal clinical OCD spectrum. Most patients had more than 1 symptom. Checking, washing, and symmetry were common obsessions. The mean total YBOCS score indicated moderate disease severity. Forty percent of the patients with positive screening results had a score at or exceeding the group mean. Dermatologic diagnoses varied and were not directly related to OCD.

Conclusions.—A substantial proportion of patients referred to the dermatology clinic may have clinically relevant OCD. These findings suggest an opportunity for improving recognition and treatment of OCD.

▶ The results would have been more convincing if the investigators had included a control group or a comparable group of patients from a non-dermatology clinic. The authors readily admit that the numbers screened were relatively small by epidemiologic standards, and the results need to be confirmed in a larger population. Moreover, the brevity of the instruments used limited the amount of information obtained about screen-positive patients.

B. H. Thiers, MD

A New Cutaneous Sign of Mercury Poisoning

Dantzig PI (Columbia Univ, New York)
Ann Intern Med 139:78-80, 2003   14–16

Introduction.—Mercury poisoning is challenging to diagnose. The evaluation of 11 patients who contracted mercury poisoning by eating seafood was discussed.

Findings.—The patients were from 25 to 75 years old. Their pretreatment blood mercury levels ranged between 29.9 nmol/L and 94.7 nmol/L (mean, 49.9 nmol/L). Prior treatments included topical steroids (n = 9), oral steroids (n = 4), antihistamines (n = 2), and cyclosporine (n = 1); all were unsuccessful. Poisoning in all 11 patients was manifested by a specific eruption characterized by nonpruritic, discrete, flesh-colored, or slightly erythematous papules and papulovesicles that were visible on the palms of all patients, on the soles of the feet in 1 patient, and on the arms and trunk in 3 patients. The lesions were small (≤1 mm in diameter) and correlated with serum mercury levels; they resolved when mercury levels decreased. The duration of the eruption before diagnosis and start of treatment ranged from 1 week to 2 years. No excoriations or crusting were noted (Figure). Pathologic examination revealed spongiosis and a perivascular and diffuse dermal lymphocytic infiltrate, with immunohistochemical findings consistent with a mixed T-cell infiltrate composed of both helper and suppressor T cells. Direct immunofluorescence demonstrated focal antinuclear staining. Indirect immunofluorescence showed basal-cell cytoplasm antibodies, findings consistent with damage to basal cells caused by a specific cytotoxic agent. All patients were treated with a seafood-free diet, and 5 underwent chelation therapy with succimer (2,3-dimercaptosuccinic acid), 200 to 300 mg 3 times daily, for 1 to 6 months. Blood mercury levels, complete blood count, and chemistry profiles were evaluated every 3 to 4 weeks. The blood mercury levels decreased, and the eruptions cleared. The treatment was well tolerated, and no adverse

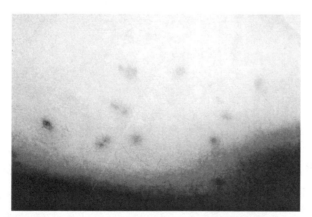

FIGURE.—The right arm of patient 11, showing discrete erythematous 1- to 2-mm papules. Note the lack of excoriations, oozing, or other eczematous changes. The crust represents a 2-mm biopsy specimen. (Courtesy of Dantzig PL: A new cutaneous sign of mercury poisoning. *Ann Intern Med* 139:78-80, 2003.)

reactions were noted. Two patients had noncutaneous symptoms that included dizziness, memory loss, and gastrointestinal bleeding.

Conclusion.—Mercury toxicity may be more prevalent than previously believed. Physicians need to be aware of the unique eruption that emerges as a specific toxic reaction to long-term mercury poisoning.

▶ The evidence for an association between mercury poisoning and the observed skin lesions may be circumstantial, but tuna fish has become a bit less popular in my house since this article appeared.

B. H. Thiers, MD

DERMATOLOGIC SURGERY AND CUTANEOUS ONCOLOGY

15 Photobiology and Photoprotection

Topical Ascorbic Acid on Photoaged Skin. Clinical, Topographical and Ultrastructural Evaluation: Double-blind Study vs Placebo
Humbert PG, Haftek M, Creidi P, et al (Univ of Franche-Comté, Besançon, France; INSERM U 346/CNRS, Lyon France; Univ of Liège, Sart Tilman, Belgium; et al)
Exp Dermatol 12:237-244, 2003   15–1

Background.—Research has demonstrated that vitamin C has antioxidant potential and activity in the collagen biosynthetic pathway. The photoprotective properties of vitamin C applied topically have also been reported, making this a possible candidate for use in preventing and treating skin aging. The efficacy and safety of a topically applied cream containing 5% vitamin C and its excipient were assessed.

Methods.—Twenty healthy women with photoaged skin on their lower neck and arms volunteered for the study. The 6-month side-by-side trial compared the action of vitamin C cream and its excipient. The women used the creams daily. Skin was assessed at baseline and at 3 and 6 months. Cutaneous biopsies were performed at the end of the study and examined by immunohistochemistry and electron microscopy.

Findings.—A dermatologist's clinical examination and the participants' self-assessment indicated a significant global improvement on the side treated with vitamin C compared with the control side. There was a highly significant increase in the density of skin microrelief and a reduction in deep furrows. Ultrastructural evidence of elastic tissue repair verified the favorable results of the clinical and skin surface examinations.

Conclusions.—The topical application of 5% vitamin C cream appears to be effective and well tolerated. In this series, improvement of photodamaged skin was apparent after 6 months. Treatment resulted in modifications of skin relief and ultrastructure, suggesting that topical vitamin C has positive effects on sun-induced skin aging.

▶ The authors report a possible role for topical application of vitamin C in the treatment of photoaging. Certainly, the results will need to be confirmed with larger studies. Explanations offered for the possible benefit of topical vitamin

C include its activity as a cofactor for enzymes, prolyl hydroxylase and lysyl hydroxylase, essential for collagen production, as well as the vitamin's ability to act as a free radical scavenger.

B. H. Thiers, MD

Assessment of Thickness of Photoprotective Lipsticks and Frequency of Reapplication: Results From a Laboratory Test and a Field Experiment

Maier H, Schauberger G, Brunnhofer K, et al (Univ of Vienna, Austria; Univ of Veterinary Medicine, Vienna, Austria)

Br J Dermatol 148:763-769, 2003   15–2

Introduction.—The thickness of the sunscreen layer applied by consumers under usual conditions has been ascertained for photoprotective lotions and creams. It has yet to be determined for photoprotective lipsticks. Lipstick thickness (area density) and frequency of application per day were evaluated for 2 commercially available photoprotective lipsticks, each having a different consistency.

Methods.—Both a laboratory test and a field experiment were performed. In the laboratory test, the applied lipstick thickness was considered to be the area density in mg/cm^2 for a group of 28 panelists under standardized conditions. In a separate group of 18 college students, the area density and frequency of application per day were evaluated for the 2 photoprotective lipsticks during a 6-day skiing course.

Results.—In the laboratory testing phase, the median of the area density for product A was 0.98 mg/cm^2 (95% confidence interval [CI], 0.66-1.65), and for product B, the median was 0.86 mg/cm^2 (CI, 0.63-1.40). Results in the field experiment showed the area density means for product A to be 1.58 mg/cm^2 (CI, 0.79-2.23) and 1.76 mg/cm^2 (CI, 1.16-3.50) for product B. Only 11% of all applications of lipstick A and 6% of all applications of lipstick B achieved the reference area density of 2.0 mg/cm^2. The difference between the median of the area density for lipstick A (firm consistency) and lipstick B (soft consistency) was not statistically significant. No statistically significant effect on the area density was seen for age, sex, photobiological skin type, or regular lipstick use. The median daily frequency of application was 2.2 and 3.0 times for lipstick A and lipstick B, respectively.

Conclusion.—Photoprotective lipsticks are applied in a much thinner layer than recommended by international guidelines (2 mg/cm^2). Sun care products with a high SPF are recommended to compensate for the influence of low-density application. Regular use and short-term reapplication should be emphasized.

▶ As with sunscreens for cutaneous use, the data suggest that frequent application of photoprotective lipsticks is desirable and that most patients do not apply the products in a thickness necessary for optimal protection.

B. H. Thiers, MD

Sunscreens Inadequately Protect Against Ultraviolet-A-Induced Free Radicals in Skin: Implications for Skin Aging and Melanoma?

Haywood R, Wardman P, Sanders R, et al (Mount Vernon Hosp, Middlesex, England)

J Invest Dermatol 121:862-868, 2003   15–3

Introduction.—The incidence of skin cancer continues to increase, even though the use of sunscreens has become more widespread. These preparations appear to reduce the incidence of basal and squamous cell tumors, but several studies suggest that sunscreen use is associated with an increased risk of melanoma. Sunscreens may be applied inadequately, and they are primarily designed to prevent UVB-associated burning and damage. A new method designed to establish the efficacy of sunscreens measures UVA-induced free-radical production.

Methods.—Because UVA-induced free-radical production is thought to contribute to UVA-related aging and malignant change, investigators applied 3 high-factor (20+) sunscreens that claim UVA protection to samples of white skin obtained at breast reduction surgery. Electron spin resonance spectroscopy was used to detect free radicals during irradiation of skin samples with UV levels comparable to solar intensities.

Results.—The 3 popular brands of sunscreen yielded similar results. At recommended application levels (≥ 2 mg/cm^2), the UV-induced free radicals were reduced by only about 55%. At the reported common usage, the reduction was only about 45%. A "free-radical protection factor" calculated on the basis of these results would be approximately 2, but less than 2 at typically used levels of application. Such a free-radical protection factor is substantially less than the erythema-based protection factors for these products.

Conclusion.—The UVA/free-radical protection currently provided by sunscreens is inadequate. High-factor sunscreens protect principally against UVB-induced erythema, and users may remain longer in the sun because of a false sense of security. White individuals, especially those with fairer skin types, should avoid prolonged sunbathing, even when a high-factor sunscreen has been applied.

▶ The results suggest that currently available sunscreens provide little protection against the damaging effects of UVA and against UVA-induced free-radical formation. The data support the argument of some dermatologists that users of high SPF factor sunscreens have an artificial sense of security that they are protected similarly against UVA, and thus may engage in outdoor activities that put them at an increased risk for skin cancer.

B. H. Thiers, MD

Prevention of Immunosuppression by Sunscreens in Humans Is Unrelated to Protection From Erythema and Dependent on Protection From Ultraviolet A in the Face of Constant Ultraviolet B Protection

Poon TSC, Barnetson RS, Halliday GM (Univ of Sydney, Australia)
J Invest Dermatol 121:184-190, 2003   15–4

Introduction.—Exposure to UV radiation results in immunosuppression, an important event in skin carcinogenesis. Sunscreens are advocated as an important means of preventing skin cancer, yet the incidence of skin cancer continues to rise. The only internationally recognized end point for the evaluation of sunscreen effectiveness is protection from erythema (primarily caused by UV-B) or sunburn as measured by the sun protection factor (SPF); however, little is known about the level of protection from immunosuppression provided by sunscreens. Six commercially available sunscreens were tested for their immune protection factor (IPF).

Methods.—A previously described in vivo human nickel contact hypersensitivity recall model of UV-induced immunosuppression was used to obtain UV dose responses (both with and without sunscreens) and to determine sunscreen IPF. Both SPF and IPF testing protocols used the same solar-simulated UV radiation source. Ninety-nine volunteers with nickel allergy and 98 volunteers without nickel allergy were studied. All sunscreens used in the study were labeled as broad spectrum, containing both UV-B and UV-A protective ingredients.

Results.—The pooled results of 15 volunteers were used to calculate IPF for each sunscreen. No correlation was observed between a sunscreen's IPF and its SPF, but IPF was significantly correlated to the UV-A protective capability of a sunscreen. Immune protection was thus independent of erythemal protection.

Discussion.—A sunscreen with exceptional UV-A protection provides better protection against immune suppression than against erythema, which is primarily caused by UV-B. All the sunscreens tested protected well in the UV-B region, but their UV-A protective abilities differed. Sunscreens should be labeled to indicate their IPF, as provided by UV-A protection, as well as their SPF.

▶ The authors demonstrate the importance of UV-A protection in guarding against immune suppression. Perhaps someday, sunscreens will be labeled with an IPF to give a more accurate assessment of protection from the damaging effects of UV light. Although it is tempting to assume that sunscreens that protect from UV-A might provide better protection against skin cancer, such a conclusion cannot be assumed without further experimental evidence.

B. H. Thiers, MD

Efficacy of Broad-Spectrum Sunscreens Against the Suppression of Elicitation of Delayed-Type Hypersensitivity Responses in Humans Depends on the Level of Ultraviolet A Protection
Moyal DD, Fourtanier AM (L'Oréal Recherche, Clichy, France)
Exp Dermatol 12:153-159, 2003   15–5

Introduction.—The issue of sunscreen protection against ultraviolet (UV)-induced immune suppression remains controversial. Previous studies emphasize that sunscreens containing both UVB and UVA filters provide better protection than those with UVB filters only. Moreover, a significant level of protection against UVA appears necessary to reach an immune protection factor as high as the sun protection factor (SPF). Two commercially available broad-spectrum sunscreens with the same SPF (15) but with different levels of UVA absorption were compared for their ability to prevent UV-induced delayed-type hypersensitivity (DTH) immunosuppression after exposure to a solar simulator.

Methods.—Volunteer participants were white men aged 18 to 40 years. All were in good health and had skin types II or III; none had had any sun exposure for at least 4 weeks prior to the study. The UV radiation dose required to induce significant DTH inhibition was first determined in several small groups of volunteers. The minimal immunosuppressive dose was found to be 2 minimal erythemal doses (2 MED), resulting in an average reduction of 36% in the DTH response. Both lower doses tested (0.5 and 1 MED) were ineffective.

Results.—Sunscreen-treated groups exposed to 1 MED × SPF doses showed no alteration in DTH response with either of the sunscreens. How-

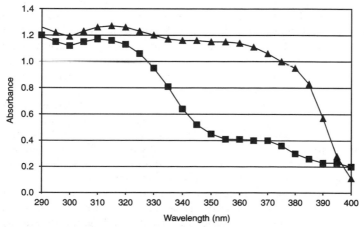

FIGURE 2.—Absorption spectra of products O (*squares*) and L (*triangles*) generated by spectroradiometric measurements between 290 and 400 nm according to the modified Diffey method. These spectra clearly show that the efficacy of product L is much higher than product O in the UVA range. (Courtesy of Moyal DD, Fourtanier AM: Efficacy of broad spectrum sunscreens against the suppression of elicitation of delayed-type hypersensitivity responses in humans depends on the level of ultraviolet A protection. *Exp Dermatol* 12:153-159, 2003.)

ever, after exposure to 2 MED × SPF, the DTH response was significantly suppressed (by 55.7%) in the group pretreated with a sunscreen offering little protection in the UVA range (product O). In contrast, the DTH response was unaltered in the group using the sunscreen with higher protection in the UVA range (product L).

Conclusion.—The SPF of a sunscreen product may not predict its ability to protect against UV-induced immune suppression. Although UV erythema may be similarly protected by products with equivalent SPFs, only products with greater efficacy in the UVA range (Fig 2) protect against immune suppression. Thus, specific information on the level of UVA protection is strongly needed.

▶ Protection against UVA, in addition to UVB, appears to be important in preventing UV-induced immunosuppression. Accurate methods of measuring UVA protection are needed, as this range of the UV spectrum, while a significant contributor to immune suppression, generates less clinically evident erythema than shorter UVB wavelengths.

B. H. Thiers, MD

A Commercial Sunscreen's Protection Against Ultraviolet Radiation-induced Immunosuppression Is More Than 50% Lower Than Protection Against Sunburn in Humans

Kelly DA, Seed PT, Young AR, et al (King's College London; St Thomas' Hosp, London)

J Invest Dermatol 120:65-71, 2003   15–6

Background.—The suppression of cutaneous cell-mediated immunity by exposure to 280 to 400 nm ultraviolet (UV) radiation plays an important role in the development of skin cancer. Sunscreens are widely advocated to protect against such cancer. However, if sunscreens' protection against immunosuppression is insufficient, an increased risk of skin cancer may result. The immunoprotection of a commercial sunscreen preparation with a sun protection factor of 15 was assessed.

Methods and Findings.—One hundred nineteen healthy, white-skinned persons volunteered for the study. Previously unexposed buttock skin was exposed to UV radiation. The sunscreen was found to absorb mainly UV-B. Absorption in the UV-A region was relatively poor. The sunscreen protected against erythema and immunosuppression. However, protection against immunosuppression was less than half that for erythema.

Conclusion.—These data support the use of sunscreen to reduce immunosuppression. However, protection against immunosuppression may be improved if sunscreens are formulated to provide equivalent protection against UV-B and UV-A.

▶ Like the article by Moyal et al (Abstract 15–5), this article emphasizes the importance of UV-A protection to maintain maximum immune responsiveness after exposure to UV radiation.

B. H. Thiers, MD

Past Exposure to Sun, Skin Phenotype, and Risk of Multiple Sclerosis: Case-Control Study

van der Mei IAF, Ponsonby A-L, Dwyer T, et al (Univ of Tasmania, Australia; Australian Natl Univ, Canberra, Australia; Canberra Hosp, Australia; et al)
BMJ 327:316-319, 2003   15–7

Background.—A striking epidemiologic characteristic of multiple sclerosis (MS) is its gradient of increasing prevalence with latitude. Whether previous high exposure to sun is associated with a decreased risk of MS was investigated in Tasmania.

Methods.—One hundred thirty-six patients with MS and 272 healthy persons chosen randomly from the community were included in the population-based study. The groups were matched by sex and year of birth. Tasmania, located at latitudes 41 to 43 degrees south, has a high MS prevalence at 75.6 per 100,000 persons. The diagnosis of MS was established by clinical and MR criteria.

Findings.—Higher sun exposure between 6 and 15 years of age correlated with a reduced risk of MS (adjusted odds ratio, 0.31). Greater exposure in winter appeared to be more important than greater exposure in summer. In addition, greater actinic damage correlated independently with a reduced MS risk (odds ratio, 0.32). There was a dose-response relation between MS and declining sun exposure between 6 and 15 years of age and with actinic damage.

Conclusions.—A decreased risk of MS appears to be associated with greater sun exposure during childhood and early adolescence. Insufficient ultraviolet radiation may affect the evolution of MS.

▶ Previous studies have shown that the prevalence of MS increases with latitude, an observation that has been attributed to differences in regional levels of ultraviolet radiation. van der Mei et al found a correlation between a reduced risk of MS, higher sun exposure during childhood and early adolescence, and greater actinic damage. They postulate that exposure to ultraviolet radiation has an inhibitory effect on autoimmune phenomena thought to play a role in the pathogenesis of the disease. Reduced levels of vitamin D in sunlight-deprived individuals might also be a contributing factor.

B. H. Thiers, MD

16 Nonmelanoma Skin Cancer

Identification of a Small Molecule Inhibitor of the Hedgehog Signaling Pathway: Effects on Basal Cell Carcinoma-like Lesions
Williams JA, Guicherit OM, Zaharian BI, et al (Curis Incorporated, Cambridge, Mass; Columbia Univ, New York; Stanford Univ, Calif)
Proc Natl Acad Sci U S A 100:4616-4621, 2003   16–1

Introduction.—The Hedgehog (Hh) protein family regulates numerous events in embryonic development, and aberrant activation of the Hh pathway in humans is associated with certain cancers. Among these is basal cell carcinoma (BCC), the most common cancer in the western world. Mutations of components of the Hh signaling pathway, including *PTCH1* and *SMO*, that activate the pathway in the absence of Hh, are present in more than 70% of sporadic BCCs. Several assay systems were developed for identification of synthetic small molecule inhibitors of the Hh signaling pathway that may be effective chemotherapeutics.

Methods and Results.—Two novel in vitro BCC culture systems were developed, one in which mouse embryonic skin punches were treated with a highly active form of Hh protein to induce basaloid nests, and another in which adult mouse skin explants containing BCC-like lesions, derived from *Ptch+/−* heterozygous mice after long-term UV irradiation, were maintained in culture. In the first system, proliferation of basal cells within the BCC-like lesions was arrested, apoptosis occurred, and complete regression of the lesions was seen after treatment with CUR61414, a potent small molecule Hh inhibitor. Histologic analysis revealed that CUR61414 significantly decreased the size and number of basaloid structures so that they were barely detectable. Investigations also showed that CUR61414 did not block other developmentally regulated signaling pathways and had no significant inhibitory effects on other G protein-coupled receptors. Lesion regression in mice exposed to UV light appeared to be the result of massive cell death, as a significant increase in apoptotic nuclei was noted after CUR61414 treatment. Skin surrounding the lesion showed no overt toxicity or noticeably increased apoptosis.

Discussion.—Prolonged and uncontrolled stimulation of the Hh signaling pathway appears to promote basal cell proliferation. The use of Hh inhibitors such as CUR61414 could effectively treat BCC. In these experiments, CUR61414 decreased the rate of proliferation of cells within the tumor and increased the rate of apoptosis of tumor cells without affecting proliferation outside the lesion or increasing apoptosis of normal skin cells.

▶ The majority of human BCCs are associated with dysfunction of the Hh protein signaling pathway, which plays an important physiologic role in normal development. When Hh binds to its receptor, *Ptch-1*, an associated receptor called Smo is permitted to trigger a signaling cascade resulting in target cell proliferation. Uncontrolled or aberrant activation of the pathway is thought to lead to the basal cell proliferation typical of BCC. In this important article, the authors describe the effect of CUR61414, a synthetic inhibitor of the Hh pathway, in murine models of BCC. This molecule has been shown to bind specifically to Smo and inhibit the downstream signaling cascade. The data clearly show that CUR61414 inhibited "basaloid nest" formation in the mouse model. In addition, the compound significantly reduced cell proliferation in existing tumor lesions, while increasing tumor cell death by apoptosis. Importantly, no evidence of toxicity was observed, and neighboring normal skin cells appeared unaffected by treatment with CUR61414. The authors suggest that such inhibitory compounds may prove to be of therapeutic value in BCC.

G. M. P. Galbraith, MD

Tumor-Selective Induction of Apoptosis and the Small-Molecule Immune Response Modifier Imiquimod
Schön M, Bong AB, Drewniok C, et al (Otto-von-Guericke Univ, Magdeburg, Germany; Univ Med Ctr "Benjamin Franklin", Berlin, Germany; Heinrich-Heine-Univ, Düsseldorf, Germany; et al)
J Natl Cancer Inst 95:1138-1149, 2003   16–2

Introduction.—The incidence of the nonmelanoma skin cancers, basal cell carcinoma (BCC), and squamous cell carcinoma (SCC) is increasing. It has been shown that impaired T lymphocyte-related immune surveillance may contribute markedly to the incidence of both tumors. Imiquimod, a topical small-molecule immune response modifier, has demonstrated efficacy toward BCC and actinic keratoses in clinical trials. However, while tumor tissue undergoes remission, the surrounding normal tissue remains mostly unaffected, despite extension of the inflammatory infiltrate to clinically uninvolved peritumoral areas. Thus, mechanisms other than immune stimulation may add to the antineoplastic effect of imiquimod. The mechanism by which imiquimod may induce apoptosis in cancer cells was analyzed.

Methods.—Apoptosis was evaluated by enzyme-linked immunosorbent assay (ELISA), Western blot analysis, and terminal deoxynucleotidyl transferase-mediated dUTP nick end labeling (TUNEL) assay in 5 SCC cell lines, HaCaT cells, and normal keratinocytes treated with imiquimod, with its analog resiquimod, or with neither. The expression of death receptors, caspases, and cytochrome *c* in the apoptotic signaling cascade was evaluated via Western blot and flow cytometric analyses. The functional relevance of imiquimod-induced cytochrome *c* release was analyzed by transfection of HaCaT cells with Bcl-2. Apoptosis in BCCs in vivo was evaluated by TUNEL assays of imiquimod-treated and untreated tumors from 3 patients. Differences between treated and untreated cells and tumors were calculated.

Results.—Imiquimod, but not resiquimod, induced apoptosis in all SCC cell lines and HaCaT cells. This induction involved activation of several caspases and Bcl-2-dependent cytosolic translocation of cytochrome *c*. It was independent of the membrane-bound death receptors, Fas, tumor necrosis factor (TNF)-associated apoptosis-inducing ligand-R1-R4 receptors, and TNF-R1 and -R2 receptors. The topical application of imiquimod to BCC tumors in vivo induced apoptosis as well.

Conclusion.—The topical application of imiquimod has the potential to induce apoptosis in SCC and BCC, possibly by circumventing mechanisms developed by malignant tumors to resist apoptotic signals.

Mechanisms Underlying Imiquimod-Induced Regression of Basal Cell Carcinoma in Vivo

Urosevic M, Maier T, Benninghoff B, et al (Univ Hosp Zurich, Switzerland; 3M Pharmaceuticals, Neuss, Germany; 3M Pharmaceuticals, St Paul, Minn)
Arch Dermatol 139:1325-1332, 2003   16–3

Introduction.—Imiquimod, a local immune response modifier with potent antiviral and antitumor activity, was found in previous studies to be effective in clearing superficial basal cell carcinoma (sBCC). The mechanisms by which topical imiquimod treatment leads to destruction of BCC were investigated.

Methods.—Eligible patients had not undergone previous biopsy or treatment and had tumors suitable for treatment by surgical excision. Lesions were located on the scalp, extremities, or trunk and ranged from 1 to 2 cm in diameter. Imiquimod cream 5% was apllied 5 times per week for up to 6 weeks. Surgical excision was performed when tumors began to show signs of erosion. Parameters evaluated before and after imiquimod treatment were those reflecting tumor apoptotic status (Bcl-2), expression of death receptors (Fas and Fas ligand [FasL]), intercellular adhesion molecule (ICAM) 1, immunosuppressive microenvironment (interleukin 10), and antigen presentation machinery (transporter associated with antigen presentation [TAP] 1). Quantitative polymerase chain reaction was used to assess changes in interferon γ messenger RNA (mRNA) levels relative to CD4 and CD8 mRNA.

Results.—In an open-label, nonrandomized manner, 6 adult patients with nonrecurrent primary sBCC participated in the study. After treatment, tumor cells became more susceptible to apoptosis through decreased Bcl-2 expression. The inflammatory infiltrate, which developed within 3 to 5 days of the start of treatment, was associated with enhanced expression of ICAM-1 and tended to be a mixed cellular response of macrophages and lymphocytes. Interferon γ was produced by CD4 and CD8 T cells. A massive increase was seen in macrophage peritumoral and intratumoral infiltration. Interleukin 10 was produced by infiltrating cells but not by tumor cells. During the first 5 days of treatment, tumor expression of TAP-1 and Fas/FasL did not appear to be affected.

Conclusion.—Clearance of sBCC after imiquimod application is thought to result from increased susceptibility of tumor cells to apoptosis. There is a marked increase in the number of peritumoral and intratumoral infiltrating cells. Macrophages appear to represent an important part of the imiquimod-induced inflammatory infiltrate.

▶ Intralesional injection of interferon-alfa into basal cell carcinoma has previously been shown to be associated with apoptosis of tumor cells.[1,2] The report by Urosevic et al extends these observations to the topical interferon inducer, imiquimod.

B. H. Thiers, MD

References

1. Buechner SA, Wernli M. Harr T, et al: Regression of basal cell carcinoma by intralesional interferon-alpha treatment is mediated by CD95 (Apo-1/Fas)-CD95 ligand-induced suicide. *J Clin Invest* 100:2691-2696, 1997.
2. Wehrli P, Viard I, Bullani R, et al: Death receptors in cutaneous biology and disease. *J Invest Dermatol* 115:141-148, 2000.

Superficial Radiotherapy for Patients With Basal Cell Carcinoma: Recurrence Rates, Histologic Subtypes, and Expression of p53 and Bcl-2
Zagrodnik B, Kempf W, Seifert B, et al (Univ Hosp Zurich, Switzerland; Univ of Zurich, Switzerland)
Cancer 98:2708-2714, 2003   16–4

Introduction.—Adequate treatment of basal cell carcinoma (BCC) requires consideration of histologic subtype in addition to factors such as patient age and health status, localization, size, and number of lesions. Predictive markers include p53, a tumor suppressor gene that when mutated is associated with aggressive behavior of BCCs, and Bcl-2, an antiapoptotic protein, high levels of which are associated with slow tumor growth. Patients with BCC who had undergone radiotherapy were reviewed for the relationship between recurrence, histologic subtype, and Bcl-2 and p53 expression levels.

Methods.—The medical records of 154 patients treated with radiotherapy between 1981 and 1991 were examined. Patients were monitored at 1, 3, 6, and 12 months after treatment, then annually for at least 5 years. Tissue samples were reclassified as nodular, superficial, and sclerosing. Sixty BCCs subjected to immunohistochemical analysis included 30 high-risk tumors of the sclerosing subtype and 30 nonaggressive tumors (12 superficial BCCs and 18 nodular BCCs).

TABLE 3.—Time to Recurrence by Histologic Subtype of Basal Cell Carcinoma

No. of Recurrences/Effective No. of Patients at Risk (%)

BCC Subtype	0-12 Mos	12-24 Mos	24-36 Mos	36-48 Mos	48-60 Mos
Nodular	5/97 (5)	3/78 (4)	0/0 (0)	0/0 (0)	0/0 (0)
Superficial	0/0 (0)	1/21 (5)	1/15 (7)	2/9.5 (21)	0/0 (0)
Sclerosing	4/43.5 (9)	2/33 (6)	3/25 (12)	0/0 (0)	1/8.5 (12)

Abbreviation: BCC, Basal cell carcinoma.
(Courtesy of Zagrodnik B, Kempf W, Seifert B, et al: Superficial radiotherapy for patients with basal cell carcinoma: Recurrence rates, histologic subtypes, and expression of p53 and Bcl 2. *Cancer* 98:2708-2714, 2003. Copyright 2003 American Cancer Society. Reprinted by permission of Wiley-Liss, Inc, a subsidiary of John Wiley & Sons, Inc.)

Results.—A total of 175 BCCs were included in the study: 103 (58.9%) of the nodular subtype, 25 (14.3%) of the superficial subtype, and 47 (26.3%) of the sclerosing subtype. Most tumors were on the head (77.1%) or trunk (17.7%). The mean age at diagnosis of the primary tumor was 69 years and the median follow-up time was 48 months. The overall estimated 5-year recurrence rate after radiotherapy was 15.8%, and the mean time to recurrence was 20 months. Nearly two thirds of the patients had 1 or more additional skin tumors develop during follow-up; 76 of 91 patients had additional BCCs. All 9 p53-positive samples were of the sclerosing subtype, whereas 21 low-risk BCCs and 10 sclerosing BCCs exhibited moderate or strong Bcl-2 expression. There was no statistically significant association between p53 or Bcl-2 expression and recurring BCCs. Recurrence was more common among patients with the sclerosing subtype (27.7%) than among those with nodular (8.2%) or superficial (26.1%) subtype (Table 3).

Conclusion.—Sclerosing BCCs have a high potential for recurrence after superficial radiotherapy, and patients with this subtype should receive an increased dose. The lack of a statistically significant correlation between recurrence rates and p53 or Bcl-2 immunoreactivity in the primary tumor may be attributed to the relatively small number of recurring tumors analyzed.

▶ It must be noted at the outset that this is not a multifactorial analysis of the recurrence rate of BCC after superficial radiotherapy. Histology is just one variable that impacts the recurrence rate of BCC, and its true role in determining whether a tumor recurs depends on how independent it is of other important variables such as anatomic location and size. Although superficial multicentric BCCs (SMBCCs) recurred with a frequency almost equal to that of sclerosing BCCs, the authors inexplicably seem to ignore this observation. SMBCCs, like sclerosing BCCs, often exhibit extensive subclinical spread, and the margins of normal skin included in the field of radiation might have been inadequate. Also, could the irradiation have been too "hard" and simply passed through the tumor? The authors suggest that with adjustment of the radiation dosage, the cure rate for sclerosing BCC might increase. Why not adjust the depth dose or increase the margin of normal skin included in the field of radiation? A 5-year cure rate of 92% for nodular BCCs is acceptable, but a 72% to 74% cure rate for sclerosing BCCs and SMBCCs is not, unless one is simply seeking palliation. While not a new observation, it should be noted that 61.5% of the patients had additional nonmelanoma skin cancers (NMSCs) develop during the follow-up period, emphasizing the importance of regular examination of patients with a history of NMSC.

Although the authors categorize one subtype as being sclerosing and accounting for 26.3% of the tumors, this reviewer would take issue with this observation and suggest that the majority of these tumors had an aggressive growth pattern and lacked a sclerotic stroma. Certainly, the photomicrograph of a "sclerosing BCC" does not demonstrate sclerosis. Finally, it is worth noting that late recurrences were more likely to be seen with "sclerosing" BCCs and SMBCCs.

P. G. Lang, Jr, MD

Seroreactivity to Epidermodysplasia Verruciformis-Related Human Papillomavirus Types Is Associated With Nonmelanoma Skin Cancer

Feltkamp MCW, Broer R, di Summa FM, et al (Leiden Univ, The Netherlands; The Netherlands Inst of Public Health, Bilthoven)
Cancer Res 63:2695-2700, 2003   16–5

Background.—Nonmelanoma skin cancer often contains DNA from epidermodysplasia verruciformis-related human papillomavirus (EV-HPV) types. Few epidemiologic studies have been performed investigating the relation between EV-HPV infection and nonmelanoma skin cancer. HPV infection in patients with a history of skin cancer and a control group was investigated.

Methods.—Five hundred forty patients with a history of skin cancer and 333 persons without skin cancer were studied. Seroreactivity to L1 viruslike particles of EV-HPV types 5, 8, 15, 20, 24, and 38 was measured. Seroreactivity to genital type HPV16 was also determined. Skin cancer risk among HPV-seropositive persons was then estimated.

Findings.—Patients with squamous cell carcinoma had significantly increased seroreactivity to 5 of the 6 EV-HPV types tested. The estimated squamous cell carcinoma relative risk was increased significantly in HPV8 and HPV38-seropositive patients after adjustment for age and sex. Patients with HPV8 seropositivity also had a significantly increased estimated relative risk for nodular and superficial multifocal basal cell carcinoma. The relative risk of developing malignant melanoma was not increased among patients seropositive for HPV. No associations were detected for HPV16. Limiting the analysis to only HPV-seropositive patients verified these findings. However, when analysis was restricted to patients with skin cancer only, EV-HPV seropositivity was not seen significantly more often in patients with nonmelanoma skin cancer than in those with melanoma skin cancer.

Conclusions.—These data indicate that EV-HPV serorecognition is nonspecifically associated with nonmelanoma skin cancer. EV-HPV-directed seroresponses appear to be induced at the time of skin cancer formation rather than upon infection.

The Prevalence of Human Papillomavirus Genotypes in Nonmelanoma Skin Cancers of Nonimmunosuppressed Individuals Identifies High-Risk Genital Types as Possible Risk Factors

Iftner A, Klug SJ, Garbe C, et al (Eberhard Karls Universitaet Tuebingen, Germany; Univ of Bielefeld, Germany; City of Hope Natl Med Ctr, Duarte, Calif)
Cancer Res 63:7515-7519, 2003   16–6

Introduction.—The known risk factors for nonmelanoma skin cancer (NMSC) include fair skin, sun exposure, male sex, and advanced age. No viral risk factors have been established for NMSC, but skin cancers associated with human papilloma virus (HPV) have been described in immunosuppressed renal transplant recipients. The association between NMSC and infection with HPV types was examined in a study of skin biopsy specimens collected from 496 nonimmunosuppressed patients.

Methods.—Patients ranged in age from 5 to 98 years and were cared for by an office-based dermatologist, a university hospital, or a cancer center. Most (352 of 496) were seen at a dermatology clinic in Germany. In all cases, a skin biopsy or resection of a nonmelanoma skin tumor was indicated for medical reasons. Samples analyzed for infection with HPV were from 209 patients with a histologically confirmed diagnosis of warts, 91 with solar keratosis or Bowen's disease, 72 with squamous cell carcinoma, and 18 with basal cell carcinoma; normal skin from 106 control subjects was also studied. Positive samples were HPV typed by sequencing. The association of certain HPV types with the occurrence of warts, precancerous lesions, and skin cancer compared with normal skin was investigated by logistic regression.

Results.—Only 5 (4.7%) histologically proven normal skin samples contained HPV DNA, and in 1 case the HPV type (HPV-12) was one found exclusively in normal skin. Although 91% of warts were positive for HPV DNA, only 3 (1.4%) warts contained DNA of the high-risk HPV types 16, 31, and 33. The finding of HPA DNA was also common in precancerous lesions (60.4%), squamous cell carcinomas (59.7%), and basal cell carcinomas (27.8%), indicating a specific link between viral infection and skin disorders. The distribution of HPV types in benign warts was clearly different from the distribution seen in solar keratoses, Bowen's disease, squamous carcinomas, and basal cell carcinomas.

Conclusion.—The adjusted odds ratio for NMSC in nonimmunosuppressed patients who were DNA positive for the high-risk mucosal HPV types (16, 31, 35, and 51) was 59 when normal skin served as the control. Thus, persistent infections of the skin with high-risk genital HPV types may also increase the risk for NMSC.

Human Papillomavirus-associated Digital Squamous Cell Carcinoma: Literature Review and Report of 21 New Cases

Alam M, Caldwell JB, Eliezri YD (Northwestern Univ, Chicago; Columbia Univ, New York)

J Am Acad Dermatol 48:385-393, 2003   16–7

Background.—Increasing evidence indicates that specific human papillomavirus (HPV) subtypes may be involved in the pathogenesis of digital and periungual squamous cell carcinomas (SCCs) in patients without epidermodysplasia verruciformis (EV). Because HPV-related SCC of the digit is so rare, little is known about its natural history, response to treatment, and prognosis. One series of in situ and invasive HPV-associated SCCs of the distal digits in patients without EV was reviewed.

Methods.—A case series of 23 patients, 21 of whom have not been reported previously, was reviewed. All had been treated during a 15-year period by 1 of the current authors. In addition, a literature search was done to identify patients previously reported. Fifty-one patients were identified in the English-language literature.

Findings.—Overall, 10% of the patients had an antecedent genital dysplasia or carcinoma containing the same HPV subtype as the digital SCC. After wide excision in 14 patients, the recurrence rate was 43%. After Mohs surgery, performed in 16 previously reported patients, the recurrence rate was 13%. In the authors' case series, however, the recurrence rate after Mohs micrographic surgery was 26%. Three percent of the tumors metastasized.

Conclusions.—Genital-digital spread may be a mechanism of tumor genesis. The current data also suggest that HPV-associated digital SCC is more likely to recur after surgery than previously believed. The recurrence rate is far higher than that for cutaneous SCCs in general and may result from residual postoperative HPV infection. However, the metastasis rate appears to be low.

▶ Alam et al present data to suggest a possible viral etiology of squamous cell carcinoma of the digit. Topical imiquimod, initially marketed as a treatment for mucocutaneous papillomavirus infections, has been reported to be effective in the treatment of nonmelanoma skin cancer. Is it possible that more of these lesions than we have previously suspected are virally induced?

B. H. Thiers, MD

A Broad Spectrum of Human Papillomavirus Types Is Present in The Skin of Australian Patients With Non-melanoma Skin Cancers and Solar Keratosis

Forslund O, Ly H, Reid C, et al (Lund Univ, Malmö, Sweden; Inst of Med and Veterinary Science, Adelaide, Australia; Royal Adelaide Hosp, Australia)
Br J Dermatol 149:64-73, 2003   16–8

Introduction.—Human papillomavirus (HPV) may have a role in the pathogenesis of non-melanoma skin cancer (NMSC) in patients with epidermodysplasia verruciformis. In the general population, no specific HPV types have been linked to these lesions. Trials examining the presence of HPV DNA in skin and NMSC are limited in both number and technological design, but recent studies that used a novel primer set (FAP) have identified many new HPV types in skin.

Thus, it may be possible to identify novel HPV types preferentially present in skin cancers. The spectrum of HPV types in tumors of patients with NMSCs or solar keratosis (SK) were examined in a high-risk Australian population and compared with perilesional skin and a body site (buttocks) not usually exposed to sun.

Methods.—Biopsy specimens from tumors and cotton swab samples of perilesional skin and buttock skin obtained from 59 Australian patients with basal cell carcinoma, squamous cell carcinoma, or SK were tested for HPV DNA by polymerase chain reaction using HPV consensus FAP primers and by type-specific primers for HPV 38 and candidate HPV 92. The identification of HPV type from consensus polymerase chain reaction was conducted by sequencing and comparison with GenBank.

Results.—Forty-nine of 59 patients (83%) harbored HPV DNA, which was identified in 28 of 64 (44%) biopsy specimens, 48 of 64 (75%; $P < .001$) perilesional swabs, and 36 of 59 (61%; $P = .04$) buttock swabs. Forty-five different HPV types/putative types were identified. Fifteen were previously characterized HPV types, 17 were earlier described putative types, and 13 were new putative types.

Additionally, 6 subtypes and 4 variants of HPV sequences were detected. HPV types within the B1 group (epidermodysplasia verruciformis HPV types) were identified in 26 of 64 (40%) lesions, 44 of 64 (69%) perilesional swabs, and 35 of 59 (59%) buttock swabs. HPV 38 was observed in 23 of 59 (39%) patients and was seen in 7 of 16 (43%) SKs; it was less common in squamous cell carcinomas (3/23 [13%]; $P = .037$) and basal cell carcinomas (4/25 [16%]; $P = .056$). Candidate HPV 92 was identified in 7 of 59 (12%) patients.

Conclusion.—A broad spectrum of HPV types, mostly from the B1 group, was detected in the skin of Australian patients with skin tumors. No specific types were linked with cancer, although HPV 38 infection was more common among patients with SK. The role of cutaneous HPV infection in the pathogenesis of NMSC requires further study.

Evidence for the Association of Human Papillomavirus Infection and Cutaneous Squamous Cell Carcinoma in Immunocompetent Individuals
Masini C, Fuchs PG, Gabrielli F, et al (Istituto Dermopatico dell'Immacolata, Rome; Universitaet zu Koeln, Cologne, Germany)
Arch Dermatol 139:890-894, 2003   16–9

Introduction.—Human papillomaviruses (HPVs) play a role in anogenital cancer and are associated with the development of skin cancer in patients with epidermodysplasia verruciformis (EV). A case-control study evaluated HPV infection as a risk factor for squamous cell carcinoma (SCC) in immunocompetent patients.

Methods.—The 46 cases were patients with histologically confirmed, cutaneous invasive SCC, newly diagnosed during the period from October 1999 through July 2000. Controls were 84 age- and sex-matched patients seen at the same referral center for unrelated dermatologic conditions. Participants were free of HPV-related skin lesions, and none had a history of SCC of the mucosae, immunosuppression, or skin diseases requiring UV radiation therapy or sun avoidance. Serum samples were obtained to test for HPV-8, HPV-15, HPV-23, and HPV-36. Known and suspected risk factors for SCC were recorded for both cases and controls.

Results.—Known risk factors for SCC (including a family history of skin cancer, sun exposure, and light eye color) and the presence of sun-induced skin lesions (such as solar keratoses) were strongly associated with the development of SCC. Both HPV-8 and HPV-36 were associated with SCC, whereas HPV-15 and HPV-23 were not, although the small number of patients positive for HPV-36 and HPV-23 did not allow for any inference. Positivity for HPV-8 was also associated with male sex (odds ratio, 3.3). In multivariate analysis, positive serologic findings for HPV-8 were independently associated with SCC (odds ratio, 3.2). There was a negative association between serologic findings positive for HPV-15 and the development of SCC (odds ratio, 0.4). In addition to previously noted risk factors for SCC, residency in radon-emitting buildings was significantly associated with SCC.

Conclusion.—Patients with positive serologic findings for HPV-8 are at increased risk for the development of SCC. The risk was strong and independent of other risk factors. Findings also suggest that whereas some HPV types increase the risk of cutaneous SCC, others may offer protection.

▶ A growing body of epidemiologic evidence suggests a possible role for HPV in cutaneous oncogenesis. Certainly, HPV may play a role in anogenital cancer and in cutaneous tumors in immunosuppressed patients. Masini et al and Forslund et al present data to suggest a possible role for HPV in cutaneous tumors in immunocompetent persons. However, the findings in published studies are quite variable, emphasizing the need for large-scale studies using standardized protocols to test for HPV in tissue and HPV reactivity in serum.

B. H. Thiers, MD

Human Papillomavirus Infection in Actinic Keratosis and Bowen's Disease: Comparative Study With Expression of Cell-Cycle Regulatory Proteins p21$^{Waf1/Cip1}$, p53, PCNA, Ki-67, and Bcl-2 in Positive and Negative Lesions

Mitsuishi T, Kawana S, Kato T, et al (Nippon Med School, Tokyo; St Luke's Internatl Hosp, Tokyo; Tokyo Women's Med Univ)

Hum Pathol 34:886-892, 2003   16–10

Introduction.—Previous studies indicate a strong link between Bowen's disease (BD) of the genitalia and fingers and infection with human papillomavirus (HPV). In addition, recent reports suggest that squamous cell carcinoma (SCC) and basal cell carcinoma (BCC) are related to HPV infection, particularly in patients who are immunosuppressed. Molecular methods were used to investigate the presence of HPV in premalignant skin lesions (BD and actinic keratosis [AK]); immunohistochemical analysis was used to characterize differences in the biological characteristics between HPV-positive and HPV-negative lesions.

Methods.—Seventy-five tissue specimens (62 BD and 13 AK) were obtained from 69 patients (66 immunocompetent and 3 renal transplant recipients). The patient group included 36 men and 33 women (mean age, 66 years). Detection and typing of HPV DNA were performed by means of polymerase chain reaction (PCR) or restriction fragment length polymorphism (RFLP), respectively.

Results.—Overall, HPV DNA was demonstrated in 44 (63.8%) patients. The positivity rates of HPV DNA in tissues were 77% for AK and 65% for BD. Twenty-seven HPV types were detected in 50 (67%) premalignant skin lesions. Rates of HPV-positivity were similar for immunocompetent patients (63.6%) and renal transplant recipients (66.7%). Among the HPV types, *Z95963, Z95968, AJ010823,* and *AJ000151* have been described as partial sequences of unknown HPV types. Two unknown types *HPVX1* and *HPVX2* were found in AK specimens; the former is related to HPV-37 (86.1% sequence homology) and the latter to HPV-38 (79.7%).

Conclusion.—Various mucosal and epidermodysplasia verruciformis-related HPV types were found to be associated with both AK and BD. The results of immunohistochemical analysis, in which cell proliferation activity did not differ significantly between HPV-positive and HPV-negative lesions, suggest that HPV infection alone does not induce cell proliferation in those lesions. It was not possible to determine whether transformation to invasive skin neoplasms occurs more often in HPV-positive than in HPV-negative premalignant skin lesions.

▶ Mitsuishi et al suggest that the mere presence of HPV is insufficient to induce cell proliferation. Other factors appear to be necessary to produce the cascade of events that may eventuate in cutaneous malignancy.

B. H. Thiers, MD

Chromosomal Aberrations in Squamous Cell Carcinoma and Solar Keratoses Revealed by Comparative Genomic Hybridization

Ashton KJ, Weinstein SR, Maguire DJ, et al (Griffith Univ–Gold Coast, Queensland, Australia; Griffith Univ–Nathan, Queensland, Australia)
Arch Dermatol 139:876-882, 2003   16–11

Introduction.—Solar keratoses (SKs) are considered premalignant precursors to cutaneous squamous cell carcinoma (SCC), but the proportion of SKs that evolve to SCC is uncertain. To examine the relationship between these entities, biopsy specimens from SKs, SCCs, and lesions with both features were examined for genetic aberrations.

Methods.—Formalin-fixed, paraffin-embedded tissue sections from 9 SCCs and 7 SKs were obtained, together with separate tissue samples from 5 SCCs arising from an adjacent SK. Five tissue sections of healthy skin were used in hybridization efficiency and dynamic range determination. Techniques used in the identification of chromosomal imbalances were comparative genomic hybridization, degenerate oligonucleotide–primed polymerase chain reaction, and DNA labeling.

Results.—The average number of aberrations in SK dysplasia was 6.3. An average of 2.8 gains and 3.5 losses were noted. Only 1 SK lesion had no detectable copy number aberrations (CNAs). Cutaneous SCCs showed an average of 8.1 aberrations, with averages of 4.1 gains and 4.1 losses per dysplasia. The total number of CNAs was significantly higher in SCC than in SK. The 2 lesion types had shared genomic imbalances. Frequent gains were located at chromosome arms 3q, 17q, 4p, 14q, Xq, 5p, 9q, 8q, 17p, and 20q; shared regional losses were detected at 9p, 3p, 13q, 17p, 11p, 8q, and 18p. Only SCC lesions demonstrated significant loss of 18q.

Conclusion.—SCCs and SKs share numerous chromosomal aberrations, a finding that suggests a clonal relationship between the 2 lesions. Loss of the chromosome 18q arm, more prevalent in SCCs, may be an important event in the progression of SK to SCC. It is not known whether SKs require further mutations for progression, or if SKs may be small SCC lesions.

▶ The authors demonstrate numerous shared chromosomal aberrations between SCCs and SKs. The findings are further evidence to support a clonal relationship between the 2 lesions; they do not, however, prove that SKs are, in fact, small SCCs. It can reasonably be argued that SKs require further mutation to progress to SCCs; indeed, the authors did find that genomic loss of 18q may be a significant event in the progression of SKs to SCCs.

B. H. Thiers, MD

The Increased Risk of Skin Cancer Is Persistent After Discontinuation of Psoralen + Ultraviolet A: A Cohort Study
Nijsten TEC, Stern RS (Harvard Med School, Boston)
J Invest Dermatol 121:252-258, 2003   16–12

Introduction.—Since its introduction in 1974, psoralen plus ultraviolet A (PUVA) has been broadly used in the treatment of psoriasis and other skin conditions. There is evidence that patients with PUVA-treated psoriasis are at increased risk for nonmelanoma skin cancer. About 50% of these tumors have occurred since 1995. The rate of persistence of cancer risk among patients who have discontinued treatment with PUVA was prospectively evaluated in a cohort of 1380 patients with psoriasis.

Findings.—A total of 27,840 person-years, of which 59.4% were considered years without PUVA, were monitored. No significant reduction in risk was seen during the initial 15 years after PUVA treatment was discontinued. Subsequently, the risk of squamous cell carcinoma was decreased (incidence rate ratio = 0.79; 95% confidence interval = 0.62, 1.01 on treatment vs more than 15 years off). After 25 years, approximately 7% of patients with 200 or less PUVA treatments and over half of patients with 400 or more treatments had developed at least 1 squamous cell carcinoma. After 25 years, approximately one third of patients exposed to 200 or more treatments developed at least 1 basal cell carcinoma.

Conclusion.—Substantial exposure to PUVA dramatically increases the risk of nonmelanoma skin cancer. Previous exposure to PUVA remains an important issue in the management of patients with psoriasis since the cancer risk linked with PUVA is persistent.

▶ The authors emphasize the need to follow PUVA-treated patients on a long-term basis. They argue that past use of PUVA may affect the choice of subsequent treatments, especially the newer immunosuppressive and immuno-modulatory agents that might heighten the risk of cutaneous carcinogenesis. The bottom line is that past use of PUVA must be considered in determining the safety of alternative therapies for psoriasis. An interesting commentary on the validity of the retrospective data presented by Nijsten and Stern accompanied their article.[1]

B. H. Thiers, MD

Reference

1. Paull CF: Treating severe psoriasis: How to navigate safely between Scylla and Charybdis. *J Invest Dermatol* 121:ix-x, 2003.

Oral Retinoid Use Reduces Cutaneous Squamous Cell Carcinoma Risk in Patients With Psoriasis Treated With Psoralen-UVA: A Nested Cohort Study

Nijsten TEC, Stern RS (Beth Israel Deaconess, Boston; Harvard Med School, Boston)

J Am Acad Dermatol 49:644-650, 2003   16–13

Introduction.—Oral retinoid use may reduce the risk of squamous cell carcinoma (SCC) of the skin in high-risk patients, such as those treated with oral psoralen-UVA (PUVA) for psoriasis. The mechanism of chemoprevention is unknown, but retinoids modulate cell growth, cell differentiation, and the immune system. Patients with psoriasis who had been exposed to PUVA were studied for the effect of oral retinoids on skin cancer risk.

Methods.—A nested cohort study included 135 patients who used retinoids for at least 26 weeks in 1 year or more during the period between 1985 and 2000. Eleven interviews administered since 1985 quantified the incidence of squamous cell carcinoma (SCC) and basal cell carcinoma (BCC) for the years of substantial retinoid use and the years of no use.

Results.—The 135 retinoid users recorded 589 person-years of retinoid use. In the 589 person-years of use, 150 SCCs occurred; in the 748 person-years of no use, 357 SCCs were documented. During the retinoid-use years, 71 BCCs were noted, in contrast to 117 BCCs that occurred during the years with no retinoid use. In a paired analysis, retinoid use was associated with a 30% reduction in SCC incidence, whereas BCC incidence was not significantly reduced. The incidence of SCC remained significantly reduced during years of substantial retinoid use in multivariate analysis that adjusted for other important predictors of SCC risk.

Conclusion.—At doses of 25 mg/day or more, retinoid use by patients treated with PUVA for psoriasis reduces SCC risk but does not significantly reduce the incidence of BCC. The benefit of retinoids in these patients at high risk for SCC is apparently limited to periods of substantial use.

► With the exception of oral retinoids, most drugs (including the new biological agents) used in the systemic treatment of psoriasis are immunosuppressive. Retinoids appear to exert their effect through modulation of cell growth and cell differentiation. This provides benefits not only in ameliorating psoriasis but also in protecting against the development of squamous cell carcinoma. The combination of oral retinoids with other systemic antipsoriatic treatments holds great promise for enhancing the therapeutic response and reducing the risk of adverse events compared to using either agent alone. The combination of systemic retinoids with UVL adds to the therapeutic effect while reducing the amount of UVL needed for clearance of psoriasis.[1-3] As demonstrated by Nijsten et al, the benefits of this combination also include a reduction of the potential carcinogenic effect of UVL treatments, especially PUVA.

B. H. Thiers, MD

References

1. Ruzicka T, Sommerburg C, Braun-Falco O, et al: Efficiency of acitretin in combination with UV-B in the treatment of severe psoriasis. *Arch Dermatol* 126:482-486, 1990.
2. Lowe NJ, Prystowsky JH, Bourget T, et al: Acitretin plus UVB therapy for psoriasis. Comparisons with placebo plus UVB and acitretin alone. *J Am Acad Dermatol* 24:591-594, 1991.
3. Tanew A, Guggenbichler A, Honigsmann H, et al: Photochemotherapy for severe psoriasis without or in combination with acitretin: A randomized, double-blind comparison study. *J Am Acad Dermatol* 25:682-684, 1991.

Acitretin Treatment of Premalignant and Malignant Skin Disorders in Renal Transplant Recipients: Clinical Effects of a Randomized Trial Comparing Two Doses of Acitretin

Sévaux RGL, Smit JV, de Jong EMGJ, et al (Univ Med Ctr, Nijmegen, The Netherlands)
J Am Acad Dermatol 49:407-412, 2003   16–14

Introduction.—The rates of premalignant and malignant skin lesions are high after renal transplantation. Treatment with acitretin improves the number and aspect of actinic keratoses and seems to decrease the incidence of squamous cell carcinomas. Treatment is thwarted by frequent side effects. No optimal long-term dosing has been determined. A randomized investigation among renal transplant recipients with histologically proven actinic keratoses was performed to compare maintenance doses of 0.2 and 0.4 mg/kg/d of acitretin. Clinical data regarding the effectiveness and side effects of treatment as well as data on patients' judgment were evaluated at regular intervals.

Methods.—Twenty-six long-term renal transplant recipients were randomly assigned to either 1 year of treatment with 0.4 mg/kg/d acitretin or 3 months of acitretin at 0.4 mg/kg, then 9 months at 0.2 mg/kg/d. At 9 different times, the numbers of actinic keratoses and tumors were counted, and erythema, the thickness of the lesions, and the severity of side effects were rated. Patients' judgment was documented by visual analogue scores.

Results.—The number of actinic keratoses decreased by almost 50% in both groups. The number of new malignant tumors during the evaluation period was similar to the number of tumors in the year before the investigation. The thickness of the keratoses diminished significantly in both groups. The acitretin dose had to be decreased in most patients due to the frequent occurrence of mucocutaneous side effects including cheilitis, excessive peeling of the skin, and hair disorders. Of 14 patients randomly assigned to continuous treatment with a dose of 0.4 mg/kg/d, only 3 patients could maintain this dose. Temporary interruption of acitretin therapy was required in 7 of 26 patients. Patients' satisfaction with their skin increased significantly, with no between-group differences.

Conclusion.—Acitretin therapy reduced the number of actinic keratoses in renal transplant recipients at a low maintenance dose of 0.2 mg/kg/d and significantly reduced the thickness of the lesions. The incidence of new skin malignancies did not change. Patients' satisfaction with their skin increased significantly, despite the high incidence of mucocutaneous side effects.

▶ Given the low dose of acitretin that was administered, the rather high incidence of adverse events necessitating temporary interruption of therapy is surprising. This fact notwithstanding, in this reviewer's opinion a more convincing analysis would require administration of the drug over a more extended time period.

B. H. Thiers, MD

Histopathologic Evaluation of Cutaneous Squamous Cell Carcinoma: Results of a Survey Among Dermatopathologists
Khanna M, Fortier-Riberdy G, Dinehart SM, et al (Univ of Arkansas)
J Am Acad Dermatol 48:721-726, 2003   16–15

Introduction.—Histopathologic features of a tumor are used for prognosis and staging. In cutaneous melanoma, depth of invasion predicts diagnosis and is usually included in the histopathologic report. In cutaneous squamous cell carcinoma (CSCC), however, histopathologic features related to prognosis are not consistently part of pathology reports. A survey of dermatopathologists asked respondents about which histopathologic features they include in their pathology reports and whether they thought these features predicted prognosis in CSCC.

Methods.—The surveys were sent to 120 members of the American Society of Dermatopathology. About two thirds were in academia and one third in private practice. Respondents were to report on their inclusion of specific histopathologic features (Table 1).

Results.—Ninety-three (78%) questionnaires were returned. Most (90%) respondents reported histologic subtype of CSSCs, but only 58% thought

---

TABLE 1.—Result of Questionnaire on Features Reported Incutaneous Squamous Cell Carcinoma

Histopathologic Feature	Percent Who Comment	Percent Who Think Predicts Prognosis
Histologic subtype	90	58
Histologic grade	54	49
Anatomic depth	63	55
Depth in millimeters	8	
Perineural invasion	96	80
Blood/lymphatic invasion	95	81
Associated actinic keratosis	43	16
Inflammation	16	4

(Reprinted by permission of the publisher from Khanna M, Fortier-Riberdy G, Dinehart SM, et al: Histopathologic evaluation of cutaneous squamous cell carcinoma: Results of a survey among dermatopathologists. *J Am Acad Dermatol* 48:721-726, 2003. Copyright 2003 by Elsevier.)

that subtype was related to prognosis. Only 54% report grade, and 49% believe that it can predict prognosis. Anatomic depth of invasion is reported by 63%, but only 8% measure depth of invasion in millimeters. Most dermatopathologists (96%) report perineural invasion and 80% believe that this feature is related to prognosis; blood or lymphatic invasion yielded similarly high responses. Nearly half (43%) include the presence of a contiguous actinic keratosis in the report, but few (16%) believe it predicts prognosis. Inflammation was the feature least likely to be reported or judged important to prognosis.

Conclusion.—Dermatopathologists in the United States and Canada do not have a uniform system for the histopathologic reporting of CSSC. Very few of those responding to the survey actually measure depth of invasion in millimeters, and slightly more than half thought depth predicted prognosis, despite studies that indicate a direct relationship between tumor thickness and depth of invasion and the prognosis of patients with CSSC. A uniform system for reporting all histopathologic features would facilitate complete evaluation of the specimen, staging, and clinical research.

▶ Evidence is accumulating in the literature that microscopic features of CSCC may be important in determining prognosis and in guiding therapy. The microscopic features that have been studied most extensively and correlate with prognosis include tumor thickness, tumor grade (degree of differentiation), tumor subtype, and perineural invasion. Of these morphologic features, perineural invasion correlates most closely with aggressive behavior. Two things seem obvious. One is the fact that more studies need to be done with greater rigor to produce the same hard data that is available for melanoma. The other is that dermatopathologists do not currently have the same conviction regarding reporting of microscopic staging for CSCC as they have for melanoma. As noted by Khanna et al, 55% of dermatopathologists believe that depth of invasion is predictive of prognosis, yet only 8% actually measure the depth of invasion in millimeters. Tumor registries reliably capture melanoma patient data but do not capture CSCC patient data. This fact makes it difficult for pathologists and dermatologists to acquire the compelling data that exists for melanoma. Hopefully, these data will be forthcoming and the microscopic staging of squamous cell carcinoma will become the standard of care.

J. C. Maize, MD

Use of Indoor Tanning Facilities by White Adolescents in the United States

Demko CA, Borawski EA, Debanne SM, et al (Case Western Reserve Univ, Cleveland, Ohio)
Arch Pediatr Adolesc Med 157:854-860, 2003   16–16

Background.—The use of indoor tanning booths increases the risk of skin cancer. The prevalence of tanning bed use by white, non-Hispanic US adolescents and the demographic and clinical characteristics of adolescents who use these facilities were examined.

Methods.—Data from Wave II of the National Longitudinal Study of Adolescent Health (Add Health) Study collected between April 1, 1996, and August 31, 1996, were examined. The data set included 6903 (of 7573 eligible respondents, or 91%) non-Hispanic, white adolescents in grades 7 to 12 enrolled from 132 schools in 80 US communities. Data of interest included age, sex, geographic region of residence, location of the school (ie, urban, suburban, or rural), maternal educational level, student income/ allowance, tobacco use, alcohol intake, marijuana use, body mass index, the lifetime frequency of tanning booth use, and the skin tan and burn types. Research subjects who had used a tanning booth at least 3 times during their life were defined as tanning booth users.

Results.—The mean age of the research subjects was 15.9 years, and 50% were female. Most research subjects (74.8%) attended urban or suburban schools, 87.6% reported skin tan types 2 to 4 (mild to deep tan), and 19.4% had skin burn types 1/2. Almost one fourth (24.1%) reported having used a tanning facility at least once; this translates to a national level of about 2.9 million. Female research subjects were more likely to use tanning booths than were their male peers (28.1% vs 6.9%). In particular, 50.8% of female tanning booth users said they had used tanning booths at least 10 times. For both sexes, the frequency of tanning booth use increased with age; in girls, the frequency increased from 11.2% of 13- to 14-year-olds to 47.0% of 18- to 19-year-olds. The frequency of tanning booth use also increased as the tanning ability increased: only 12.6% of poor tanners used tanning booths compared with 38.1% of research subjects with a strong tan response. Multivariate logistic regression analyses identified the following factors as significantly and independently correlated with an increased use of tanning booths: age (adjusted odds ratio [aOR], 1.46 per year); residence in the South (aOR, 2.91) or Midwest (aOR, 2.38); being able to achieve at least a mild tan (aOR, 5.27 for deep tan vs no tan); attending a rural high school (aOR, 1.80); using alcohol, tobacco, or marijuana (aOR, 1.57 for 1 substance, 3.06 for 2-3 substances); having a personal allowance or income (aOR, 1.27); and trying to lose weight (aOR, 1.26). Factors negatively associated with tanning booth use included having a higher cognitive ability (aOR, 0.89 per 10-point increase on the Add Health Picture Vocabulary Test), having a mother with a college degree (aOR, 0.68), and having a body mass index greater than the 85th percentile (aOR, 0.68). Also, among females only, considering oneself more physically mature than others increased the likelihood of tanning booth use (aOR, 1.56), whereas regular physical activity decreased the likelihood of indoor tanning (aOR, 0.91).

Conclusion.—This nationally representative sample of white, non-Hispanic US teenagers indicates tanning booth use is common in this population, particularly among girls. Tanning booth use correlates significantly with certain risk behaviors and appearance-related factors. These findings may help target strategies to reduce tan-seeking behavior among adolescents.

▶ The authors note that adolescents living in the Midwest and South, where natural sunlight is prevalent, are 2 to 3 times more likely to use tanning beds than are adolescents in the rest of the country. This is the first study to reveal a strong positive association between tanning bed use and other health risk behaviors. Incorporating information on the risks of artificial tanning into comprehensive health promoting messages might be of benefit to some adolescents.

S. Raimer, MD

Selenium Supplementation and Secondary Prevention of Nonmelanoma Skin Cancer in a Randomized Trial
Duffield-Lillico AJ, Slate EH, Reid ME, et al (Mem Sloan-Kettering Cancer Ctr, New York; Med Univ of South Carolina, Charleston; Roswell Park Cancer Inst, Buffalo, NY; et al)
J Natl Cancer Inst 95:1477-1481, 2003   16–17

Introduction.—The Nutritional Prevention of Cancer Trial, designed to test whether selenium supplementation could prevent nonmelanoma skin cancer in patients who previously had the disease, unexpectedly found that selenium reduced the incidences of several other cancers and of total cancer mortality. However, results from September 15, 1983, through December 31, 1993, showed no effect on the incidence of basal and squamous carcinomas of the skin. The entire blinded treatment period, which ended on January 31, 1996, was then summarized.

Methods.—The double-blind, randomized, placebo-controlled clinical trial enrolled 1312 patients. Those in the selenium supplementation group received selenized yeast, 200 µg daily. The association between treatment and time to first nonmelanoma skin cancer diagnosis and between treatment and time to multiple skin tumors was evaluated for the study group as a whole and for various subgroups. Data from 1250 patients were included in statistical analyses.

Results.—Estimates from the 1983-1993 analysis found more cases of basal cell and squamous cell carcinoma in the group supplemented with selenium than in the placebo group, but the difference was not statistically significant. Results through January 31, 1996, indicated a statistically significant increased risk for both squamous cell carcinoma and total nonmelanoma skin cancer (Fig 1) among selenium-treated individuals. Patients with baseline selenium in the upper tertile showed a 60% increase in the probability of a new skin cancer as a result of selenium supplementation.

Discussion.—Previous studies reported a protective association between plasma selenium level and the risk of nonmelanoma skin cancer, but the Nutritional Prevention of Cancer Trial failed to confirm this finding. Instead, selenium supplementation increased the risk of squamous cell carcinoma and total nonmelanoma skin cancer in patients with a history of these cancers.

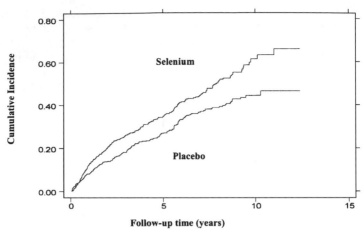

FIGURE 1.—Nelson-Aalen cumulative incidence estimates (95% CIs) for both treatment groups at 5 years and 10 years of follow-up. Placebo group: 5-year follow-up = 0.27 (0.23 to 0.32); 10-year follow-up: 0.44 (0.38 to 0.52). Treatment groups: 5-year follow-up = 0.34 (0.30 to 0.40); 10-year follow-up = 0.61 (0.53 to 0.71). Log-rank test P value = .004. (Courtesy of Duffield-Lillico AJ, Slate EH, Reid ME, et al: Selenium supplementation and secondary prevention of nonmelanoma skin cancer in a randomized trial. *J Natl Cancer Inst* 95:1477-1481, 2003. By permission of Oxford University Press.)

▶ Not only did selenium supplementation fail to reduce the risk of basal cell carcinoma, it was associated with a statistically significantly increased risk of squamous cell carcinoma and nonmelanoma skin cancer in general. These results contrast with previous findings suggesting a protective effect of plasma selenium levels on the risk of nonmelanoma skin cancer,[1,2] and reports that topical application of selenium protects humans against the damaging effects of UVB radiation.[3]

B. H. Thiers, MD

References

1. Breslow RA, Alberg AJ, Helzlsouer KJ, et al: Serological precursors of cancer: Malignant melanoma, basal and squamous cell skin cancer, and prediagnostic levels of retinal, betacarotene, lycopene, alpha-tocopherol, and selenium. *Cancer Epidemiol Biomarkers Prev* 4:837-842, 1995.
2. Karagas MR, Greenberg ER, Nierenberg D, et al: Risk of squamous cell carcinoma of the skin in relation to plasma selenium, alpha-tocopherol, beta-carotene, and retinal: A nested case-control study. *Cancer Epidemiol Biomarkers Prev* 6:25-29, 1997.
3. Burke KE, Burford RG, Combs GF Jr, et al: The effect of topical L-selenomethionine on minimal erythema dose of ultraviolet irradiation in humans. *Photodermatol Photoimmunol Photomed* 9:52-57, 1992.

Sentinel Lymph Node Analysis in Patients With Sweat Gland Carcinoma

Delgado R, Kraus D, Coit DG, et al (Mem Sloan-Kettering Cancer Ctr, New York)
Cancer 97:2279-2284, 2003   16–18

Background.—Sweat gland carcinomas are derived from the epithelium of the sweat gland apparatus. Many types of sweat gland carcinoma exist, and some of them (notably, eccrine duct carcinoma, hidradenocarcinoma, and porocarcinoma) carry a significant risk of regional lymph node metastasis. The utility of lymphatic mapping and sentinel lymph node (SLN) biopsy in patients with these uncommon cutaneous neoplasms was investigated.

Methods.—The medical records of 6 patients (2 men, 4 women; age range, 41-72 years) with sweat gland carcinoma were reviewed. All patients had undergone lymphatic mapping with SLN biopsy. Biopsy specimens were examined by routine hematoxylin and eosin (H&E) staining and by immunohistochemistry (IHC) with antibodies against epithelial membrane antigen and cytokeratins. Patients were monitored for 2 to 19 months (mean, 12 months) to determine outcomes.

Results.—Histologic evaluation identified hidradenocarcinoma in 3 patients, eccrine duct carcinoma in 2 patients, and porocarcinoma in 1 patient. Four tumors were present on the head and neck, and 2 tumors were present on the lower extremity. Tumor thickness ranged from 2.6 to 8.5 mm, and all tumors were centered in the dermis. Five tumors extended into the subcutis, and 3 tumors were associated with lymphatic tumor emboli.

The SLN biopsy specimen was positive for metastasis in 4 of the 6 patients (66.7%), including all 3 patients with lymphatic tumor emboli. Additionally, 1 patient with a primary tumor of the neck had bilateral positive SLNs. H&E staining detected tumor deposits in 3 of the 5 positive SLNs, while 2 SLNs were negative by H&E staining but positive by IHC. The amount of positive tissue in the lymph nodes varied, from less than 1% in the patient with hidradenocarcinoma to almost 50% in a patient with poorly differentiated eccrine duct carcinoma.

ICH with antibody to epithelial membrane antigen was best for identifying metastatic tumor deposits from hidradenocarcinoma (Fig 1; see color plate XIII) or porocarcinoma (Fig 3; see color plate XIV); 34BE12 was also useful in identifying micrometastasis in porocarcinoma. ICH with antibod-

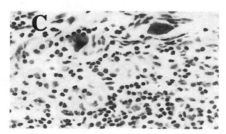

FIGURE 1.—Hidradenocarcinoma. C, Rare tumor cells were noted in the sentinel lymph node and were positive for epithelial membrane antigen. (Courtesy of Delgado R, Kraus D, Coit DG, et al. Sentinel lymph node analysis in patients with sweat gland carcinoma. *Cancer* 97(9): 2279-2284, 2003. ©2003 American Cancer Society. Reprinted by permission of Wiley-Liss, Inc, a subsidiary of John Wiley & Sons, Inc.)

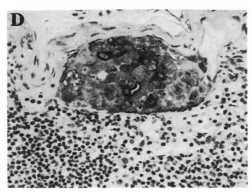

FIGURE 3.—Porocarcinoma. D, The tumor cells were immunoreactive for epithelial membrane antigen. (Courtesy of Delgado R, Kraus D, Coit DG, et al. Sentinel lymph node analysis in patients with sweat gland carcinoma. *Cancer* 97(9): 2279-2284, 2003. ©2003 American Cancer Society. Reprinted by permission of Wiley-Liss, Inc, a subsidiary of John Wiley & Sons, Inc.)

ies to cytokeratins CK7 and Cam5.2 was best for identifying metastatic tumor deposits from eccrine duct carcinoma (Fig 2; see color plate XIII). Two of the 4 patients with metastases underwent complete regional lymph node dissection and were found to have positive non-SLNs as well. The other 2 patients with a positive SLN did not undergo lymph node dissection. At last follow-up, all patients were alive and free of disease.

Conclusion.—Four of these 6 patients had a positive SLN(s), which suggests SLN biopsy is useful for staging disease in patients with sweat gland carcinoma. ICH appears to be superior to routine H&E staining for identifying micrometastases in these patients.

▶ Lymphatic mapping with SLN biopsy has come to play a major role in the staging and management of patients with melanoma and breast carcinoma. It also has been successfully used for Merkel cell carcinoma and squamous cell carcinoma. Sweat gland carcinoma is not a single entity but consists of a number of histologic subtypes that vary in their potential to metastasize.

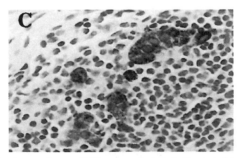

FIGURE 2.—Eccrine duct carcinoma. C, The tumor deposits in the contralateral sentinel lymph node became apparent only on the immunostain for cytokeratins (Cam5.2). (Courtesy of Delgado R, Kraus D, Coit DG, et al. Sentinel lymph node analysis in patients with sweat gland carcinoma. *Cancer* 97(9): 2279-2284, 2003. ©2003 American Cancer Society. Reprinted by permission of Wiley-Liss, Inc, a subsidiary of John Wiley & Sons, Inc.)

Three subtypes—hidradenocarcinoma, eccrine duct carcinoma, and porocarcinoma—exhibit a significant predilection for metastasis.

In this study, the authors report their experience with SLN biopsy in these 3 subtypes of sweat gland carcinoma. Not unexpectedly, patients with deeply invasive tumors were more likely to have a positive SLN biopsy specimen, as were patients with tumors that had invaded the lymphatics. Although tumor deposits within the SLN were readily seen with H&E staining, there were several instances in which minute deposits of tumor were detected only by IHC. Moreover, a battery of immunostains was required to consistently demonstrate tumor deposits. Cytokeratin stains Cam5.2 and CK7 best demonstrated eccrine duct carcinoma whereas epithelial membrane antigen and 34BE12 best demonstrated porocarcinoma and hidradenocarcinoma.

Despite the small number of patients included, this study does illustrate the potential usefulness of the SLN biopsy for the staging and management of patients with sweat gland carcinoma. However, whether or not it would impact survival remains to be demonstrated.

P. G. Lang, Jr, MD

Lymphatic Mapping and Sentinel Lymph Node Biopsy in the Detection of Early Metastasis From Sweat Gland Carcinoma
Bogner PN, Fullen DR, Lowe L, et al (Univ of Michigan, Ann Arbor)
Cancer 97:2285-2289, 2003   16–19

Background.—Digital papillary adenocarcinoma, hidradenocarcinoma, and eccrine duct carcinoma are subtypes of sweat gland carcinoma that have a propensity for regional lymph node and systemic metastases. The utility of lymphatic mapping and sentinel lymph node (SLN) biopsy in patients with these uncommon cutaneous neoplasms was investigated.

Methods.—The medical records of 5 patients (1 man, 4 women; age range 31-78 years) with sweat gland carcinoma were reviewed. All patients had undergone lymphatic mapping with SLN biopsy between 1999 and 2002. Biopsy specimens were examined by routine hematoxylin and eosin staining, with immunohistochemistry reserved for confirming metastatic disease. Patients were monitored for 1 to 25 months (mean, 10.2 months) to determine outcomes.

Results.—Histologic evaluation identified aggressive digital papillary adenocarcinoma in 2 patients (both of which occurred on a finger), hidradenocarcinoma in 2 patients (present on the knee in 1 case and the foot in the other), and eccrine duct carcinoma (on the scalp) in 1 patient. Tumor size ranged from 5 to 35 mm, and depth ranged from 3.5 to 18 mm. SLN biopsy speciments were positive for metastasis in 3 of the 5 patients (60%), including 4 of the 13 SLNs that were removed.

The amount of positive tissue in the lymph nodes varied from less than 5% in a patient with hidradenocarcinoma to about 20% in patients with digital papillary adenocarcinoma or eccrine duct carcinoma. Each of these 3 patients subsequently underwent regional lymphadenectomy, which revealed no evidence of further metastasis. At last follow-up, all patients were alive and free of disease.

Conclusion.—Three of these 5 patients had 1 or 2 positive SLNs, which suggests that SLN biopsy at the time of resection would be useful for detecting subclinical metastases in patients with these types of sweat gland tumors.

▶ Sweat gland carcinomas are rare tumors that are histologically diverse and vary in their potential for metastasis. In one study, there was a 43% incidence of lymph node involvement, a 38% incidence of distant metastases, and a 37% mortality rate.[1] This retrospective study included 5 patients who underwent lymphatic mapping and SLN biopsy for sweat gland carcinoma.

Three different histologic subtypes were represented—syringoid carcinoma, hidradenocarcinoma, and aggressive digital papillary adenocarcinoma. Tumor size and depth of invasion did not appear to correlate with SLN positivity. Staining with hematoxylin and eosin was often adequate to demonstrate tumor in the SLN, although occasionally this required the use of immunostains for cytokeratin AE1/AE3 and Cam5.2. This study, like that of Delgado et al (Abstract 16–18), again demonstrates the usefulness of SLN biopsy for detecting occult metastases in patients with sweat gland carcinoma. However, whether this will eventuate in better survival or a lower incidence of recurrence remains to be determined.

P. G. Lang, Jr, MD

Reference

1. El-Domeiri AA, Brasfield RD, Huvos AG, et al: Sweat gland carcinoma: A clinico-pathology study of 83 patients. *Ann Surg* 173:270-274, 1971.

17 Nevi and Melanoma

Prevalence and Anatomical Distribution of Naevi in Young Queensland Children
Whiteman DC, Brown RM, Purdie DM, et al (PO Royal Brisbane Hosp, Queensland, Australia)
Int J Cancer 106:930-933, 2003   17–1

Background.—The primary environmental cause of melanoma is sunlight. It has also been implicated in the pathogenesis of melanocytic nevi. In childhood, melanocytes appear to be susceptible to the effects of sunlight. However, little is known about the development of nevi in infancy. The current survey of child-care centers was performed to document the prevalence and anatomic distribution of melanocytic nevi in young children in Brisbane, Australia.

Methods.—One hundred ninety-three children, aged 1 to 3 years, were examined. Brisbane is at latitude 27 degrees south. All skin surfaces except the scalp, buttocks, and genitalia were examined for nevi.

Findings.—Nearly 90% of children had at least 1 nevus of any size. More than 30% had 10 or more. Total counts ranged from 0 to 45. Age was a strong determinant of total count. Nevus densities were highest on exposed body sites, such as the face and limbs. The density of nevi 5 mm or greater in size, however, was significantly greater on the trunk than on the face, neck, and ears.

Conclusions.—These findings support the notion that melanocytic neoplasia begins early in life. The evolution of nevi appears to be influenced by the anatomic cite of the target cell.

▶ In this study, 193 Queensland children aged 12 to 47 months were examined for the presence of nevi. Only 3 of 133 2- and 3-year-olds had no nevi. By age 3 the nevi of boys were most numerous on the face, ears, and neck, while those of girls were primarily on the upper extremities. Large nevi were most common on the trunk. The significance of these findings is uncertain.

S. Raimer, MD

Sun Exposure and Number of Nevi in 5- to 6-Year-Old European Children

Dulon M, Weichenthal M, Blettner M, et al (Univ of Bielefeld, Germany; Univ of Kiel, Germany; Dermatology Ctr, Buxtehude, Germany; et al)
J Clin Epidemiol 55:1075-1081, 2002   17–2

Background.—Occurrence and number of melanocytic nevi are important risk factors for malignant melanoma. The causes of nevi were studied to develop successful strategies for preventing melanoma.

Methods and Findings.—A cohort of 11,478 white German preschool-aged children was studied. The relation between benign melanocytic nevi and numerous risk factors for skin cancer was determined. Whole-body examinations revealed 0 to 120 nevi, with a median of 11 nevi. In each subgroup of skin phototype, the regular use of sunscreens did not significantly reduce nevi. Mean nevus counts increased with number and severity of sunburns and with number of holidays spent in foreign countries with sunny climates (Table 3).

Conclusions.—In this study, children with a reported history of increased sun exposure and an increased number of holidays in sunny climates had significantly greater nevus counts than children without such histories. The current data suggest that nevus counts result from increased exposure to ultraviolet radiation as well as a genetic predisposition. Strategies for decreasing melanoma incidence should begin with young children.

TABLE 3.—Whole-Body Number of Melanocytic Nevi by Sun Exposure Variables and Phenotypic Characteristics (n = 11,478)

	N	Adjusted Geometric Means (95% Confidence Intervals)		
		Model 1*	Model 2†	Model 3‡
Sunburn				
None	3,684	9.9 (9.6-10.2)	9.0 (8.7-9.3)	11.4 (11.0-11.7)
Light	5,837	11.4 (11.1-11.7)	10.6 (10.3-10.9)	12.9 (12.7-13.2)
Painful	1,957	12.2 (11.8-12.7)	11.4 (11.0-11.8)	13.5 (13.1-14.0)
Holidays in the south				
0	6,862	9.7 (9.5-10.0)	8.9 (8.7-9.2)	10.9 (10.7-11.2)
1	2,942	11.4 (11.0-11.7)	10.5 (10.1-10.9)	12.8 (12.5-13.2)
2+	1,674	12.6 (11.0-13.1)	11.6 (11.1-12.0)	14.2 (13.7-14.7)
Skin phototype				
I	419	8.7 (8.1-9.3)		
II	4,021	12.1 (11.8-12.4)		
III	5,428	12.4 (12.2-12.7)		
IV	1,610	11.9 (11.4-12.4)		
Hair color				
Red	462		7.1 (6.7-7.6)	
Fair	4,840		12.3 (12.0-12.6)	
Brown	6,176		12.4 (12.1-12.7)	
Freckles				
None	8,895			11.6 (11.4-11.8)
Some/many	2,583			13.6 (13.2-14.0)

*Each factor is adjusted in multivariate analysis for amount of sunburn, holidays in the south, skin phototype, and sex.
†Each factor is adjusted in multivariate analysis for amount of sunburn, holidays in the south, hair color, and sex.
‡Each factor is adjusted in multivariate analysis for amount of sunburn, holidays in the south, freckles, and sex.
(Courtesy of Dulon M, Weichenthal M, Blettner M, et al: Sun exposure and number of nevi in 5- to 6-year-old European children. *J Clin Epidemiol* 55:1075-1081, 2002.)

▶ Surprisingly, German children with skin phototype I actually had fewer nevi at age 5 or 6 years than did their counterparts with skin types II, III, or IV. There was no correlation between the amount of daily sun exposure in their home region and the number of nevi. However, nevi did appear to be increased in number in children who had vacationed in the south, suggesting that intense intermittent sun exposure might encourage nevus formation. The number of nevi was also increased in children who had had painful sunburns and in those who had freckles.

S. Raimer, MD

Evaluation of Aid to Diagnosis of Pigmented Skin Lesions in General Practice: Controlled Trial Randomised by Practice
English DR, Burton RC, del Mar CB, et al (Cancer Council Victoria, Carlton, Australia; National Cancer Control Initiative, Carlton, Australia; Univ of Queensland, Herston, Australia)
BMJ 327:375-378, 2003   17–3

Introduction.—A previously reported melanoma screening trial with Australian general practitioners (GPs) revealed high sensitivity and low specificity in the diagnosis of melanoma. Whether an algorithm can be used as an aid to diagnosis of pigmented skin lesions and can decrease the excision rate of benign lesions versus melanomas in general practice was investigated in another controlled randomized trial.

Methods.—The study included 468 general practitioners from 223 practices who were on the mailing lists of the divisions of general practice in Perth, Western Australia, and who were given national guidelines on melanoma management. Physicians selected randomly to the intervention group were educated in the use of an algorithm (Fig 1) and in the use of an instant camera. Assessment was based on the ratio of benign to malignant pigmented skin lesions excised. A malignant lesion was considered to be an in situ or invasive melanoma, and a benign lesion was considered to be a nevus (including dysplastic nevus) or a seborrheic keratosis. The latter was included because it is commonly mistaken for melanoma. All pathology reports related to excisions of pigmented skin lesions between November 1, 1998, and August 31, 2000, were obtained and reviewed. The primary outcome measures were the ratio of benign pigmented lesions to melanomas excised. Analyses were performed with and without inclusion of seborrheic keratoses.

Results.—At baseline, the ratios of benign to malignant lesions were less in the intervention group than they were in the control group. During the evaluation period, the ratios were higher in the intervention group (without seborrheic keratoses [19:1 vs 17:1]; with seborrheic keratoses [29:1 vs 26:1]). After adjusting for patients' age, sex, and socioeconomic status, the ratio was 1.02 times higher (95% confidence interval [CI], 0.68-1.51; $P =$ .94) in the intervention group when seborrheic keratoses were not included and 1.03 times higher (CI, 0.71 to 1.50; $P =$ .88) when seborrheic keratoses

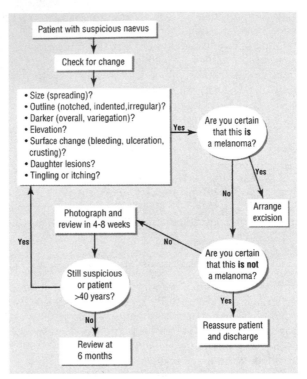

FIGURE 1.—Algorithm to assist with the management of patients with pigmented skin lesions. (Courtesy of English DR, Burton RC, del Mar CB, et al: Evaluation of aid to diagnosis of pigmented skin lesions in general practice: Controlled trial randomised by practice. *BMJ* 327:375-378, 2003. Reprinted with permission from the BMJ Publishing Group.)

were included. General practitioners in the intervention group were less likely than those in the control group to excise the most recent pigmented skin lesion (22% vs 48%; $P < .001$) and to refer the patient to a specialist (16% vs 27%; $P = .06$).

Conclusion.—The provision of an algorithm and camera to GPs to assist them in managing patients with suspicious pigmented lesions did not reduce the ratio of benign lesions to melanomas they excised.

▶ A previous study from Australia showed that the use of an instant camera and an algorithm for the management of pigmented lesions could reduce the ratio of excisions of benign lesions to melanomas without reducing the number of melanomas diagnosed. The current study, which failed to confirm those findings, is more supportive of those in a report published in the 2003 YEAR BOOK OF DERMATOLOGY AND DERMATOLOGIC SURGERY that demonstrated the difficulty primary care physicians have in differentiating benign from malignant skin lesions.[1]

B. H. Thiers, MD

Reference

1. Offidani A, Simonetti O, Bernardini ML, et al: General practitioners' accuracy in diagnosing skin cancers. *Dermatology* 205:127-130, 2002. (2003 YEAR BOOK OF DERMATOLOGY AND DERMATOLOGIC SURGERY, pp 389-390.)

The Transformation Rate of Moles (Melanocytic Nevi) Into Cutaneous Melanoma: A Population-Based Estimate

Tsao H, Bevona C, Goggins W, et al (Massachusetts Gen Hosp, Boston; Univ of Kansas, Kansas City; Hong Kong Baptist Univ, China; et al)
Arch Dermatol 139:282-288, 2003   17–4

Background.—Early detection and ongoing surveillance of moles for malignant degeneration comprise a strategy for reducing the burden of advanced cutaneous melanoma. The underlying assumption of this approach is that moles show a certain risk of transformation into melanoma. However, this risk is not known. The risk of moles transforming into cutaneous melanoma was estimated.

Methods.—A model of transformation was developed. The minimal number of moles transforming into cutaneous melanoma per year was assumed to be roughly equal to the number of melanomas diagnosed annually with associated nevic components. Annual risk was calculated as the number of mole-related melanomas diagnosed in 1 year in a 10-year age group. The cumulative risk during the lifetime of an individual mole was also estimated by using a modified standard life table method.

Findings.—For men and women younger than 40 years, the annual transformation rate of any single mole into melanoma was 0.0005% or less. For men older than 60 years, this rate was 0.003%. This transformation rate, comparable between women and men younger than 40 years, was markedly greater for men older than 40 years. A 20-year-old man had an approximate 0.03% lifetime risk of any selected mole transforming to melanoma by 80 years of age. This risk for a 20-year-old woman was 0.009%.

Conclusions.—This model suggests that the risk of any individual mole transforming into melanoma is low, especially among younger persons. Because moles can disappear, those that persist to older age have an increased risk of malignant transformation. Systematic excision of benign-appearing lesions would have a limited benefit in young persons with many moles and no other risk factors.

▶ This reviewer is always reluctant to draw conclusions from studies based on numerous assumptions and complex mathematical models. However, as the authors concede, to perform a prospective study that assesses the frequency with which melanomas arise in pre-existing melanocytic lesions would be difficult. On the basis of their calculations several conclusions can be drawn: (1) Patients younger than 30 years are more likely (up to 50%) to have their melanoma arise in association with a pre-existing melanocytic lesion than older patients (less than 20%). (2) Dysplastic or atypical nevi are not the only lesions that can coexist with or serve as precursors to melanoma; common nevi and congenital nevi may do so as well. (3) The risk of a melanocytic lesion transforming into melanoma increases with age, especially in men; however, the risk is extremely small, thus reinforcing this reviewer's long-held opinion that wholesale removal of moles to prevent melanoma is not justified. Finally, with regard to the pathogenesis of melanoma, there may be 2 populations of patients: (1) those with genetically unstable moles that, in combination with intermittent sun exposure, may evolve into melanoma at a relatively young age, and (2) those patients who require years of sun exposure to develop melanoma. In the latter group, the melanomas are less likely to arise in pre-existing melanocytic lesions.

P. G. Lang, Jr, MD

Melanocytic Nevi, Solar Keratoses, and Divergent Pathways to Cutaneous Melanoma
Whiteman DC, Watt P, Purdie DM, et al (Queensland Inst of Medical Research, Australia)
J Natl Cancer Inst 95:806-812, 2003   17–5

Introduction.—There is a divergent pathway model for melanomas that suggests that persons with an inherently low propensity for melanocyte proliferation need chronic sun exposure to drive clonal expansion of transformed epidermal melanocytes. Thus, melanomas in this group should arise on habitually sun-exposed body sites. Among persons with an inherently high propensity for melanocyte proliferation, exposure to sunlight is required early in the process of carcinogenesis, after which various factors drive melanoma development. This group would be expected to have less solar damage on habitually sun-exposed sites and to develop their tumors on body sites with unstable melanocyte populations. This divergent pathway theory was assessed for the development of melanoma according to anatomical site in a population-based epidemiologic investigation.

Methods.—Patients were randomly selected from 3 prespecified groups reported to the Queensland (Australia) Cancer Registry as follows: 154 patients with superficial spreading or nodular melanomas of the trunk (reference group), 77 patients with such melanomas on the head and neck (main comparison group), and 75 patients with lentigo maligna melanoma (LMM) (the chronic sun-exposed group). All participants completed a questionnaire, and a research nurse counted melanocytic nevi and solar keratoses. Exposure odds ratios (ORs) and 95% confidence intervals (CIs) were determined to quantify the relationship between factors of interest and each melanoma group.

Results.—Patients with head and neck melanomas, compared with those with melanomas of the trunk, were significantly less likely to have over 60 nevi (OR, 0.34; 95% CI, 01.5-0.79), yet were significantly more likely to have over 20 solar keratoses (OR, 3.61; 95% CI, 1.42-9.17) and also tended to have a past history of excised solar skin lesions (OR, 1.87; 95% CI. 0.89-

3.92). Those with LMM were also less likely than patients with truncal melanomas to have over 60 nevi (OR, 0.32; 95% CI, 0.14-0.75) and tended toward more solar keratoses (OR, 2.14; 95% CI, 0.88-5.16).

Conclusion.—The prevalences of nevi and solar keratoses vary substantially between patients with head and neck melanomas or LMM and patients with melanomas of the trunk. Cutaneous melanomas may arise through either an inherent propensity for melanocyte proliferation or as a result of chronic sunlight exposure.

▶ Although there is no doubt that ultraviolet light (UVL) is important in the pathogenesis of melanoma, it has never been clear exactly how this effect is mediated. For example, many melanomas occur on the trunk, a site that is often exposed to the sun only intermittently. Many epidemiologists believe that the initiating events in the development of melanoma begin early in life.

In keeping with this hypothesis, the authors propose that 2 different pathways can lead to the development of melanoma. In patients with a normal number of moles and presumably stable melanocytes that are not easily stimulated to proliferate, they suggest that chronic UVL exposure is required to bring about the development of melanoma. In such patients, the melanoma is usually located on chronically sun-exposed skin. These individuals usually have other evidence of chronic sun damage, ie, solar keratoses and non-melanoma skin cancer.

In contrast, the authors argue that patients with numerous moles might have less stable melanocytes that are more easily stimulated to proliferate. In this population, UVL exposure early in life, with or without intermittent UVL exposure later in life, would be sufficient to bring about the development of melanoma on relatively sun-protected areas such as the trunk.

For the second pathway to be plausible, melanocytes on the trunk—the usual location for numerous moles—would have to be more unstable and more susceptible to the effects of the sun than melanocytes located on chronically sun-exposed skin. This remains to be determined. Also uncertain is whether patients with numerous moles who develop melanoma are more likely to have tumors on the trunk as opposed to chronically sun-damaged skin. This article would suggest so, but a larger epidemiologic study is needed to confirm this.

P. G. Lang, Jr, MD

***BRAF* Mutation: A Frequent Event in Benign, Atypical, and Malignant Melanocytic Lesions of the Skin**
Uribe P, Wistuba II, González S (P. Universidad Catolica de Chile, Santiago)
Am J Dermatopathol 25:365-370, 2003   17–6

Introduction.—A recent study reported a high frequency (66%) of *BRAF* mutations in cutaneous melanoma. The mutations were within the kinase domain, with a single substitution in exon 15 (T1796A) at codon 599 (V599E) accounting for 5 of 6 *BRAF* mutations in primary melanoma and

19 of 20 in melanoma cell lines. To investigate the stage in which *BRAF* mutations occur in the malignant transformation of melanocytes, benign and atypical nevi and primary cutaneous melanomas were examined for *BRAF* mutations at codon 599.

Methods.—Included in the analysis were 23 benign melanocytic nevi, 23 atypical melanocytic nevi, and 25 primary cutaneous melanoma from 63 different patients. The examination for *BRAF* mutations used DNA extracted from microdissected formalin-fixed and paraffin-embedded tissues and a strategy that was based on a 2-round polymerase chain reaction restriction fragment length polymorphism (PCR-RFLP).

Results.—All 3 groups of melanocytic lesions examined were found to have *BRAF* mutations at codon 599; the overall incidence was 60%. The frequencies were 72% in benign melanocytic nevi, 52% in atypical melanocytic nevi, and 56% in primary melanomas. Microdissected epidermal keratinocytes adjacent to melanocytic lesions having the specific *BRAF* mutations (4 benign nevi, 4 atypical nevi, and 3 melanomas) exhibited no *BRAF* mutations at codon 599. In malignant melanoma, no correlation was observed between *BRAF* mutational status and patient age, sun exposure, or Clark level. However, among atypical nevi and melanoma lesions, the frequency of *BRAF* mutation was significantly greater in male (78%) than in female (35%) patients.

Conclusion.—Because of the high frequency of *BRAF* mutation at codon 599 in benign and atypical melanocytic lesions of the skin, the *BRAF* mutation should not be considered a feature of malignant melanocyte transformation. However, the mutation may play an important role in initial melanocytic proliferation.

▶ Cancer results from an accumulation of mutations in critical genes that affect normal programs of cell proliferation, differentiation, and death. An article in the 2003 YEAR BOOK OF DERMATOLOGY AND DERMATOLOGIC SURGERY suggested an important role for the BRAF gene in the pathogenesis of melanoma.[1] However, as demonstrated by Uribe et al, *BRAF* mutations can be seen in benign as well as malignant melanocytic proliferations. It is perhaps more likely that *BRAF* plays a key role in the development of melanocytes, and this may account for its high frequency in all types of melanocytic lesions.[2,3]

B. H. Thiers, MD

References

1. Davies H, Bignell GR, Cox C, et al: Mutations of the *BRAF* gene in human cancer. *Nature* 417:949-954, 2002. (2003 YEAR BOOK OF DERMATOLOGY AND DERMATOLOGIC SURGERY, pp 428-429.)
2. Busca R, Abbe T, Mantoux S, et al: Ras mediates cAMP-dependent activation of extracellular single-related kinases (ERKs) in melanocytes. *EMBO J* 19:2900-2910, 2000.
3. Pollock PM, Meltzer PS: Lucky draw in the gene raffle. *Nature* 417:906-907, 2002.

Suppression of BRAF^V599E in Human Melanoma Abrogates Transformation

Hingorani SR, Jacobetz MA, Robertson GP, et al (Univ of Pennsylvania; Pennsylvania State Univ, Hershey)

Cancer Res 63:5198-5202, 2003   17–7

Background.—More than 70% of human melanomas demonstrate activating mutations in the *BRAF* serine/threonine kinase. More than 90% are *BRAF^V599E*. The role of the *BRAF^V599E* allele in malignant melanoma was investigated.

Methods and Findings.—In cultured human melanoma cells, the suppression of *BRAF^V599E* expression by RNA interference inhibited the mitogen-activated protein kinase cascade, arrested growth, and promoted apoptosis. Knockdown of *BRAF^V599E* expression abrogated the transformed phenotype completely, as assessed by colony formation in soft agar. Similar targeting of *BRAF^V599E* or wild-type *BRAF* in human fibrosarcoma cells lacking the *BRAF^V599E* mutation did not recapitulate these effects. These findings were specific for *BRAF*. Targeted interference of *CRAF* in melanoma cells did not significantly change their biological properties.

Conclusions.—When present, *BRAF^V599E* appears to be essential for melanoma cell viability and transformation. Thus, *BRAF^V599E* may be an attractive therapeutic target in melanomas that harbor the mutation.

▶ Although perhaps not sufficient by itself for malignant transformation (see Abstract 17–6), mutations in the *BRAF* gene may nonetheless represent an attractive chemopreventive or chemotherapeutic target. The BRAF gene product is a protein kinase, and protein kinase inhibitors, such as imatinib mesylate, have been an active area of oncologic research. Beneficial effects have been reported in a number of myeloproliferative disorders[1,2] and even metastatic dermatofibrosarcoma protuberans.[3] Inhibitors of *BRAF* will quite likely be tested for their ability to halt the spread of melanoma as well.

B. H. Thiers, MD

References

1. Druker BJ, Talpaz M, Resta DJ, et al: Efficacy and safety of a specific inhibitor of the BCR-ABL tyrosine kinase on chronic myeloid leukemia. *N Engl J Med* 344:1031-1037, 2001.
2. Apperley JF, Gardembas M, Melo JV, et al: Response to imatinib mesylate in patients with chronic myeloproliferative diseases with rearrangements of the platelet-derived growth factor receptor beta. *N Engl J Med* 347:481-487, 2002.
3. Maki RG, Awan RA, Dixon RH, et al: Differential sensitivity to imatinib of two patients with metastatic sarcoma arising from dermatofibrosarcoma protuberans. *Int J Cancer* 100:623-626, 2002.

Are En Face Frozen Sections Accurate for Diagnosing Margin Status in Melanocytic Lesions?

Prieto VG, Argenyi ZB, Barnhill RL, et al (Univ of Texas, Houston; Univ of Seattle; George Washington Univ, Washington, DC; et al)
Am J Clin Pathol 120:203-208, 2003   17–8

Introduction.—The presence of scattered atypical melanocytes secondary to actinic damage complicates the evaluation of frozen sections to determine surgical margin status in pigmented lesions of the head and neck. In en face sections, an isolated, atypical melanocyte may represent either lentigo maligna at the margin or a background of sun-damaged skin. The diagnostic accuracy of en face frozen sections was compared with that of standard paraffin-embedded sections in cases of malignant melanomas (MMs) and nonmelanocytic lesions (NMLs).

Methods.—Twenty-four blocks from 23 cases in which en face frozen sections were used to examine the surgical margins included 13 MMs and 10 NMLs. The blocks were thawed, processed in paraffin, and stained with hematoxylin and eosin. Slides of frozen and paraffin-embedded sections were randomly coded and reviewed by 15 dermatopathologists who were unaware of clinical histories and of MM or NML status. Margin status was categorized as positive, negative, or indeterminate.

Results.—Two cases, 1 of MM and 1 of NML, had to be excluded, leaving 330 possible diagnoses (22 cases × 15 dermatologists). Discrepancies in diagnoses between frozen and permanent sections were analyzed by case and by dermatologist. A total of 132 discrepancies (40.0%) occurred, 66 for MM and 66 for NML cases. In 80 instances, the dermatopathologist classified margin status as indeterminate in either frozen or paraffin sections. In 43 instances, the diagnosis was changed from negative in the frozen section to positive in the permanent section. A positive margin in the frozen section was changed to negative in the permanent section in 9 instances. There was slightly better agreement between frozen- and permanent-section diagnoses in NML cases. Agreement was also slightly better among dermatopathologists who routinely studied frozen sections than among those who did not.

Discussion.—Frozen sections provide a quick diagnosis, but their quality usually is lower than that obtained with routinely processed, formalin-fixed tissue. In this series of MMs and NMLs, there was a general lack of agreement among dermatopathologists regarding correlation of en face frozen- and paraffin-section diagnoses. Perpendicular sections or quick paraffin processing may be preferable in the evaluation of melanocytic lesions.

▶ This study has 2 objectives, one to compare the analysis of frozen section with paraffin-embedded material, and the second to compare perpendicular margins with "en face" margins. The authors found that paraffin-embedded material is superior to frozen-section material for the analysis of subtle melanocytic proliferations. They observed "a drawback of the method of perpendicular sections is that the entire margin is not examined." They also note that performing en face margins permits the examination of the entire margin with a relatively low number of sections, yet they conclude that the use of perpendicular sections is the preferable option in most cases. Unfortunately, the data to support this conclusion are soft. One problem that is always faced when determining the margins of excision of melanoma in situ on chronically sun-damaged skin is the challenge of distinguishing tumor cells from background melanocytes that may show atypical features. The technique of Mohs surgery is based on the fact that en face margins examined by experienced Mohs surgeons enable a much higher cure rate for nonmelanoma skin cancer than do margins determined by the traditional breadloaf technique. Mohs surgeons have now used the same rationale for treating melanoma in situ on the face with excellent long-term results. Many if not most Mohs surgeons prefer the "slow Mohs'" procedure utilizing paraffin-embedded rather than frozen sections for analyzing the adequacy of melanoma margins because of the superior morphologic detail present in permanent sections.

J. C. Maize, MD

Repair of UV Light-Induced DNA Damage and Risk of Cutaneous Malignant Melanoma
Wei Q, Lee JE, Gershenwald JE, et al (Univ of Texas, Houston)
J Natl Cancer Inst 95:308-315, 2003   17–9

Background.—UV exposure can induce cutaneous malignant melanoma (CMM), and some evidence suggests DNA repair capacity (DRC) plays a role in the pathogenesis of sunlight-induced CMM. A case-control study was undertaken to explore the role of DRC in the development of CMM.

Methods.—The cases were 312 hospitalized non-Hispanic white patients with CMM (51% men; mean age, 48.0 years) and no prior chemotherapy or radiation therapy. The controls were 324 cancer-free subjects matched to the cases by age, sex, and race. All subjects completed a questionnaire to collect demographic data and information on risk factors for CMM. They also provided blood samples for a host-cell reactivation assay to measure DRC in lymphocytes.

Results.—The mean DRC was significantly lower in the cases than in the controls (8.5% vs 10.5%, or a 19.0% decrease). The mean DRC was also significantly lower in patients with tumors on sun-exposed skin than in patients whose tumors were on unexposed skin (8.2% vs 9.5%, or a 13.7% decrease). In multivariate analyses, controls whose DRC was at or below the median value of 9.4% had a significantly increased risk of CMM (odds ratio, 2.02). There was a significant dose-response relationship between a decreased DRC and an increased risk of CMM.

Conclusion.—A reduced DRC is independently associated with an increased risk of CMM. There is a dose-response relationship between a decreased DRC and an increased risk of CMM, and patients whose tumors were on sun-exposed skin had a significantly lower DRC. These results suggest that a reduced DRC may contribute to the development of sun-induced CMM.

▶ Wei et al present data to suggest that a reduced DRC is an independent risk factor for CMM. The results contrast with a recent case-control study from Italy that compared 132 CMM patients and 145 control subjects from a population with high risk familial dysplastic nevi. In that study, DRC was not found to be an independent risk factor for CMM.[1]

B. H. Thiers, MD

Reference

1. Landi MT, Baccarelli A, Tarone RE, et al: DNA repair, dysplastic nevi, and sunlight sensitivity in the development of cutaneous malignant melanoma. *J Natl Cancer Inst* 94:94-101, 2002.

Mortality From Cancer and Other Causes Among Male Airline Cockpit Crew in Europe
Blettner M, Zeeb H, Auvinen A, et al (Univ of Bielefeld, Germany; Univ of Tampere, Finland; STUK Radiation and Nuclear Safety Authority, Helsinki; et al)
Int J Cancer 106:946-952, 2003   17–10

Background.—Airline pilots and flight engineers comprise an occupational group exposed to ionizing radiation of cosmic origin and other factors that may affect their health and mortality. The mortality rate in such workers in 9 European countries was reported in the current cohort study.

Methods.—Cohorts of cockpit crews were studied in Denmark, Finland, Germany, Great Britain, Greece, Iceland, Italy, Norway, and Sweden. The study included 28,000 persons with 547,564 person-years at risk.

Findings.—Among male crew members, 2244 deaths were recorded, for a standardized mortality ratio (SMR) of 0.64. Overall, death from cancer was reduced (SMR = 0.68). Mortality from lung cancer was decreased, but that from malignant melanoma was increased. Neither employment period nor duration correlated with cancer mortality rate. Cardiovascular mortality rate was low. The mortality rate from aviation accidents was increased.

Conclusions.—Cockpit crew members have a low mortality rate overall. However, their risk of malignant melanoma is increased.

▶ The results are similar to those reported in an article reviewed in the 2000 YEAR BOOK OF DERMATOLOGY AND DERMATOLOGIC SURGERY, in which an increased risk of melanoma was observed among those in a cohort of 485 men commercial pilots who had the highest radiation exposure.[1]

B. H. Thiers, MD

Reference

1. Rafnsson V, Hrafnkelsson J, Tulinius H: Incidence of cancer among commercial airline pilots. *Occup Environ Med* 57:175-179, 2000. (2000 YEAR BOOK OF DERMATOLOGY AND DERMATOLOGIC SURGERY, pp 327-328.)

Melanomas in Prepubescent Children: Review Comprehensively, Critique Historically, Criteria Diagnostically, and Course Biologically

Mones JM, Ackerman AB (Ackerman Academy of Dermatopathology, New York City)
Am J Dermatopathol 25:223-238, 2003   17–11

Introduction.—There has been considerable controversy regarding the matter of primary cutaneous melanoma in young children. This review represents the largest series reported to date of de novo, metastasis-proven melanomas in prepubescent (younger than 10 years) children. Excluded were lesions that arose in association with a nevus of any kind, in children with xeroderma pigmentosa, in conjunction with another malignant neoplasm in a child who was immunocompromised, or in a zone of previous irradiation.

Findings.—Eleven children, 4 girls and 7 boys aged 1 to 10 years (mean 5.2 years), were studied. Two melanomas were located on the head and neck, 2 on the trunk, 2 on an arm, and 5 on a lower extremity. Most lesions were initially thought to be nevi, with none suspected to be melanoma on the basis of clinical features. The most common diagnoses offered by the original histopathologist were Spitz nevus or atypical Spitz nevus. Melanoma was mentioned as a possibility in 3 cases. These lesions have many findings in common, yet melanoma in prepubescent children and Spitz nevus have major differences in architectural pattern and in cytopathologic features (Table 5). The vertical orientation of the melanocytic neoplasm, its only slightly asymmetric shape, and its uneven distribution of melanin characterize mel-

---

TABLE 5.—Major Criteria for Differentiating Melanoma in Prepubescents From Spitz Nevus Histopathologically

Architectural
  Striking confluence of fascicles of melanocytes in the reticular dermis (and subcutaneous fat) with formation of a sheet of cells
  Extensive involvement of the subcutaneous fat often
  Peculiar geometric shapes assumed by aggregations of neoplastic melanocytes, i.e., neither stereotypical nests nor fascicles usually
  Perivascular infiltrates of lymphocytes at the periphery of the neoplasm and especially the base of it
Cytopathological
  Many nuclei of melanocytes small as well as large, and nuclei, irrespective of size, heterochromatic
  Cytoplasm of many melanocytes scant and cytoplasm of others abundant
  Many mitotic figures and many of them in the lower part of the neoplasm

(Courtesy of Mones JM, Ackerman AB: Melanomas in prepubescent children: Review comprehensively, critique historically, criteria diagnostically, and course biologically. *Am J Dermatopathol* 25:223-238, 2003.)

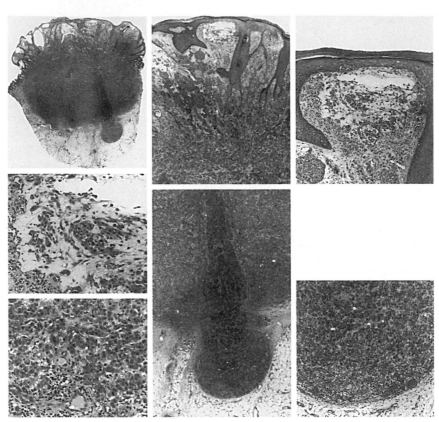

FIGURE 3.—Melanoma in a 2-year-old (our Case 4). At scanning magnification, some features in the neoplasm are reminiscent of Spitz nevus, namely, vertical orientation, hyperkeratosis, focal hypergranulosis, adnexal hyperplasia, and edema in the upper part of the dermis. Even at scanning magnification, however, this neoplasm can be gauged to be a melanoma by virtue of its asymmetry, uneven base, and crowding of aggregations of neoplastic cells that give the impression of diffuseness. At higher magnification, definitive signs of melanoma are more apparent, namely, marked variation in size and shape of aggregations of neoplastic cells, the assumption of peculiar geometric shapes by some of those aggregations, confluence to form a sheet of neoplastic cells, and nuclei of neoplastic cells that are crowded, heterochromatic, and pleomorphic. In the lower part of the neoplasm, many cells are in mitosis. The diagnosis of the original histopathologist was not recorded. (Courtesy of Mones JM, Ackerman AB: Melanomas in prepubescent children: Review comprehensively, critique historically, criteria diagnostically, and course biologically. *Am J Dermatopathol* 25:223-238, 2003.)

anoma in prepubescent children (Fig 3). Every melanoma in this series was very thick, and metastasis occurred in all 11 children (to regional lymph nodes in 10). One child had died of disease; 10 were alive at the time of publication with follow-up ranging from 2 to 37 months, but all have a grave prognosis.

Discussion.—Primary cutaneous melanomas can arise de novo in prepubescent children and may easily be confused with a Spitz nevus. The neoplasm is often thick at the time of biopsy, an indication of its rapid growth, and is characterized by vertical orientation, diffuse infiltration throughout the dermis, and often extensive involvement of the subcutaneous fat. An accurate diagnosis requires application of criteria established for the histopathologic differentiation of melanoma from Spitz nevi. The ABCD criteria (asymmetry, border irregularity, color variability, and diameter >6 mm) are inadequate in children.

▶ Melanomas in childhood are rare but have been a subject of considerable interest ever since Sophie Spitz described "juvenile melanoma" more than a half a century ago. This benign melanocytic proliferation now bears her name, despite the fact that she was mistaken in her interpretation of it. In this article by Mones and Ackerman, 11 cases of malignant melanoma in childhood are reviewed. Interestingly, none of them was diagnosed prospectively by the physicians who removed them. This suggests that the clinical criteria used to diagnose melanoma in adults may not be as useful in the evaluation of childhood melanoma. Mones and Ackerman offer histopathologic criteria for differentiating melanoma in children from Spitz nevus. Hopefully, these criteria will be reproducible and can be applied prospectively.

J. C. Maize, MD

Acral Lentiginous Melanoma Mimicking Benign Disease: The Emory Experience

Soon SL, Solomon AR Jr, Papadopoulos D, et al (Emory Univ, Atlanta, Ga; Bethesda Dermatopathology Lab, Silver Spring, Md)
J Am Acad Dermatol 48:183-188, 2003   17–12

Introduction.—Plantar and subungual melanomas have a higher incidence of misdiagnosis, compared with other anatomical sites. Misdiagnosis and delay in diagnosis are statistically correlated with poor patient outcome. The awareness of atypical manifestations of acral melanoma may be important in reducing the rate of misdiagnosis and improving patient outcome.

Methods.—A retrospective case review of patients with plantar or lower-extremity subungual melanoma seen between 1985 and 2001 was performed. Clinical and demographic data were recorded. The histopathology of case biopsy specimens was examined by an experienced dermatologist.

Results.—Fifty-three cases of plantar or lower-extremity subungual melanoma were detected. Of these, 18 were initially misdiagnosed. The misdiagnoses included wart, callous, fungal disorder, foreign body, crusty lesion, sweat gland condition, blister, nonhealing wound, mole, keratoacanthoma, subungual hematoma, onychomycosis, ingrown toenail, and defective/infected toenail. Nine of the 18 misdiagnosed cases were clinically amelanotic.

Conclusion.—Awareness that amelanotic variants of acral melanoma may assume the morphology of benign hyperkeratotic dermatoses may increase the incidence of correct diagnosis and improve outcome in patients with atypical manifestations of acral melanoma.

▶ It has long been recognized that acral lentiginous melanoma often has a poor prognosis because of a delay in diagnosis and advanced disease at the time of correct diagnosis. For the most part, this article simply repeats the observations of others; however, several points are worth mentioning. Over 50% of the lesions were amelanotic, which would increase the likelihood of misdiagnosis. In addition a significant number of the lesions were hyperkeratotic, which would increase the likelihood of confusion with benign entities such as callous or wart. Finally, the authors present some evidence that African Americans with acral lentiginous melanoma may have a worse prognosis, although this possibility needs further study before any final conclusions are drawn.

P. G. Lang, Jr, MD

Conjunctival Melanoma: Is It Increasing in the United States?
Yu G-P, Hu D-N, McCormick S, et al (New York Med College; EyeCare Foundation Inc., New York)
Am J Ophthalmol 135:800-806, 2003   17–13

Introduction.—The incidence of cutaneous melanoma has increased rapidly and continuously in the Western world. A relatively large cancer registry database in the United States was used to ascertain whether any changes had occurred in the rate of conjunctival melanoma.

Methods.—Population-based registry data from the Surveillance, Epidemiology, and End Results program of the National Cancer Institute were used to identify 206 newly diagnosed patients with conjunctival melanoma from 1973 to 1999. Unique characteristics of this analysis are the calculations of age-adjusted rate and the descriptions of trends using a joinpoint regression model.

Results.—The overall estimated biannual percent change (EBAPC) was 5.5 (95% confidence interval [CI], 2.3-8.8; $P < .001$). The significant elevated trend was observed in white males (EBAPC = 11.2; 95% CI, 6.3-16.3; $P < .001$) but not in white females (EBAPC = 0.3; 95% CI, -4.1 to 4.9; $P < .05$). In white males, the rate rose 295% in 27 years. A significant upward trend was seen in patients aged 60 years or older (EBAPC = 7.6; 95% CI, 3.9-11.3; $P < .001$). The incidence was nonsignificantly increased in the group aged 40 to 59 years (EBAPC = 4.4; 95% CI, -2.3 to 11.6; $P = .1536$).

Conclusion.—Marked temporal changes in the incidence of conjunctival melanoma have occurred in the United States. The changing incidence patterns parallel those observed in cutaneous melanoma, indicating a possible link to a sunlight-associated etiology.

▶ Previous studies have suggested a stable trend in the incidence of conjunctival melanoma. In contrast, Yu et al observed an overall increase in the incidence of conjunctival melanoma from 1973 to 1999. This rising trend was observed in white men but not in white women. The changing incidence patterns coincide with those seen in cutaneous melanoma, suggesting a possible etiologic link to sun exposure.

B. H. Thiers, MD

Melanoma-Associated Retinopathy: High Frequency of Subclinical Findings in Patients With Melanoma

Pföhler C, Haus A, Palmowski A, et al (Saarland Univ Hosp, Homberg/Saar, Germany; Univ of California, Sacramento)

Br J Dermatol 149:74-78, 2003   17–14

Introduction.—Melanoma-associated retinopathy (MAR) is a paraneoplastic syndrome characterized by symptoms of night blindness, light sensations, visual loss, visual field defects, and diminished b-waves in the electroretinogram. Patients with MAR frequently experience a sudden onset of ocular symptoms considered to result from antibody production against melanoma-associated antigens that cross-react with corresponding epitopes on retinal depolarizing bipolar cells. The incidence of subclinical symptoms suggestive of MAR in patients with melanoma was correlated with the various stages of disease, patient age, type and thickness of the primary tumor, form of therapy, S-100 level, and tumor burden.

Methods.—Twenty-eight patients with melanoma in stages I to IV (according to the American Joint Committee on Cancer tumor classification) were evaluated for the presence of subclinical MAR symptoms with the use of scotopic electroretinography, static and kinetic perimetry, and nyctometry.

Results.—Seven patients had clinical signs and symptoms consistent with MAR, 18 had some indications, and 3 had no indications. No association was observed between clinical symptoms and disease stage, tumor burden, or S-100 level. Findings suggestive of MAR were seen more frequently in advanced stages of disease.

Conclusion.—Subclinical retinal involvement representative of MAR seems to be more common than previously suspected in patients with cutaneous malignant melanoma. An unexpectedly high percentage of patients had abnormal ophthalmologic findings, yet only 1 patient reported subjective symptoms.

▶ The paraneoplastic syndrome, MAR, is characterized by symptoms of night blindness and progressive loss of vision. Typical symptoms include a sudden onset of shimmering, flickering, or pulsating lights and often begin suddenly, months after tumor diagnosis. Pföhler et al report that subclinical MAR may occur more often than previously suspected and that the condition may be more common in patients with advanced stages of melanoma.

B. H. Thiers, MD

Enhanced Survival in Patients With Multiple Primary Melanoma

Doubrovsky A, Menzies SW (Univ of Sydney, Australia)
Arch Dermatol 139:1013-1018, 2003   17–15

Background.—Patients with melanoma are at an increased risk of a second primary melanoma. The survival probabilities of patients with 3 or more multiple primary melanomas were reported.

Methods.—This retrospective cohort study included 5250 patients treated for stage I or II melanoma between 1983 and 1999. Two hundred sixty-four patients (5%) had 2 primary melanomas and 34 (0.6%) had 3 or more primary melanomas.

Findings.—The estimated 10-year risk for the development of a second primary melanoma was 12.7%. Patients with 2 primary melanomas had a 27.7% 10-year risk of developing a third lesion. A proportional hazards regression model, controlling for known prognostic factors, indicated that the number of primary melanomas significantly and favorably predicted survival when the thickest or first tumor was modeled. Thirty-one patients with 3 or more primary melanomas survived, compared with an expected number of 25. Multiple primary melanomas may have had greater opportunity to develop in longer-term survivors, whereas patients with all primary lesions developing within 2 years may not have been subject to this bias. Eleven patients with 3 or more melanomas had all primary lesions within 2 years. All 11 survived, compared with an expected number of 9.

Conclusions.—Patients with 3 or more primary melanoma lesions survived longer than expected. This increase in survival may be consistent with the phenomenon of an "immunization effect" in animals inoculated with multiple tumors.

▶ For years, investigators have studied the role of the immune system in the growth and development of melanoma in hopes that the information obtained could be used to improve survival of affected patients. Melanoma vaccines are an outgrowth of this effort. In this study from Australia, the authors found that patients with 3 or more primary melanomas experienced a better than expected survival rate. Based on animal studies, the authors propose that the development of 3 or more melanomas immunizes patients against the tumor, thus accounting for their improved survival. However, as a caveat, such patients without doubt are genetically predisposed to the disease, and this same genetic predisposition that renders them susceptible to melanoma may also influence the biological behavior of their tumors; that is, perhaps their melanomas have a reduced propensity to metastasize.

P. G. Lang, Jr, MD

Pancreatic Carcinoma Surveillance in Patients With Familial Melanoma
Parker JF, Florell SR, Alexander A, et al (Univ of Utah, Salt Lake City; Salt Lake
City Veterans Affairs Med Ctr, Utah)
Arch Dermatol 139:1019-1025, 2003   17–16

Introduction.—There is growing evidence that cyclin-dependent kinase inhibitor 2A (*CDKN2A*) mutations, which are associated with familial melanoma, may also predispose to pancreatic carcinoma. One study of 19 families with familial atypical multiple mole melanoma syndrome (FAMMM) and a specific 19–base-pair deletion in exon 2 of the *CDKN2A* gene (the p16-Leiden deletion) found pancreatic cancer to be the second most frequent cancer in these families. No cases of pancreatic cancer were found among persons from families with FAMMM without the p16-Leiden deletion. A patient from a kindred with familial melanoma and an established functional germline *CDKN2A* mutation was described. In addition, the most recent literature surrounding screening methods for early detection of pancreatic tumors was reviewed, with the goal of evaluating the role of traditional and more innovative surveillance methods in patients with familial malignant melanoma and *CDKN2A* mutations.

> *Case Report.*—Man, 32, had a clinically atypical melanocytic lesion excised from the right side of his back in 1978. Pathologic evaluation confirmed superficial spreading malignant melanoma (Clark level IV). Fourteen months later, right axillary node dissection revealed metastatic malignant melanoma. Nodules were also resected from the right lung, and the patient underwent 21 courses of chemotherapy during a 2-year period. New primary lesions were excised when the patient was 39 and 46. At the age of 57, after enrolling in the Familial Melanoma Research Clinic at the University of Utah, the patient received a diagnosis of FAMMM syndrome. His family history was positive for melanoma, numerous atypical nevi, and pancreatic carcinoma. Two months later, numerous tests to investigate the cause of chronic low back pain and abdominal pain confirmed pancreatic carcinoma with widespread metastases. The patient died 11 days later.

Discussion.—Pedigree analysis of data from the Utah Population Database led to construction of a 6-generation, 2-founder pedigree of 179 persons. In this kindred with familial melanoma, the observed-expected ratio for melanoma was 16.4 to 20.8, and the observed-expected ratio for pancreatic adenocarcinoma was 8.9 to 12.6. An algorithm for surveillance of patients with familial melanoma and known *CDKN2A* mutations was proposed. At-risk patients should undergo spiral CT, endoscopic US, and measurement of CA 19-9 levels as initial screening tests at age 50 or sooner.

▶ *CDKN2A* has been identified as the major melanoma susceptibility gene in the familial melanoma syndrome. Mutations in that gene are found in 20% to

40% of melanoma-prone families and are associated with FAMMM. Patients carrying this gene also appear to be predisposed to pancreatic carcinoma, as illustrated in the pedigree reported by Parker et al.

B. H. Thiers, MD

Evidence for an Association Between Cutaneous Malignant Melanoma and Lymphoid Malignancy: A Population-Based Retrospective Cohort Study in Scotland

McKenna DB, Stockton D, Brewster DH, et al (Royal Infirmary of Edinburgh, Scotland; Trinity Park House, Edinburgh, Scotland)
Br J Cancer 88:74-78, 2003   17–17

Background.—The risk of melanoma and nonmelanoma skin cancer is increased in patients with cutaneous malignant melanoma (CM). In addition, second cancers, including CM, have been documented in patients with lymphoid cancers such as non-Hodgkin lymphoma (NHL) and chronic lymphatic leukemia (CLL). The possible association between CM and NHL or CLL was investigated with the use of a population-based cancer registry.

Methods.—Cohorts in whom CM, NHL, or CLL was diagnosed between 1975 and 1997 were identified from the Scottish national cancer registry. Data on 9385 patients with CM, 4016 with CLL, and 13,857 with NHL were obtained. These cohorts were then followed through the registry for subsequent diagnoses.

Findings.—The risks of both CLL and NHL were increased after a diagnosis of CM, with standardized incidence ratios of 2.3 and 1.5, respectively. The risk of CM was also increased after a diagnosis of CLL or NHL, with a ratio of 2.3 and 2.1, respectively. The risks of CLL developing in patients with CM and of CM developing in NHL survivors were increased to a level that reached statistical significance ($P < .05$).

Conclusions.—These data indicate an association among CM, CLL, and NHL in the same patient. Immunosuppression, exposure to UV radiation, and genetic factors may contribute to a host environment that supports the development of these cancers.

▶ McKenna et al report an association between CM, CLL, and NHL. Future studies are needed to determine the influence of treatment effects and survival bias and to determine what role, if any, shared environmental or genetic factors play in this association.

B. H. Thiers, MD

Vascular Endothelial Growth Factor-C Expression Correlates With Lymph Node Localization of Human Melanoma Metastases

Schietroma C, Cianfarani F, Lacal PM, et al (Istituto Dermopatico Dell'Immacolata-Istituto di Ricovero e Cura a Carattere Scientifico, Rome; Ed Herriot Hosp, Lyon, France)
Cancer 98:789-797, 2003   17–18

Introduction.—Melanoma metastasizes by different mechanisms that involve direct invasion of the surrounding tissue and spreading via the lymphatic or vascular system. The molecular mechanisms that guide the route of spreading and localizing metastases in various tissues are not well understood. Recent trials of various tumor types have reported that vascular endothelial growth factor-C (VEGF-C), which demonstrates a high specificity for lymphatic endothelium, is involved in tumor-induced lymphangiogenesis and lymphatic metastatic spread. The expression of VEGF-C in cultured human melanoma cells derived from cutaneous and lymph node metastases, along with metastatic melanoma tissue specimens, was evaluated to ascertain a possible involvement of this growth factor in lymph node localization of melanoma metastases.

Methods.—The VEGF-C expression was assessed in vitro on human melanoma cell lines established from cutaneous and lymph node metastasis specimens by reverse transcriptase–polymerase chain reaction, Northern blot analysis, and immunofluorescence analysis. Forty-two tissue specimens of melanoma metastases and 10 tissue samples of primary skin melanomas also underwent immunohistochemical analysis.

Results.—Preferential expression of VEGF-C was identified in lymph-node–derived tumor cells at both the messenger RNA and protein levels. The correlation between VEGF-C production and lymph node localization of metastases was verified by the in vivo analysis. Analysis of 10 patients from whom specimens of both the primary skin melanoma and melanoma metastases were available indicated an association between VEGF-C expression in the primary tumor and lymph node localization of metastases.

Conclusion.—A preferential expression of VEGF-C messenger RNA and protein in lymph node–derived versus cutaneous-derived metastatic tumor cells was observed. The VEGF-C expression is associated with localization of melanoma metastases in the lymph nodes. Expression of VEGF-C in primary skin melanoma may be predictive of lymph node metastatic dissemination.

Differential Expression of Vascular Endothelial Growth Factor–A Isoforms at Different Stages of Melanoma Progression

Gorski DH, Leal AD, Goydos JS (UMDNJ-Robert Wood Johnson Medical School, New Brunswick, NJ)
J Am Coll Surg 197:408-418, 2003   17–19

Introduction.—Melanomas have a consistent pattern of spreading from the primary tumor to the regional lymphatic bed to distant metastatic sites. It is unusual for a melanoma to metastasize to a distant site without first passing through the regional lymphatics. The factors involved in this specific pattern of spread are mostly unknown. It is apparent that melanoma cells have to undergo progressive phenotypic changes to develop the ability to form a vertical growth phase and spread to the dermal lymphatic bed, the regional lymph nodes, and to distant metastatic sites.

The development of the ability to express proangiogenic factors is likely to be one of the changes that permit melanoma cells to spread and grow in the regional lymph nodes. A strong relationship has been reported between levels of vascular endothelial growth factor-A (VEGF-A) and melanoma progression and metastasis. Message levels for the 3 major isoforms of VEGF-A were compared in melanoma specimens from various stages of progression.

Methods.—Eighteen, 5, 11, 12, 18, and 9 samples, respectively, from primary melanomas, primary recurrences, regional dermal metastases, nodal metastases, normal lymph nodes, and distant metastases were prospectively obtained. Samples from the horizontal and vertical growth phases of primary tumors were also obtained from 5 additional patients. Message levels for the 3 major VEGF-A isoforms were determined by real-time quantitative reverse transcriptase–polymerase chain reaction and normalized to β-actin messenger RNA levels.

Results.—There was a substantial increase in the expression of all 3 VEGF-A isoforms from the vertical growth phase tissue compared with the horizontal growth phase tissue. Primary tumors, local recurrences, regional dermal metastases, nodal metastases, and distant metastases all produced more $VEGF_{121}$ and $VEGF_{165}$, compared with negative nodes. Nodal metastases produced the highest level of these 2 isoforms, which was even higher than that observed in distant metastases. There were no significant between-group differences in $VEGF_{189}$ expression.

Conclusion.—Melanomas in the vertical growth phase produce more VEGF-A (all isoforms) than tumors in the horizontal growth phase. Nodal metastases create the highest levels of $VEGF_{121}$ and $VEGF_{165}$, but not $VEGF_{189}$, compared with other stages of disease progression. The soluble forms of VEGF-A may be important in melanoma metastasis to regional lymph nodes.

▶ The findings suggest that cell-specific factors may determine the metastatic potential of melanoma cells. The observation that metastasis may not be a random event is not new. In a landmark article published 25 years ago, Nicolson observed that murine melanoma cells metastatic to the lung, when injected into a second animal, would localize to the lung.[1] Similar specificities were observed for other organs. These findings suggest that, as inferred by Schietroma et al (Abstract 17–18), certain factors unique to a tumor cell and its target organ may be important in determining the propensity for tumor dissemination.

B. H. Thiers, MD

Reference

1. Nicolson GL: Cancer metastasis. *Sci Am* 240:66-76, 1979.

Investigation of the Growth and Metastasis of Malignant Melanoma in a Murine Model: The Role of Supplemental Vitamin A
Weinzweig J, Tattini C, Lynch S, et al (Brown Univ, Providence, RI)
Plast Reconstr Surg 112:152-158, 2003   17–20

Introduction.—The wound-healing and antitumor qualities of vitamin A suggest its potential benefit in the treatment of human disease. Previous studies have shown that vitamin A inhibits the proliferation and differentiation of preneoplastic and neoplastic cells. A melanoma-inoculated murine model was used to determine whether vitamin A supplementation might result in fibroplasia and tumor encapsulation, thereby suppressing melanoma growth.

Methods.—Sixty DBA/2J male mice were inoculated intracutaneously with 1×10^6 Cloudman S91 melanoma cells and divided into 3 study groups. Controls received a basal control chow that contained approximately 15,000 IU of vitamin A and 6.4 mg of beta-carotene per kilogram. The experimental diet given to the second and third groups added vitamin A

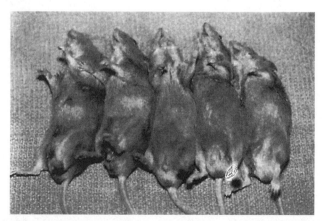

FIGURE 3.—The pre-vitamin A group. All animals remained tumor-free at the time of death 60 days after inoculation. (Courtesy of Weinzweig J, Tattini C, Lynch S, et al: Investigation of the growth and metastasis of malignant melanoma in a murine model: The role of supplemental vitamin A. *Plast Reconstr Surg* 112:152-158, 2003.)

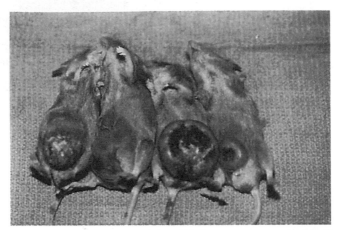

FIGURE 1.—The control group. All mice developed local tumors; one mouse developed liver and lung metastases. (Courtesy of Weinzweig J, Tattini C, Lynch S, et al: Investigation of the growth and metastasis of malignant melanoma in a murine model: The role of supplemental vitamin A. *Plast Reconstr Surg* 112:152-158, 2003.)

palmitate (150,000 IU/kg chow) to the basal control chow. The second group received the supplemented diet starting at 10 days before inoculation (pre–vitamin A group), and the third started vitamin A supplementation on the day of inoculation (post–vitamin A group). Tumor growth was assessed on days 4, 7, 10, 14, 21, and 60 after inoculation. Randomly selected mice were killed at each period for histologic assessment.

Results.—No group of mice killed before day 60 had metastases. At 60 days, the survival rate was 60% in the remaining 5 control group mice versus 100% in the 10 vitamin A–supplemented mice. The mean tumor size was 26.1 mm in controls versus 5.7 mm in the post–vitamin A group. There was

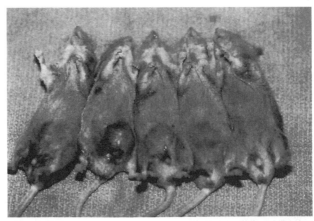

FIGURE 2.—The post-vitamin A group. Two mice developed local tumors; neither of these mice developed metastases. (Courtesy of Weinzweig J, Tattini C, Lynch S, et al: Investigation of the growth and metastasis of malignant melanoma in a murine model: The role of supplemental vitamin A. *Plast Reconstr Surg* 112:152-158, 2003.)

no tumor growth (Fig 3) in the pre–vitamin A group, whereas 40% of animals in the post–vitamin A group had tumor growth. One control (Fig 1) animal, but none of the vitamin A–supplemented animals (Fig 2), had distant metastases at day 60. In the treated mice, a thin collagenous capsule surrounding the tumor was observed histologically.

Conclusion.—Supplemental vitamin A may have prophylactic and therapeutic potential in the treatment of malignant melanoma.

▶ Studies reviewed in the 2003 YEAR BOOK OF DERMATOLOGY AND DERMATOLOGIC SURGERY detailed the inhibitory effects of vitamin E on melanoma growth.[1,2] The current report suggests that vitamin A may have a similar beneficial effect. The real question that must be answered is whether administration of vitamin A to melanoma patients enhances prognosis. As demonstrated by Weinzweig et al, this does appear to be true in an animal model. Unfortunately, administration of vitamin A in human trials has not been successful.[3]

B. H. Thiers, MD

References

1. Malafa MP, Fokum FD, Mowlavi A, et al: Vitamin E inhibits melanoma growth in mice. *Surgery* 131:85-91, 2002.
2. Malafa MP, Fokum FD, Smith L, et al: Inhibition of angiogenesis and promotion of melanoma dormancy by vitamin E succinate. *Ann Surg Oncol* 9:1023-1032, 2002.
3. Evans GRD: Investigation of the growth and metastasis of malignant melanoma in a murine-model: The role of supplemental vitamin A. *Plast Reconstr Surg* 12:159-161, 2003.

The Antitumor Effects of IFN-α Are Abrogated in a STAT1-deficient Mouse

Lesinski GB, Anghelina M, Zimmerer J, et al (Ohio State Univ, Columbus; Children's Hosp, Columbus, Ohio)
J Clin Invest 112:170-180, 2003

17–21

Introduction.—Interferon-α (IFN-α) is used in the treatment of metastatic melanoma, but whether its antitumor effects are mediated by the host or by direct antitumor action is not clear. IFN-α signaling leads to formation of a DNA-binding complex, interferon-stimulated gene factor 3 (ISGF3), which is composed of STAT1-α, STAT2, and interferon regulatory factor 9 (IRF9). The role of STAT1-mediated gene regulation both in the tumor and in the host was investigated in a murine model.

Methods and Results.—A murine melanoma cell line (AGS-1) was derived from STAT1 −/− mice. This cell line did not express STAT1 nor respond to IFN-α. When this cell line was treated with IFN, there was no proliferation inhibition. When mice were challenged with the AGS-1 cell line, IFN treatment significantly enhanced survival. This suggested that IFN had antitumor effects even when the tumor was STAT1 deficient. When the mice were STAT1 deficient, but the tumor contained STAT1, IFN treatment did not enhance survival. When wild type mice were depleted of natural killer (NK) cells, IFN also did not have a survival enhancement effect.

Conclusions.—Results with a murine melanoma model suggest that IFN-α–mediated activation of STAT1 in the host, not the tumor, is sufficient for its antitumor effect. This effect appears to be mediated, at least in part, through the activation of NK cells.

▶ IFN-α is a potent immunomodulatory cytokine that also exhibits antitumor activity. Its therapeutic efficacy has been investigated in several human cancers, including malignant melanoma, where it has been shown to be beneficial in up to 20% of patients with advanced disease. These authors previously reported that exposure of patient-derived melanoma cells to IFN-α resulted in activation of the transcription factors STAT1 and STAT2, which are involved in downstream gene regulation. These data suggested that IFN-α exerted a direct effect on the tumor cells. In this study, the investigators used a murine model to determine the relative roles of host immune modulation and direct antitumor effect of IFN-α therapy in melanoma. STAT-deficient and normal mice were injected intraperitoneally with murine melanoma cells that were either STAT1 positive or negative, and treated with IFN-α. The results showed that the cytokine prolonged survival of the tumor-bearing normal mice, whether or not the tumor cells possessed functional STAT1. In contrast, STAT-deficient mice challenged with STAT1-positive melanoma cells experienced no therapeutic benefit from treatment with IFN-α. Further studies showed that the response to treatment was NK cell–dependent. These findings suggest that, in this model of melanoma, the response to IFN-α is mediated by the host immune system.

G. M. P. Galbraith, MD

Use of Tamoxifen in the Treatment of Malignant Melanoma: Systematic Review and Metaanalysis of Randomized Controlled Trials

Lens MB, Reiman T, Husain AF (Univ of Oxford, England; Cross Cancer Inst, Edmonton, Ontario, Canada; Univ of Toronto)
Cancer 98:1355-1361, 2003   17–22

Background.—Tamoxifen has been used to treat metastatic malignant melanoma as a single agent or combined with other chemotherapeutic drugs. Clinical studies of tamoxifen in different combination chemotherapy regimens have yielded inconclusive findings. In this study, available clinical evidence on the role of tamoxifen in different combination chemotherapy regimens was summarized.

Methods and Findings.—A systematic review and meta-analysis of published randomized controlled studies were conducted. Six studies involving a total of 912 patients met inclusion criteria. Four hundred fifty-five patients were assigned randomly to tamoxifen added to chemotherapy or biochemotherapy regimens. Four hundred fifty-seven patients were assigned to chemotherapy or biochemotherapy without tamoxifen. The analyses indicated that the overall response rate was not significantly improved by adding tamoxifen to the chemotherapy regimens. Results for complete responses between groups did not differ significantly.

Conclusions.—Tamoxifen added to combined chemotherapy regimens does not seem to significantly improve the overall response rate, the complete response rate, or the survival rate in patients with metastatic melanoma. Current evidence does not support the use of tamoxifen combined with other systemic chemotherapies in this patient population.

▶ The possibility that the estrogen receptor (ER) antagonist, tamoxifen, could be a viable treatment for melanoma was suggested by early reports that ERs were present on melanoma cells derived from metastatic tumors. Later studies using more sensitive and specific techniques failed to confirm those observations. Other investigators[1] have suggested that induction of apoptosis and inhibition of angiogenesis might be other mechanisms by which tamoxifen suppresses tumor growth. Unfortunately, the study by Lens et al leaves little optimism that tamoxifen may be a useful agent for treating this disease.

B. H. Thiers, MD

Reference

1. Toma S, Ugolini D, Palumbo R: Tamoxifen in the treatment of metastatic malignant melanoma: Still a controversy? *Int J Oncol* 15:321-337, 1999.

Evaluating Invasive Cutaneous Melanoma: Is the Initial Biopsy Representative of the Final Depth?

Ng PC, Barzilai DA, Ismail SA, et al (Case Western Univ, Cleveland, Ohio)
J Am Acad Dermatol 48:420-424, 2003   17–23

Introduction.—The accuracy of biopsy in the assessment of invasive cutaneous melanomas depends on the expertise of the clinician. The accuracy and predictive value of initial biopsy specimens of cutaneous melanoma were examined, along with the value of punch versus superficial or deep shave biopsy. The accuracy of these biopsy approaches was compared with that of excisional biopsy alone. The determinants of biopsy success and the choice of biopsy method among physicians were evaluated.

Methods.—Data on cases of invasive cutaneous melanoma in which a biopsy and subsequent excision were performed between September 1996 and April 2001 were obtained from a database and assessed retrospectively. A total of 145 cases were reviewed. The Breslow depth on preliminary biopsy was compared with Breslow depth on subsequent excision to ascertain whether the initial diagnostic biopsy was performed on the deepest segment of the melanoma.

Results.—In 95 of the 108 (88%) initial shave or punch biopsies (excluding excisional biopsies and unknown biopsy technique), the physician's clinical evaluation of the melanoma for biopsy was accurate, with the Breslow

TABLE 1.—Accuracy Rates with Biopsy Depth Greater than or Equal to Subsequent Excision Breslow Depth for Each Combination of Breslow Depth and Biopsy Method

Biopsy Method	<1 mm (% Accurate)	1-2 mm (% Accurate)	>2 mm (% Accurate)	All Depths (% Accurate)
Superficial shave (n = 30)	26/27 (96.3)	1/2 (50)	1/1 (100)	28/30 (93.3)
Deep shave (n = 37)	6/6 (100)	21/22 (95.5)	7/9 (77.8)	34/37 (91.9)
Punch biopsy (n = 41)	18/23 (78.3)	5/5 (100)	10/13 (76.9)	33/41 (80.5)
All methods* (n = 108)	50/56 (89.3)	27/29 (93.1)	18/23 (78.3)	95/108 (88.0)
Excisional biopsy (n = 30)	15/15 (100)	6/6 (100)	9/9 (100)	30/30 (100)

Note: In thin melanomas less than 1 mm Breslow depth, measured Breslow depth in a superficial or deep shave biopsy is a reliable predictor of final melanoma depth. In intermediate melanoma 1 to 2 mm Breslow depth, measured Breslow depth in a deep shave biopsy is a reliable predictor of final depth. Punch biopsies were generally less accurate than superficial or deep shave biopsies.

*Excludes excisional biopsy (30 patients) and unknown biopsy method (7 patients).

(Reprinted by permission of the publisher from Ng PC, Barzilai DA, Ismail SA, et al: Evaluating invasive cutaneous melanoma: Is the initial biopsy representative of the final depth? *J Am Acad Dermatol* 48:420-424, 2003. Copyright 2003 by Elsevier.)

depth on biopsy greater than or equal to the Breslow depth detected on subsequent wide local excision ($P < .0001$). Both the superficial and deep shave biopsy techniques were more accurate than the punch biopsy technique for melanomas thinner than 1 mm. Excisional biopsy was the most accurate biopsy technique (Table 1).

Conclusion.—Deep shave biopsy is preferable to superficial shave or punch biopsy for thin and intermediate depth (<2 mm) melanomas when an initial sample is obtained for diagnosis rather than complete excision. Overall, this group of experienced dermatologists accurately evaluated the depth of invasive melanoma via a variety of initial biopsy types.

▶ Because the ultimate margin of excision and whether the patient requires sentinel lymph node biopsy depends on lesion thickness, the preferable method of biopsy for a suspicious pigmented lesion is excision with a narrow margin of clinically normal skin. Thus, the more material the pathologist has for study, the more likely the true thickness of the lesion can be determined.

There have been a number of articles demonstrating that a single, small biopsy of a large lesion is often quite inaccurate in determining whether the tumor is invasive and its true depth of invasion. This article essentially confirms these previous observations. Unfortunately, the authors did not have information regarding the size of the lesions that were biopsied. Not surprisingly, a shave biopsy specimen, which often samples a larger portion of the lesion, was more likely to give a better estimate of Breslow thickness. Also not surprising was the fact that the thicker or deeper the lesion, the less likely the shave biopsy was to reflect the true depth of invasion, ie, many of these lesions probably were transected by the biopsy procedure.

There was some inconsistency in the data. For example, why would a superficial shave biopsy give more accurate information than a deep shave biopsy for deeply invasive disease? Also why would a punch biopsy give accurate information for lesions 1 to 2 mm thick but not for lesions less than 1 mm thick or for lesions more than 2 mm thick? It was also clear from this study that experienced clinicians were more likely to select the best biopsy method for the lesion in question. Although one could view this article in the context of shave versus punch biopsy in the diagnosis of melanoma, a broader conclusion might be that when dealing with a large pigmented lesion that may be invasive, if an excisional biopsy is not practical, the biopsy technique selected should remove a significant portion of the lesion and extend down to and into the subcutaneous tissue.

P. G. Lang, Jr, MD

The Potential Impact on Melanoma Mortality of Reducing Rates of Suboptimal Excision Margins

Barzilai DA, Singer ME (Case Western Reserve Univ, Cleveland, Ohio; Louis Stokes Cleveland Dept of Veterans Affairs Med Ctr, Ohio; MetroHealth Med Ctr, Cleveland, Ohio)
J Invest Dermatol 120:1067-1072, 2003   17–24

Background.—Some research has shown correlations or trends between greater rates of local melanoma recurrence and narrow excision margins, especially when those margins are less than 1 cm. Other research has reported a markedly worse prognosis when local recurrence of melanoma follows surgical excision. The impact of suboptimal excision margins was determined in patients with localized invasive melanoma.

Methods.—A hypothetical cohort of 55-year-old white patients in a community setting newly diagnosed with localized invasive melanoma was included in a computer-simulated Markov decision analytical model. Patients were followed from diagnosis until death. The 2 scenarios considered were the standard of care and a hypothetical intervention to reduce the proportion of suboptimal excision margins. The Markov states generated were recurrence free, local recurrence, cured, and dead. Rates of optimal excision margins, local recurrence, and mortality were obtained from published population-based data. Melanoma-related death and life expectancy were the 2 outcome measures. The major assumptions were local recurrence within 10 years of diagnosis and reversion to general population mortality rates 10 years after melanoma excision or subsequent local recurrence.

Findings.—The model estimated an 8.2% melanoma-related mortality rate among patients receiving usual care. Intervention with 100% optimal excision margins decreased this to 6.2%, for a 25% relative mortality reduction. This intervention increased average life expectancy by 0.44 years, equivalent to approximately 11 additional years in the 4% of patients who would not have a local recurrence because of improved excision margins. Increasing the percentage of optimal excision margins to 80% was also associated with marked improvement, with a 6.8% melanoma-related mortality rate or 0.29 life-years saved compared with baseline values.

Conclusions.—In patients with localized invasive melanoma, suboptimal excision margins may be responsible for approximately one fourth of all melanoma-related deaths. Interventions adhering even modestly to optimal excision margins may markedly decrease mortality rate.

▶ This is yet another study based on assumptions and a mathematical model. While it would be difficult to do a comprehensive prospective study on the relationship of margins of excision and melanoma mortality, there have been several large studies that have addressed this issue. These investigations have determined that margins more than 2 cm offer no benefit regardless of the thickness of the melanoma.[1-3] The major assumption or variable that flaws the current study and older studies of margin size is the lumping together of satellite lesions, which represent metastases, with true local recurrences due to inadequate excisions. Satellite lesions are associated with regional and systemic metastases and portend a worse prognosis. Thus, combining them with true local recurrences yields skewed data and false conclusions. This reviewer agrees that adequate margins of resection are critical in the management of melanoma, but wide margins are unlikely to encompass satellite lesions and improve survival.

P. G. Lang, Jr, MD

References

1. Balch CM, Urist MM, Karakousis CP, et al: Efficacy of 2-cm surgical margins for intermediate-thickness melanomas (1-4 mm). Results of a multi-institutional randomized surgical trial. *Ann Surg* 218:262-269, 1993.
2. Cohn-Cedermark G, Rutqvist LE, Andersson R, et al: Long term results of a randomized study by the Swedish Melanoma Study Group on 2-cm versus 5-cm resection margins for patients with cutaneous melanoma with a tumor thickness of 0.8-2.0 mm. *Cancer* 89:1495-1501, 2000.
3. Karakousis CP, Balch CM, Urist MM, et al: Local recurrence in malignant melanoma: Long-term results of the multiinstitutional randomized surgical trial. *Ann Surg Oncol* 3:446-452, 1996.

Prognosis for Patients With Thin Cutaneous Melanoma: Long-term Survival Data From the New South Wales Central Cancer Registry and the Sydney Melanoma Unit
McKinnon JG, Yu XQ, McCarthy WH, et al (Univ of Calgary, Alta, Canada; Cancer Council, Woolloomooloo, Australia; Sydney Melanoma Unit, Sydney, Australia; et al)
Cancer 98:1223-1231, 2003   17–25

Background.—Estimates of long-term survival vary greatly among patients with primary cutaneous melanomas of 1 mm thickness or less. In this study, 2 separate methods were used to determine survival among such patients.
Methods.—Between 1983 and 1998, data on all 18,088 patients from New South Wales (NSW), Australia, diagnosed as having cutaneous melanoma 1 mm thick or less were obtained from the NSW Central Cancer Registry (NSWCCR). Patients with metastases at diagnosis were excluded. In

TABLE 4.—Cox Regression Analysis for Patients in the Sydney Melanoma Unit (Sydney, Australia) Melanoma-Specific Survival

Variable	Hazard Ratio	95% CI	P Value
Gender	1.081646	0.63-1.86	0.777797
Age	1.028663	1.01-1.05	0.002912
Thickness	15.20981	2.69-86.0	0.002086
Ulceration	2.883081	1.39-5.99	0.004577
Mitoses	1.15566	1.02-1.31*	0.026617
Clark level	1.441801	0.95-2.19	0.086532

Abbreviation: CI, Confidence interval.
*Number of mitoses per mm².
(Courtesy of McKinnon JG, Yu XQ, McCarthy WH, et al: Prognosis for patients with thin cutaneous melanoma: Long-term survival data from the New South Wales Central Cancer Registry and the Sydney Melanoma Unit. *Cancer* 98:1223-1231, 2003. Copyright 2003 American Cancer Society. Reprinted by permission of Wiley-Liss, Inc, a subsidiary of John Wiley & Sons, Inc.)

addition, the Sydney Melanoma Unit (SMU) database was consulted, and information on 2746 patients meeting the above criteria, diagnosed from 1979 to 1998, was obtained.

Findings.—Analysis of the NSWCCR data demonstrated a 96.4% survival rate at 10 years. The 10-year survival rate for the SMU patients was 92.7%. The median time to recurrence among nonsurvivors at SMU was 49.8 months. The median time to their death was 65.9 months. Patients at SMU with lesions 0.75 mm thick or less had a 10-year survival rate of 96.9%, compared with 84.3% for those with lesions 0.76 to 1 mm thick. Patients with ulcerated melanomas 1 mm thick or less had a 10-year survival rate of 83%, compared with 92.3% for those with nonulcerated melanomas (Table 4).

Conclusions.—Patients with thin melanomas have an excellent 10-year survival rate. Subgroups of patients at higher risk can be identified, enabling aggressive investigation and treatments.

▶ The findings in this article are somewhat similar to those reported by Zapas et al (see Abstract 17–32). However, on multivariate analysis, age, but not gender, was associated with a worse prognosis for patients with melanomas less than 1 mm thick. A higher mitotic rate, ulceration, and a greater thickness also had an adverse effect on prognosis, although Clark level of invasion did not. Regression also adversely affected survival. The overall 10-year survival rate for this group of patients was estimated to be between 92.7% and 96.4%. The median time to recurrence was 49.8 months. The 10-year survival rate for patients with ulcerated lesions was 83% compared with 92.3% for patients with nonulcerated lesions. Patients with lesions less than .75 mm thick had a 10-year survival rate of 96.9% compared with 84.3% for patients with lesions .76 to 1.00 mm thick. Based on their observations, the authors suggest that sentinel lymph node biopsy be offered to patients with 1 or more adverse prognostic factors.

P. G. Lang, Jr, MD

Revised American Joint Committee on Cancer Staging Criteria Accurately Predict Sentinel Lymph Node Positivity in Clinically Node-Negative Melanoma Patients

Rousseau DL, Ross MI, Johnson MM, et al (Univ of Texas, Houston)
Ann Surg Oncol 10:569-574, 2003   17–26

Introduction.—The American Joint Committee on Cancer (AJCC) has recently revised staging criteria for primary melanoma patients. Lymphatic mapping and sentinel lymph node (SLN) biopsy have become standard in ascertaining the pathologic status of the regional lymph node basin in many patients with primary cutaneous melanoma. The incidence of SLN metastasis was correlated with revised AJCC staging to better understand which of the known clinicopathologic prognostic factors could be used to predict the risk of SLN metastasis in a large cohort of patients who underwent successful SLN biopsy.

Methods.—A prospective surgical melanoma database was used to identify 1375 patients with primary cutaneous melanoma who underwent successful intraoperative lymphatic mapping and SLN biopsy between 1991 and May 2001. Univariate and multivariate analyses were performed to determine predictors of a positive SLN. Patients were stratified by means of revised AJCC criteria to ascertain whether such groups also predicted positive SLNs.

Results.—A positive SLN was identified in 16.9% of patients. Multivariate analysis revealed that tumor thickness (relative risk, 3.4) and ulceration (relative risk, 2.2) were dominant independent predictors of SLN metastases, and that there was an increasing risk of SLN metastases with successive stage groups (Tables 4 and 5).

Conclusion.—Given the significant correlation between SLN status and survival, the ability of the revised AJCC staging system to predict survival is probably due to its ability to predict the risk of occult nodal disease.

TABLE 4.—Multivariate Analysis of Prognostic Factors for Predicting Sentinel Lymph Node Metastases

Prognostic Factor	OR	95% CI	P Value
Tumor thickness	3.42	2.54-4.61	<.0001
Ulceration	2.21	1.57-3.13	<.0001
Age ≤50 y	1.81	1.31-2.51	.0003
Axial location	1.45	1.05-2.02	.026
Clark level IV/V	1.34	.94-1.92	.107
Male sex	1.09	.78-1.52	.629

Note: 1351 patients.
Abbreviations: OR, Odds ratio; *CI*, confidence interval; *SLN*, sentinel lymph node.
(Courtesy of Rousseau DL, Ross MI, Johnson MM, et al: Revised American Joint Committee on Cancer staging criteria accurately predict sentinel lymph node positivity in clinically node-negative melanoma patients. *Ann Surg Oncol* 10(5):569-574, 2003.)

TABLE 5.—The Effect of Ulceration on Sentinel Lymph Node Metastases for a Given Tumor Thickness

Tumor Thickness (mm)	Total Patients (%)	All (%)	Positive SLN				
			Not Ulcerated		Ulcerated		
			%	AJCC Stage*	%	AJCC Stage*	P Value (Ulcerated vs. not)†
≤1.00	28	4	3	IA	16	IB	.026
1.01-2.00	38	12	11	IB	22	IIA	.007
2.01-4.00	23	28	25	IIA	34	IIB	.115
>4.00	11	44	33	IIB	53	IIC	.021
All patients	100	17	12		35		<.0001

Note: 1375 patients
*Stage groupings calculated with tumor thickness and ulceration data only.
†Fisher's exact test for each tumor thickness group.
Abbreviations: SLN, Sentinel lymph node; AJCC, American Joint Committee on Cancer.
(Courtesy of Rousseau DL, Ross MI, Johnson MM, et al: Revised American Joint Committee on Cancer staging criteria accurately predict sentinel lymph node positivity in clinically node-negative melanoma patients. *Ann Surg Oncol* 10(5):569-574, 2003.)

▶ In this study, the authors verify that the new revised AJCC staging criteria[1] are quite reliable for predicting SLN positivity in patients with melanoma. Consequently, since SLN positivity correlates with survival, it should follow that this staging system can also be useful for predicting survival. As previously shown, the 2 most powerful predictors of SLN positivity were tumor thickness and ulceration. However, an axial location of the lesion and age less than 50 years also correlated with SLN positivity.

P. G. Lang, Jr, MD

Reference

1. Balch CM, Buziad AC, Soong S-J, et al: Final version of the American Joint Committee on Cancer staging system for cutaneous melanoma. *J Clin Oncol* 19:3635-3648, 2001.

Review and Evaluation of Sentinel Node Procedures in 250 Melanoma Patients With a Median Follow-up of 6 Years
Estourgie SH, Nieweg OE, Valdés Olmos RA, et al (The Netherlands Cancer Inst/Antoni van Leeuwenhoek Hosp, Amsterdam)
Ann Surg Oncol 10:681-688, 2003   17–27

Background.—The current trend is to include sentinel node biopsy in the standard management of patients with clinically localized melanoma. The results of sentinel node biopsy in cutaneous melanoma at 1 center were reported.

Methods.—Two hundred fifty patients with cutaneous melanoma were investigated prospectively. Preoperatively, patients were injected with ^{99m}Tc-nanocolloid intradermally around the primary tumor or biopsy site before

TABLE 3.—A Total of 105 Recurrences in 59 of 250 Patients (24%)

Variable	Sentinel Node Tumor/ Negative (N = 190)		Sentinel Node Tumor/ Positive (N = 60)		Total (N = 250)	
	n	%	n	%	n	%
Lymph node recurrence	12	6	5	8	17	7
Local recurrence	6	3	3	5	9	4
Satellite metastasis	5	3	0	0	5	2
In-transit metastasis	13	7	14	23	27	11
Distant metastasis	22	12	25	42	47	19
Total number of recurrences	58		47		105	

(Courtesy of Estourgie SH, Nieweg OE, Valdés Olmos RA, et al: Review and evaluation of sentinel node procedures in 250 melanoma patients with a median follow-up of 6 years. *Ann Surg Oncol* 10(6):681-688, 2003.)

lymphoscintigraphy. Sentinel nodes were identified surgically with patent blue dye and a gamma ray detection probe. Patients were monitored for a median of 72 months.

Findings.—Lymphoscintigraphic visualization was 100%. Surgical identification was 99.6%. In 24% of the patients, 1 or more sentinel nodes were tumor-positive at the initial pathologic assessment. Recurrences were observed in 59 patients (Table 3). Late complications, including leg edema and infection, occurred in 18% of the remaining 190 patients after sentinel node biopsy. Results were false-negative in 9% of patients. In-transit metastases were documented in 7% of patients with negative sentinel nodes and in 23%

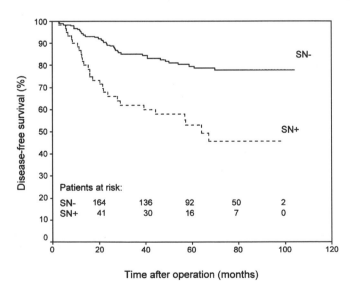

FIGURE 2.—Kaplan-Meier plot of disease-free survival in patients with a tumor-negative or a tumor-positive sentinel node ($P < .001$; log-rank test). *Abbreviation: SN*, Sentinel node. (Courtesy of Estourgie SH, Nieweg OE, Valdés Olmos RA, et al: Review and evaluation of sentinel node procedures in 250 melanoma patients with a median follow-up of 6 years. *Ann Surg Oncol* 10(6):681-688, 2003.)

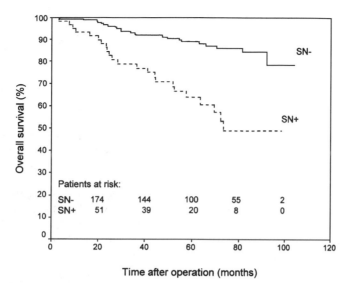

FIGURE 3.—Kaplan-Meier plot of overall survival in patients with a tumor-negative or a tumor-positive sentinel node ($P < .001$; log-rank test). *Abbreviation: SN,* Sentinel node. (Courtesy of Estourgie SH, Nieweg OE, Valdés Olmos RA, et al: Review and evaluation of sentinel node procedures in 250 melanoma patients with a median follow-up of 6 years. *Ann Surg Oncol* 10(6):681-688, 2003.)

of those with positive nodes. Estimated survival rates at 5 years were 89% and 64%, respectively (Figs 2 and 3 and Table 4).

Conclusion.—The status of the sentinel node is a strong independent prognostic variable in patients with melanoma. However, the false-negative rate and incidence of in-transit metastases in patients with positive sentinel nodes are high and must be weighed against the possible survival benefit of early nodal metastasis removal.

▶ A number of interesting questions and observations can be gleaned from this article. The false-negative rate (ie, recurrence of tumor in a nodal basin determined to be negative by sentinel lymph node biopsy) for sentinel lymph

TABLE 4.—Cox Multivariate Regression Analysis for Overall Survival of All 250 Patients: Results of Backward Elimination Method

Variable	P	Hazard Ratio (95% Confidence Interval)
Tumor-positive sentinel node	.001	2.87 (1.52-5.45)
Breslow thickness (mm)	.016	1.15 (1.03-1.30)
Age (y)	.006	1.01 (1.00-1.02)
Male sex	.032	1.98 (1.06-3.70)

(Courtesy of Estourgie SH, Nieweg OE, Valdés Olmos RA, et al: Review and evaluation of sentinel node procedures in 250 melanoma patients with a median follow-up of 6 years. *Ann Surg Oncol* 10(6):681-688, 2003.)

node biopsy (SLNB), in these investigators hands, was determined to be 9%. In some series, this figure has been as high as 32%, raising questions about the reliability of the procedure. Although several explanations may account for false negative SLNBs, certainly one that accounts for a significant number of these is lack of experience on the part of the surgeon(s) and pathologist(s), along with inadequate examination of the SLN. Another proposed explanation is that there may be tumor cells in transit at the time of SLNB, which reach the nodal basin after the SLNB has been performed. If this were shown to be true, one could make an argument for delaying SLNB; however, one then would have to address how long to delay the procedure and what effect the excision of the primary lesion might have on lymphatic mapping and identification of the SLN.

The authors state that only 24% of their patients undergoing SLNB had positive findings. Although complications associated with SLNB are not common, this suggests that 76% of patients underwent an unnecessary procedure with its inherent risks. Moreover, of those undergoing complete lymph node dissection (CLND), only 12% had positive nodes, adding unnecessary morbidity in 88% of these patients.

Although the 5-year survival for patients with a negative SLNB specimen was significantly better (89% vs 64%), a significant number of these patients did experience a recurrence of various types. This was even more true for patients with a positive SLNB specimen who had undergone CLND, raising the age-old question of whether SLNB followed by CLND affects prognosis. Because definitively proven adjuvant therapy is not available, the authors speculate as to whether we have anything to offer patients at high risk for recurrence and thus whether SLNB is justified. Although a number of questions were raised about the value of SLNB, it was demonstrated again that the procedure is a powerful staging tool and prognostic indicator. Only ulceration had an additional effect on prognosis in patients with a positive SLNB specimen.

P. G. Lang, Jr, MD

Preoperative Ultrasonographic Identification of the Sentinel Lymph Node in Patients With Malignant Melanoma
Kahle B, Hoffend J, Wacker J, et al (Heidelberg Univ, Germany)
Cancer 97:1947-1954, 2003   17–28

Introduction.—Identification of the sentinel lymph node (SLN) by lymphoscintigraphy with radiolabeled colloids is the most widely used method for mapping the SLN in patients with malignant melanoma (MM). Seventy-six patients with MM located on the trunk or extremities were evaluated to determine whether the SLN could be mapped by US and to ascertain whether US of the SLN is of clinical value in patients with MM.

Methods.—All patients had tumors with a Breslow thickness greater than 1.0 mm (range, 1.08-5.5 mm) and a Clark level greater than III, and thus wide excision and SLN biopsy were indicated. The average patient age was 48.8 years. All participants underwent US of the regional lymph nodes before preoperative lymphoscintigraphy. The MM was located on the legs, arms, and trunk in 30, 14, and 23 patients, respectively.

During regional US, the location of the lymph nodes that differed in the cortex/medulla ratio from the surrounding lymph nodes was marked on the skin in correspondence with the planes of insonation when the probe was positioned vertical to the skin surface (M1). After lymphoscintigraphy with ^{99m}Tc, the position of a gamma probe at which the highest count rate vertical to the skin surface was documented was also marked (M2).

Results.—The agreement between M1 and M2 in the inguinal region was 100% (40/40 SLNs) (Fig 4), and in the axilla it was 72.5% (29/40 SLNs). In patients with MM on the leg, the location of M1 and M2 agreed in 97% of cases (36/37 lymph nodes in 30 patients). In patients with MM on the arms, the agreement was 76% (13/17 lymph nodes in 14 patients). In participants with MM on the trunk, the agreement was 75% (21/28 lymph nodes in 23 patients).

The position documented by US relative to the neighboring structures of the SLN was verified intraoperatively in all patients. In 58 patients, an increase of the cortex in a peripheral direction in the longitudinal dimension (corresponding to the location of the sonographic "cap" and also corre-

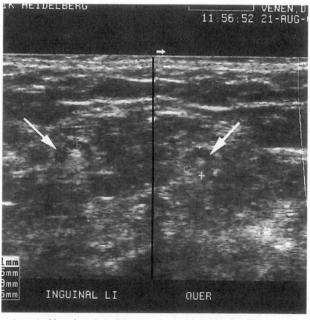

FIGURE 4.—A sentinel lymph node in the inguinal area of a patient with malignant melanoma with a Breslow index of 1.8 mm and Clark level IV located on the left abdomen. The *left half* of the picture is in longitudinal section, the *right half* is in cross-section. The cap-like cortical thickening is marked with an *arrow*. The dimensions of the lymph node were 9.45 mm × 8.19 mm (a × b) in the longitudinal section and 8.25 mm × 6.31 mm (c × d) in the cross-section. (Courtesy of Kahle B, Hoffend J, Wacker J, et al: Preoperative ultrasonographic identification of the sentinel lymph node in patients with malignant melanoma. *Cancer* 97 (8):1947-1954, 2003. ©2003 American Cancer Society. Reprinted by permission of Wiley-Liss, Inc, a subsidiary of John Wiley & Sons, Inc.)

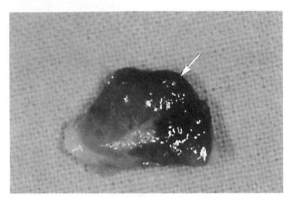

FIGURE 3.—Longitudinal section through a sentinel lymph node. Staining of the pole by Patent Blue V, which corresponds to the "cap," was marked with an arrow. (Courtesy of Kahle B, Hoffend J, Wacker J, et al: Preoperative ultrasonographic identification of the sentinel lymph node in patients with malignant melanoma. *Cancer* 97(8):1947-1954, 2003. ©2003 American Cancer Society. Reprinted by permission of Wiley-Liss, Inc, a subsidiary of John Wiley & Sons, Inc.)

sponding to the point of maximum Patent Blue V staining) was observed on inspection of SLNs after extirpation (Fig 3; see color plate XIV).

Conclusion.—The SLN in patients with MM on the limbs, particularly the legs, are characterized by a specific sonomorphologic pattern. Preoperative sonography may be an important addition to lymphoscintigraphy in planning SLN biopsy.

▶ In Europe, US is commonly used to assess lymph node status in patients with MM. In this study, the authors investigated whether US is a reliable tool to identify the SLN in patients with MM. When compared to lymphoscintigraphy, US was quite reliable if the SLN was located in the inguinal area; however, if the SLN was located in the axilla, it was less reliable, especially in obese patients. With US, the identifying feature of an SLN was an asymmetric thickening of the cortex of the lymph node, giving the appearance of a "cap." One of the advantages of preoperative US was its ability to demonstrate the location of the SLN in relation to other important anatomical structures and to determine its depth below the surface of the skin. These features help in planning the surgery and in determining whether local or general anesthesia is necessary.

P. G. Lang, Jr, MD

Sentinel Lymph Node Biopsy in Patients With Thin Melanoma
Lowe JB, Hurst E, Moley JF, et al (Washington Univ, St Louis)
Arch Dermatol 139:617-621, 2003   17–29

Background.—The number of "thin" (1 mm thick or less) melanomas has increased in the past few years. These patients generally have an excellent prognosis, but thin lesions occasionally recur and metastasize. The incidence of positive sentinel lymph nodes (SLNs) in patients with thin melanomas was examined, along with risk factors for regional node involvement.

Methods.—The medical records of 46 patients (26 men, 20 women; age range, 20-75 years), with melanoma 1 mm deep or less who underwent lymphatic mapping and SLN biopsy between 1996 and 2002, were reviewed. Biopsy specimens were examined by routine hematoxylin and eosin staining and (beginning in 2000) by immunohistochemistry (IHC).

Results.—Eight of the 46 patients (17.4%) had in situ lesions; the mean lesion depth in the remaining 38 patients was 0.74 mm. Twelve tumors (26.1%) were Clark level I or II, 19 lesions (41.3%) were Clark level III, and 15 lesions (32.6%) were Clark level IV. Tumors were present on the trunk (22 cases, or 47.8%), extremities (18 cases, or 39.1%), head and neck (5 cases, or 10.9%), and the sole of the foot (1 case, or 2.2%).

Histologic subtypes included 32 (70%) superficial spreading tumors, 7 (15%) lentigo maligna, 2 (4%) acral lentiginous lesions, and 5 (11%) lesions not otherwise specified. The SLN biopsy specimen was positive for metastasis in 3 patients (6.5%), all 3 of whom had Clark level III/IV tumors ($P < .07$). In 1 of these 3 patients, only IHC findings were positive for disease. None of the primary lesions associated with positive SLNs had regression or ulceration. These 3 patients underwent lymph node dissection, which revealed no further extension of disease. The 3 patients, as well as the other 43 patients with negative SLN findings, were alive and free of disease at the last follow-up examination.

Conclusion.—Current recommendations call for SLN biopsy of patients with thin lesions that are ulcerated or invasive at a Clark level of IV or greater. These findings suggest SLN biopsy of patients with thin melanoma is warranted when the Clark level is III or greater, regardless of whether ulceration or invasion is present.

▶ Several previous studies have reported that 4.7% to 5.6% of patients with melanoma thickness of less than 1 mm will have a positive SLN specimen.[1,2] This correlates with the presence of ulceration and a Clark level of IV or greater. In this study, the authors report their experience with SLN biopsies in patients with melanomas less than 1 mm thick. In their group of 46 patients, the incidence of SLN metastasis was 7%, more than in previous studies. The authors found no correlation with ulceration, regression, vertical growth phase, or Clark level of invasion. Interestingly, some patients with positive SLN biopsy specimens had Clark level III tumors. Although the data confirm that patients with thin melanomas can develop metastasis, the study was flawed in several ways: (1) patients with lesions 1 mm thick were included; (2) the amount of regression observed was not defined; (3) patients with in situ melanoma were included; and (4) patients with residual disease on re-excision were excluded without a detailed explanation as to why this was done.

P. G. Lang, Jr, MD

References

1. Gershenwald JE, Thompson W, Mansfield PF, et al: Multi-institutional melanoma lymphatic mapping experience: The prognostic value of sentinel lymph node status in 612 stage I or II melanoma patients. *J Clin Oncol* 17:976-983, 1999.
2. Bedrosian I, Faries MB, Guerry D, et al: Incidence of sentinel node metastasis in patients with thin primary melanoma (< or = 1 mm) with vertical growth phase. *Ann Surg Oncol* 7:262-267, 2000.

Role of Sentinel Lymph Node Biopsy in Patients With Thin (<1 mm) Primary Melanoma
Jacobs IA, Chang CK, DasGupta TK, et al (Univ of Illinois at Chicago)
Ann Surg Oncol 10:558-561, 2003   17–30

Introduction.—Thin melanomas are considered highly curable when treated solely with wide local excision. There may be a subset of high-risk patients with thin melanomas who may be more effectively managed with sentinel lymph node biopsy (SLNB) and/or adjuvant therapy with interferon α-2b vs wide excision alone. The chance of regional lymph node involvement and, therefore, whether it is appropriate to perform the sentinel lymph node (SLN) biopsy depends on the Breslow thickness of the primary tumor. A Breslow thickness cutoff has yet to be established. Melanoma patients who underwent SLN biopsy were examined to ascertain which patients would most benefit from the procedure.

Methods.—During a 5-year evaluation, 259 patients with cutaneous malignant melanoma underwent 266 lymphatic mapping and SLNB procedures using both radioisotope and blue dye. Sixty-five of the 266 invasive melanomas were thin (thickness ≤ 1 mm) and underwent wide excision and SLNB.

Results.—Two (3%) of the 65 thin melanomas had a positive SLN biopsy specimen. No positive SLN was identified in melanomas thinner than 0.75 mm.

Conclusion.—Sentinel lymphadenectomy is not indicated for melanomas less than 0.75 mm in thickness. Patients whose melanomas are over 0.75 mm and under 1.0 mm thickness have a 3% incidence of nodal metastasis. SLNB may be useful in these patients.

► This is another report addressing the role of SLNB in the management of patients with thin (<1 mm) melanomas. In this group of 65 patients, the authors found the incidence of a positive SLNB to be 3%, the thinnest positive lesion being 0.75 mm thick. Of note is that this patient had a Clark level III tumor. In summarizing their findings, the authors state that patients with lesions less than 0.75 mm thick do not require SLNB. Although their conclusion may be correct, upon what is it based—a single patient with a 0.75-mm-thick lesion? Unfortunately, the reader is not told how many patients in the study had lesions less than 0.75 mm thick.

P. G. Lang, Jr, M D

Cost-Effectiveness of Sentinel Lymph Node Biopsy in Thin Melanomas

Agnese DM, Abdessalam SF, Burak WE Jr, et al (Ohio State Univ, Columbus)
Surgery 134:542-548, 2003   17-31

Background.—Sentinel lymph node biopsy (SLNB) is generally considered for patients with thin melanomas with poor prognostic features. However, few metastases are identified. The cost-effectiveness of SLNB in this patient population was investigated.

Methods.—One hundred thirty-eight patients with melanomas less than 1.2 mm thick who had SLNB between 1994 and 2002 were included in the study. Physician and hospital charges were obtained for analysis.

Findings.—Sentinel lymph nodes were identified in 1.4% of the patients. One of the 2 patients with positive SLNs had a melanoma less than 1 mm thick. Patient charges for SLBN were $10,096 to $15,223. By comparison, the cost for wide excision on an outpatient basis was $1000 to $1740. The estimated cost to identify a single positive SLN was $696,6000 to $1,051,100. The estimated cost for wide excision was $69,000 to $120,100. The cost per life saved would be $627,000 to $931,000, assuming that all patients with a positive SLN would die of melanoma.

Conclusions.—The authors conclude that the cost of SLNB in patients with thin melanomas is high. Further research is needed.

▶ Although there is universal agreement that the SLNB is an excellent procedure for staging patients and for determining prognosis in patients with primary cutaneous melanoma, there are several points of controversy. First, does performing a complete node dissection in patients with a positive SLNB alter their prognosis? Second, is there truly effective adjuvant therapy to offer patients with positive SLNBs? Finally, does the benefit of the procedure justify the additional cost? There have been a number of studies that have addressed the frequency of positive SLNBs in patients with melanomas less than 1 mm thick. Those studies have also looked at what other clinical and histological variables might predict the likelihood of a positive SLNB in this group of patients, since performing a SLNB on all patients with lesions less than 1 mm thick would not be cost effective because of the low yield of positive results. Agnese et al address the cost effectiveness of SLNBs in patients with thin melanomas. Despite the fact that only "high-risk" patients underwent SLNB and that a thickness of 1.2 mm rather than 1.0 mm was used as a cut-off, the authors were unable to demonstrate that SLNB was cost effective in this subset of patients. However, it should be noted that their incidence of positive SLNB findings was much lower than has been reported in other series. Thus, further data need to be collected before one can say with certainty whether SLNB is justified in this subset of patients.

P. G. Lang, Jr, MD

The Risk of Regional Lymph Node Metastases in Patients With Melanoma Less than 1.0 mm Thick: Recommendations for Sentinel Lymph Node Biopsy

Zapas JL, Coley HC, Beam SL, et al (Franklin Square Hosp Ctr, Baltimore, Md)
J Am Coll Surg 197:403-407, 2003   17–32

Background.—Among patients with melanoma of intermediate thickness, 1 to 4 mm, lymphatic mapping and sentinel lymph node biopsy (SLNB) can upstage disease. No strict guidelines currently exist for SNLB in patients with melanoma less than 1 mm thick. The risk of regional lymph node metastases in such patients was investigated.

Methods.—In this retrospective analysis, the records of 598 patients seen at 2 centers between 1970 and 2002 were reviewed. Those with primary cutaneous melanoma of less than 1 mm thick, disease recurrence, and follow-up for at least 5 years were identified. Patients with primary melanoma of similar thickness and follow-up, in whom disease did not recur, comprised a comparison group.

Findings.—Of 114 patients with primary cutaneous melanoma less than 1 mm thick, 17 had a disease recurrence. The site of first recurrence was the regional lymph nodes in 13 patients. In 4 patients, disease recurred with distant metastases. The median time to lymph node recurrence was 55 months. The median primary tumor thickness was significantly greater in patients with regional lymph node recurrence than in those without recurrence, those thicknesses being 0.8 mm and 0.45 mm, respectively (Table 3). Recurrence was unassociated with Clark level of invasion. Overall, 35% of patients initially seen with melanoma 0.80 to 0.99 mm in thickness had a lymph node recurrence at a median 41 months after surgery.

Conclusions.—These data suggest that SNLB is justified for patients with melanoma 0.8 mm thick or greater. The justification for this approach relies on the procedure's ability to detect metastatic disease years before it becomes apparent clinically.

TABLE 3.—Comparison of Disease Status by Breslow Thickness

Breslow Depth (mm)	Lymph Node Recurrence (n = 13) n (%)	No Recurrence (n = 97) n (%)	P Value*
0.00-0.19	0 (0)	3 (3)	
0.20-0.39	3 (23)	33 (34)	
0.40-0.59	2 (15)	31 (32)	
0.60-0.79	1 (8)	17 (18)	
0.80-0.99	7 (54)	13 (13)	0.01
Breslow depth (mm), median (range)	0.80 (0.30-0.99)	0.45 (0.00-0.96)	0.02†

*Cochran-Armitage trend test.
†Wilcoxon rank sum test.
(Courtesy of Zapas JL, Coley HC, Beam SL, et al: The risk of regional lymph node metastases in patients with melanoma less than 1.0 thick: Recommendations for sentinel lymph node biopsy. *J Am Coll Surg* 197:403-407, 2003. Copyright 2003 American College of Surgeons.)

▶ It is well recognized that thin melanomas (< 1.0 mm thick) can metastasize, most commonly to the regional lymph nodes. This usually occurs a number of years after the diagnosis and treatment of the primary lesion. Previous studies have suggested that certain variables may be associated with metastatic disease in such patients; these include male gender, truncal location, regression, large size, and Clark level of invasion. Zapas et al assessed the risk of metastasis for thin melanomas and attempted to determine which clinical and pathological variables were associated with metastatic disease. Similar to previous studies, they found that male gender, location on the head and neck and torso, and ulceration were associated with metastases. In contrast to a number of previous studies, Clark level of invasion did not appear to correlate with regional or systemic spread, although a Breslow thickness greater than .80 mm did. No recurrences or metastases were noted in patients with lesions less than .30 mm thick. Metastases occurred a median of 55 months after diagnosis of the primary lesion. Although the majority of tumors recurred in the regional lymph nodes, systemic metastases developed in several patients in the absence of regional metastases. The overall metastatic rate for this group of patients with thin melanomas was 15%. The mortality in those patients developing metastases was 46%. Based on their observations, the authors recommend that sentinel lymph node biopsy be offered to patients with melanomas more than .80 mm thick, to those with ulcerated lesions, and to males with .30- to .79-mm thick lesions of the trunk and head and neck.

P. G. Lang, Jr, MD

Delayed Harvesting of Sentinel Lymph Nodes After Previous Wide Local Excision of Extremity Melanoma
Leong SPL, Thelmo MC, Kim RP, et al (Univ of California, San Francisco)
Ann Surg Oncol 10:196-200, 2003   17–33

Introduction.—The optimal time to perform selective sentinel lymphadenectomy (SSL) in patients with malignant melanoma is simultaneously with wide local excision (WLE) of the primary melanoma site. Patients who had undergone a WLE of extremity melanoma were reviewed to determine the value of delaying SSL for detection of micrometastasis to the regional basin.

Methods.—The study included 24 patients who were referred for SSL after WLE of primary melanoma on an upper or lower extremity. Patients with primary melanoma at other sites were excluded because the drainage pattern in the extremities is more predictable. Twelve patients had primary closure, and 12 had skin grafting; the median Breslow thickness was 2.0 mm. After preoperative lymphoscintigraphy, SSL was performed to assess micrometastasis in the regional lymph node basin.

Results.—All 24 patients had drainage from the injection site to a regional lymph node basin and had at least 1 sentinel lymph node (SLN) harvested. The mean number of nodal basins per patient was 1.13 and the mean number of SLNs per patient was 3.25. Two patients exhibited SLNs, all in the inguinal area, with occult metastases. With a median follow-up time of 3 years, 21 of 22 patients with negative SLNs had no evidence of recurrence, and 1 had died of non-melanoma–related causes. One patient with a positive SLN had no evidence of disease with a follow-up time of 1.9 years; the other was alive with no evidence of disease 1.6 years after excision of a popliteal recurrence.

Conclusion.—Delayed SSL was performed successfully in a select group of patients who had undergone WLE of extremity melanoma. When this delayed group was compared with a simultaneous group, no difference was found in mean Breslow thickness, number of nodal basins per patient, number of SLNs per patient, or percentage of positive SLNs. Patients with head and neck or trunk melanoma probably should not undergo SSL after WLE.

Lymphoscintigraphy and Sentinel Node Biopsy Accurately Stage Melanoma in Patients Presenting After Wide Local Excision

Evans HL, Krag DN, Teates CD, et al (Univ of Virginia, Charlottesville; Univ of Vermont, Burlington; Academisch Ziekenhuis van de Vrije Universiteit, Amsterdam; et al)
Ann Surg Oncol 10:416-425, 2003   17–34

Background.—Sentinel lymph node (SLN) biopsy is often used to evaluate nodal status before proceeding with wide local excision (WLE) of cutaneous melanoma. Might SLN biopsy also be useful for staging patients after prior WLE? Given that more patients are seen at tertiary referral centers after WLE for melanoma, the utility of SLN biopsy after WLE was examined.

Methods.—The subjects were 76 patients who had undergone standard WLE of melanoma up to 252 days earlier; most patients (87%) had undergone WLE less than 2 months earlier. At study entry, patients had no clinical evidence of regional or distant metastases.

Radiolabeled colloid was injected 1 cm from the edge of the melanoma excision scar at 1-cm intervals around the scar's circumference. Lymphoscintigraphy was then performed with a handheld gamma probe to identify SLNs. SLNs were excised and examined by hematoxylin and eosin staining, with immunohistochemistry reserved for confirming areas of suspected disease identified by histopathology. Patients were followed for a median of 38 months to determine recurrences.

Results.—At least 1 SLN could be identified in 75 (38 men, 37 women; mean age, 49 years) of the 76 patients (98.6%); 63 patients (84.0%) had SLNs confined to 1 basin, 10 patients (13.3%) had SLNs in 2 basins, and 2 patients (2.7%) had SLNs in 3 basins. SLN biopsy findings were positive for disease in 11 patients (14.6%) and negative in 67 patients (85.4%). During follow-up, of the 11 patients with positive SLN findings, 3 patients (27.3%) had recurrences. Two of these died 4 to 5 years after diagnosis (the third patient was lost to follow-up).

Of the 64 patients with negative findings on SLN biopsy, 3 (4.7%) had systemic metastasis develop simultaneous with nodal recurrences in a basin that had been negative for disease. Additionally, 1 patient (1.6%) had an isolated recurrence in a lymph node contralateral to the primary tumor (this may represent a failure of lymphatic mapping).

Conclusion.—Lymphatic mapping with SLN biopsy can accurately stage regional lymph nodes in patients after prior standard WLE. Even with conservative estimates, the negative predictive value of SLN biopsy in these patients was 95%. These findings suggest that melanoma patients with prior WLE need not be excluded from SLN biopsy.

▶ Although it is acknowledged that lymphatic mapping and SLN biopsy should be performed before definitive removal of a melanoma, there are times when a patient who has already had a melanoma widely excised presents for further evaluation. A frequently asked question is whether lymphatic mapping and SLN biopsy are reliable in such patients. Several prior studies have addressed this issue and the conclusions drawn have been that they are, especially if the primary lesion was on an extremity and a flap had not been used to repair the defect.

This study confirms these findings and suggests that if a simple advancement flap was used to repair the surgical defect or if the lesion was not on the head and neck, lymphatic mapping and SLN biopsy are as reliable as if these had been performed at the same time as definitive removal of the primary lesion. If the primary lesion was located on the head or neck, which are notorious for their unpredictable lymphatic drainage patterns, or if the primary lesion was located in skin overlying a nodal basin, delayed lymphatic mapping and SLN biopsy might be less reliable.

P. G. Lang, Jr, MD

The Impact of Immunohistochemistry on Sentinel Node Biopsy for Primary Cutaneous Malignant Melanoma
Ross GL, Shoaib T, Scott J, et al (Canniesburn Hosp, England; Glasgow Royal Infirmary, England; Univ of Glasgow, England)
Br J Plast Surg 56:153-155, 2003   17–35

Background.—Sentinel node biopsy (SNB) is an accurate way to identify nodal disease in patients with malignant melanoma. Accurate selecting of pathologic nodes permits improved pathologic disease staging. The effect of immunohistochemical analysis on the pathologic staging of sentinel nodes was investigated.

Methods.—The study included 100 consecutive patients undergoing SNB for primary cutaneous malignant melanoma. Sentinel node harvesting involved preoperative lymphoscintigraphy, intraoperative gamma probes and blue dye. When a sentinel node was found to contain tumor on routine pathologic or immunohistochemical analysis, therapeutic lymph node dissection (TLND) was performed. When the sentinel node was free of metastases, no other treatment was delivered to the primary lymph node basin.

Findings.—At least 1 node was identified in 95 patients. Twenty-five were staged as SNB positive and offered TLND. Seventy-six percent of SNB-positive patients were found to be positive on routine pathologic analysis, and 24% with immunohistochemical staining. In 8% of the patients, immuno-histochemical findings upstaged disease. Twenty-one patients who staged positive with SNB underwent TLND. Fifty percent who were staged sentinel node positive on routine pathologic analysis were found to have no further disease in the TLND, compared with all 5 of those staged as sentinel node positive with immunohistochemical results. Recurrence developed in the nodal basin in 3 patients after a negative SNB. At a mean 24 months of fol-low-up, the procedure had a sensitivity of 89%.

Conclusions.—Immunohistochemical staining is essential for identifying micrometastases in sentinel nodes. Differentiating patients with micrometa-static disease from those with occult disease is important for determining the prognostic effects of micrometastases.

▶ Immunohistochemical staining is necessary to maximize the detection of melanoma cells in a sentinel lymph node (SLN). This study confirms the find-ings of similar studies done previously. In the series reported here, immuno-histochemical stains detected melanoma cells in an additional 8% of patients. However, despite the use of immunohistochemical analysis, 11% of patients with negative SLB biopsy specimens had a recurrence in the nodal basin from which the SLN had been taken. Although the use of polymerase chain reaction (PCR) technology probably would have increased the sensitivity of the SLN bi-opsy in these patients, previous studies have shown that even with this sen-sitive technology, there are still patients with negative reports who will have a recurrence in the sampled nodal basin. This could be because PCR might not be sufficiently sensitive to always detect melanoma cells, because of errors in the identification and sampling of the SLN(s), or because melanoma cells may sometimes bypass the SLN.

P. G. Lang, Jr, MD

Prognostic Significance of Reverse Transcriptase-Polymerase Chain Reaction–Negative Sentinel Nodes in Malginant Melanoma
Ribuffo D, Gradilone A, Vonella M, et al ("La Sapienza" Univ, Rome; Policlinico "Mater Domini," Catanzaro, Italy; Mediterranean Inst of Neurosciences, Pozzilli, Italy)
Ann Surg Oncol 10:396-402, 2003 17–36

Background.—Hematoxylin and eosin staining and immunohistochem-istry (IHC) are the standards for evaluating melanoma metastasis in sentinel lymph nodes (SLNs). However, some patients with negative findings by these methods have positive findings when examined by reverse transcriptase–polymerase chain reaction (RT-PCR). Whether the identifica-tion of residual disease by RT-PCR is associated with a higher risk of devel-opment of recurrence was examined.

Methods.—The subjects were 137 patients with primary stage I or II cu-taneous melanoma (Breslow thickness, 0.75-4 mm). All patients underwent

TABLE 1.—Detection of Nodal Micrometastasis by Immunohistochemistry and Reverse Transcriptase–Polymerase Chain Reaction

	No. Patients (%)			
	Immunohistochemistry		RT-PCR	
	Positive	Negative	Positive	Negative
Sentinel nodes	15 (11)	119 (89)	85 (63)	49 (37)

Abbreviation: RT-PCR, Reverse transcriptase–polymerase chain reaction.
(Courtesy of Ribuffo D, Gradilone A, Vonella M, et al: Prognostic significance of reverse transcriptase–polymerase chain reaction–negative sentinel nodes in malignant melanoma. *Ann Surg Oncol* 10(4):396-402, 2003.)

lymphoscintigraphy and intraoperative lymphatic mapping; the radioactive colloid was injected perilesionally and activity was read by a handheld gamma probe. SLN specimens were divided and examined by hematoxylin and eosin and IHC (using antibodies against HMB-45 antigen and S-100 protein), and by RT-PCR (with markers for tyrosinase and MART-1 [melanoma antigen recognized by T cells]). Patients were followed for a median of 42 months to identify recurrent or metastatic disease.

Results.—At least 1 SLN was identified in 134 (69 men, 65 women; median age, 55.5 years) of the 137 patients (98%), and 287 SLNs were dissected and analyzed. IHC detected nodal micrometastasis in 15 of these 134 patients (11%). In comparison, RT-PCR detected nodal micrometastasis in 85 patients (63%; $P < .001$) (Table I). All IHC-positive nodes were also positive on RT-PCR. Additionally, RT-PCR was positive in 59 of 119 patients (50%) with negative IHC findings. Disease-free survival differed significantly according to IHC and RT-PCR status (Fig 2).

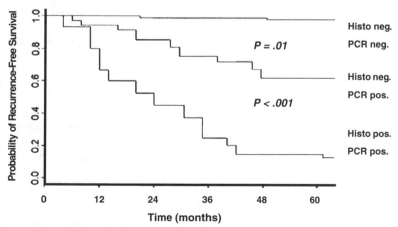

FIGURE 2.—Kaplan-Meier disease-free survival rate. Probability of disease-free survival rate for immunohistochemistry (IHC)-negative and reverse transcriptase-polymerase chain reaction (RT-PCR)-negative patients (Histo neg. PCR neg.), for patients IHC negative but RT-PCR positive(Histo neg. PCR pos.), and for patients IHC and RT-PCR positive (Histo pos. PCR pos.). (Courtesy of Ribuffo D, Gradilone A, Vonella M, et al: Prognostic significance of reverse transcriptase-polymerase chain reaction–negative sentinel nodes in malignant melanoma. *Ann Surg Oncol* 10(4):396-402, 2003.)

Among patients with negative IHC findings, recurrences were significantly more common in those with positive RT-PCR findings than in those with negative findings. Additionally, among patients with positive RT-PCR findings, recurrences were significantly more common in patients whose IHC findings were also positive, compared with IHC-negative patients. Of note, none of the patients with RT-PCR–negative findings had recurrence during follow-up. In multivariate analyses, RT-PCR status did not correlate significantly with Breslow tumor thickness.

Conclusion.—RT-PCR with markers for tyrosinase and MART-1 is sensitive and specific for detecting melanoma cells, and negative RT-PCR findings are highly predictive of disease-free survival. Patients with positive findings on RT-PCR have poorer disease-free survival, even when IHC results are negative. Still, the impact of positive RT-PCR findings on treatment strategies remains to be determined.

▶ Some patients with a negative SLN biopsy specimen will develop recurrent melanoma in the same nodal basin. When the SLNs from these patients are re-examined using PCR technology, melanoma cells are detected in a significant number of patients. Several questions arise as the result of these observations: (1) Should PCR technology routinely be employed in the examination of SLNs? (2) What is the significance of SLNs that are positive by PCR alone, and how should such patients be managed? This study addresses these questions.

Based on the authors' observations, several conclusions can be drawn: (1) To maximally detect melanoma cells in SLNs, at least 2 markers need to be used (in this study, tyrosinase and MART-1); (2) PCR is reliable and specific when performed properly with appropriate controls; (3) PCR is more sensitive than IHC in detecting melanoma cells; and (4) patients positive by PCR alone fare worse than patients who are PCR-negative. Unfortunately, the authors were not able to definitively answer the most important question; ie, how should patients positive by PCR alone be managed? However, they do argue that not all of these patients should be subjected to a complete node dissection.

P. G. Lang, Jr, MD

Patterns of Recurrence in Patients With Melanoma and Histologically Negative But RT-PCR–Positive Sentinel Lymph Nodes
Goydos JS, Patel KN, Shih WJ, et al (UMDNJ-Robert Wood Johnson Med School, New Brunswick, NJ; Cancer Inst of New Jersey, New Brunswick)
J Am Coll Surg 196:196-205, 2003   17–37

Introduction.—Reverse transcriptase polymerase chain reaction (RT-PCR) of lymph nodes can identify minute amounts of melanoma that are unidentifiable by routine histopathologic examination. The patterns of recurrent disease in patients with only RT-PCR evidence of regional nodal

TABLE 1.—Distribution of First Recurrences

Nodal Status	In Transit Mets	Regional Nodal Mets	Distant Mets	Total Recurrence
Positive histology (n)	8	0	9	17
Positive RT-PCR (n = 34) (%)	24	0	26	50
Negative histology (n)	6	2	6	14
Positive RT-PCR (n = 68) (%)	9	3	9	21

Note: Recurrence rate was significantly higher for histologically positive patients, compared with histologically negative but reverse transcriptase–polymerase chain reaction (*RT-PCR*)-positive patients (50% vs 21%; P = .002). Given recurrence, though, the pattern of recurrence was not significantly different between these patients (P = .92).

(Courtesy of Goydos JS, Patel KN, Shih WJ, et al: Patterns of recurrence in patients with melanoma and histologically negative but RT-PCR–positive sentinel lymph nodes. *J Am Coll Surg* 196:196-205, 2003. Copyright 2003, American College of Surgeons.)

spread were examined to ascertain whether proposed treatment interventions are likely to be effective.

Methods.—A total of 175 patients who underwent selective lymphadenectomy for clinical stage I or II melanoma were included. A proportion of each sentinel lymph node (SLN) was preserved in liquid nitrogen in the operating room. Specimens underwent RT-PCR analysis to identify the melanoma/melanocyte-specific marker tyrosinase. The pattern of recurrence (regional dermal metastases, regional nodal recurrence, or distant metastatic spread) of patients with histologically positive SLNs were compared with that of patients with histologically negative SLNs.

Results.—The mean follow-up time was 33.83 months (range, 6.21-62.95 months). Of 34 patients with a minimum of 1 histologically positive SLN, 17 (50%) had a recurrence. Of 141 patients with histologically negative SLNs, 73 had SLNs that were also negative for tyrosinase by RT-PCR; none had recurrent disease. Of 68 patients with histologically negative but RT-PCR positive SLNs, 14 had recurrence (20.6%) (P = .002). The pattern of recurrence was not significantly different between the 2 groups (P = .92) (Table 1).

Conclusion.—The pattern of recurrence of patients with only RT-PCR evidence of melanoma in SLNs was identical to that of patients with histologically evident melanoma in the SLN who underwent subsequent completion lymphadenectomy. Thus, completion lymphadenectomy may be ineffective in reducing the recurrence rate of patients with only RT-PCR evidence of melanoma in SLNs.

▶ A number of interesting observations come from this study, as follows:

1. As demonstrated previously, patients whose SLN biopsy specimens are positive only by PCR fare worse than those who are negative both by PCR and histology. In this study, patients who were negative by both histology and PCR did not develop a recurrence, whereas those positive by PCR alone experienced a 21% recurrence rate. However, this recurrence rate was less than that for patients positive by both assays (50% recurrence rate).

2. The pattern of recurrence for patients positive by PCR alone was similar to that for patients with histologically positive SLN biopsy specimens, ie, in

transit metastases and distant metastases. In very few of the patients posi-tive by PCR alone was there recurrence in the nodal basin. At first glance, this would appear surprising since none of those patients had a complete lymph node dissection; however, it is worth remembering that only a small percentage of patients with positive SLN biopsy specimens have positive non-SLNs when subjected to a complete lymph node dissection.

3. The fact that many of the recurrences seen in both groups with positive SLN biopsy specimens occurred outside the regional nodal basin(s) raises the question whether patients with positive SLN biopsy specimens benefit from a complete lymph node dissection. There are ongoing studies that hopefully will answer this question.

4. Since a number of studies have now documented that an SLN biopsy posi-tive by PCR alone is prognostically significant, the question arises as to whether PCR analysis should be performed on histologically negative SLNs.[1] This would allow for better prognostication and also eventually could be important in the selection of patients for adjuvant therapy.

P. G. Lang, Jr, MD

Reference

1. Shivers SC, Xiangning W, Weiguo L, et al: Molecular staging of malignant mela-noma: Correlation with clinical outcome. *JAMA* 280:1410-1415, 1998.

Predicting Residual Lymph Node Basin Disease in Melanoma Patients With Sentinel Lymph Node Metastases
Salti GI, Das Gupta TK (Univ of Illinois at Chicago)
Am J Surg 186:98-101, 2003   17–38

Background.—Patients with melanoma whose sentinel lymph node (SLN) biopsy specimen is positive for disease typically undergo complete lymph node dissection (CLND) to rule out residual disease in the basin. In most cases, however, the SLNs are the only positive nodes detected. Factors that might predict which patients with a positive SLN will have non-SLN in-volvement were investigated.

Methods.—The subjects were 200 patients with melanoma (Breslow thickness greater than 1.0 mm) and clinically negative regional lymph nodes who were evaluated between August 1996 and June 2000. SLNs were iden-tified via lymphoscintigraphy with perilesional radiotracer injection and a handheld gamma probe; positive SLN biopsy specimens were examined with hematoxylin and eosin staining and by immunohistochemistry. All pa-tients with positive SLNs underwent CLND, and non-SLNs were examined by hematoxylin and eosin staining. Multivariate logistic regression analyses were performed to identify demographic and clinical factors associated with positive non-SLNs.

Results.—Lymphoscintigraphy identified 56 patients (39 males and 17 fe-males 7-79 years of age) with a total of 68 SLN-positive nodal basins (1 basin

TABLE 2.—Multivariate Logistic Regression of Factors
Associated With Non–Sentinel Lymph Node Positivity

Factor	P Value
Number of positive sentinel nodes	
1 vs. >1	0.586
≤2 vs. >2	0.028
Characteristic of sentinel lymph node metastases	0.427
Breslow thickness (mm)	0.702
Clark level	0.877
Histological subtype	0.814
Location of primary	0.541
Ulceration	0.537
Mitoses/mm^2	0.193
Age (years)	0.320
Sex	0.773
Number of draining nodal basins	0.673

(Reprinted from Salti GI, Das Gupta TK: Predicting residual lymph node basin disease in melanoma patients with sentinel lymph node metastases. *Am J Surg* 186:98-101, 2003. Copyright 2003, with permission from Excerpta Medica Inc.)

in 42 patients, 2 in 11 patients, 3 in 2 patients, and 4 in 1 patient). CLND revealed that 8 patients (14%) had 13 (19%) residual positive non-SLNs. In multivariate analyses, the only significant and independent predictor of positive non-SLNs was having more than 2 positive SLNs (Table 2). None of the patients whose SLNs were positive by immunohistochemisty alone (4 patients) or who had only 1 microscopic focus of disease (9 patients) had non-SLN disease.

Conclusion.—In all, 56 of the 200 patients with melanoma (28%) had positive SLNs, and 8 of the 56 patients with positive SLNs (14%) had positive non-SLNs. The only factor that predicted the presence of positive non-SLNs was the presence of more than 2 positive SLNs. Nevertheless, until better methods are available for identifying which patients are at increased risk for residual lymph node basin disease, all patients with positive SLNs should undergo CLND.

▶ In patients with a positive SLN biopsy specimen, it is customary to perform a CLND. In the majority of these patients, the nodal basin contains no additional disease. Thus, a significant number of patients are subjected to an unnecessary procedure that is sometimes associated with significant morbidity. In addition, there is controversy as to whether performing a CLND alters prognosis. To avoid performing an unnecessary CLND in patients with a positive SLN biopsy specimen, efforts have been made to predict which patients are most likely to have residual disease in the nodal basin(s). To date, these attempts have either been unsuccessful or the findings inconsistent from study to study.

This study represents yet another attempt to predict which patients might have residual disease in their nodal basin(s). In contrast to some previous studies, here the authors report that the only significant predictor of non-SLN involvement was the number of positive SLNs. Patients with more than 2 positive SLNs were more likely to have positive non-SLNs. Patients with SLN biopsy specimens positive by immunohistochemistry alone or who had only a single focus of tumor in their SLN were less likely to have non-SLN involvement, but this was not statistically significant. The authors conclude that despite their observations, there is no reliable way to predict which patients will have residual tumor in their nodal basin(s), and thus all patients with a positive SLN biopsy specimen should undergo CLND.

P. G. Lang, Jr, MD

The Amount of Metastatic Melanoma in a Sentinel Lymph Node: Does It Have Prognostic Significance?
Carlson GW, Murray DR, Lyles RH, et al (Emory Univ, Atlanta, Ga)
Ann Surg Oncol 10:575-581, 2003   17–39

Introduction.—Sentinel lymph node (SLN) mapping and biopsy has revolutionized the operative management of primary malignant melanoma. Nodal staging in the new version of the American Joint Committee on Cancer (AJCC) is based in part on the presence of micrometastases after sentinel lymphadenectomy. The amount of metastatic disease in the SLN was evaluated as a predictor of residual nodal disease and prognosis.

Methods.—A total of 592 patients with clinical AJCC stage I or II malignant melanoma who received dynamic lymphoscintigraphy and gamma probe–guided SLN biopsy between January 1, 1994, and December 31, 1999, were retrospectively evaluated. One hundred four patients had 134 SLNs that contained metastatic melanoma.

The slides were reviewed and the size of the metastatic lesion in each SLN was determined. The size of the metastatic deposit was defined as either macrometastatic (>2 mm), micrometastatic (≤2 mm), a cluster of cells (10-30 grouped cells) in the subcapsular space or interfollicular zone, or isolated melanoma cells (1-20 or less individual cells) in subcapsular sinuses.

Results.—Pathologic information included only patients who underwent successful SLN mapping and biopsy. The mean follow-up time was 39.6 months. Of 592 patients evaluated, 104 had positive SLNs. There were 45 relapses and 31 deaths. The tumor site was strongly correlated with tumor thickness ($P = .002$), with a higher proportion of head and neck tumors classified as T4. Ulceration was highly correlated with tumor thickness and SLN positivity ($P < .001$ for both).

The number of metastatic deposits in each SLN was as follows: isolated melanoma cells, 5 (3.7%); cluster of cells, 35 (26.1%); 2 mm or less, 45 (33.6%); and more than 2 mm, 49 (36.7%). The size of the largest nodal metastasis was used to stratify patients who had multiple positive SLNs. The overall 3-year survival rate in patients with SLN micrometastases was 90%, compared to 58% for patients with SLN macrometastases ($P = .004$).

Conclusion.—The amount of metastatic melanoma in the SLN is independently predictive of survival. Patients with SLN metastatic deposits larger than 2 mm in diameter have significantly reduced survival.

▶ Two important pieces of information came from this study: (1) there is no reliable way to predict which patients with a positive SLN biopsy specimen will have non-SLN involvement; even patients with a few cells in their SLN may be found to have non-SLN involvement after a complete node dissection; and (2) the amount of tumor in the SLN predicts overall survival but not relapse-free survival.

P G. Lang, Jr, MD

Sentinel Lymph Node Biopsy for Patients With Cutaneous Desmoplastic Melanoma

Gyorki DE, Busam K, Panageas K, et al (Memorial Sloan-Kettering Cancer Ctr, New York)

Ann Surg Oncol 10:403-407, 2003   17–40

Background.—Desmoplastic melanoma (DM) is a distinct variant of malignant melanoma characterized by a high incidence of local recurrence and a low incidence of lymph node metastasis. Sentinel lymph node (SLN) biopsy can accurately identify nodal involvement in patients with other types of melanoma. Whether lymphatic mapping with SLN biopsy is useful for staging patients with DM was investigated.

Methods.—The subjects were 27 patients (20 men, 7 women; median age, 64 years) with cutaneous DM treated between 1996 and 2001. Tumors were present on the head and neck (14 patients), trunk (8 patients), and the extremities (5 patients). Breslow thickness ranged from 0.7 to 20 mm (median, 2.2 mm), and lesions were Clark level IV (20 patients) or V (7 patients). All patients underwent wide local excision and lymphatic mapping via a handheld gamma probe, followed by SLN biopsy. Patients were followed for a median of 27 months to identify recurrences.

Results.—SLN biopsy was successful in 24 of the 27 patients (88.9%). None of these 24 patients had evidence of SLN involvement. Five (20.8%) patients had a recurrence 6 to 43 months after SLN biopsy. Four of these recurrences were systemic, and 1 was local. Two patients are alive with disease and 2 have died. The fifth patient (with the local recurrence) is free of disease 9 months after re-excision. The other patients are alive without evidence of disease.

Conclusion.—Regional lymph node metastases are uncommon in patients with DM, both at presentation and during follow-up. Given the rarity of nodal involvement, the utility of SLN biopsy in patients with DM is questionable.

▶ DM, an unusual variant of melanoma, constitutes 4% of all melanomas. It is more common in men and usually occurs on the head and neck. Perineural involvement is not unusual. Local recurrences are common. Because the lesion is often not pigmented, diagnosis is sometimes delayed and by the time the correct diagnosis is made, the tumor is often quite thick. Unlike other types of melanoma, when DM metastasizes it often bypasses the nodal basin and spreads systemically.

A number of studies, including this one, have documented that SLN biopsy is frequently negative in patients with DM. A review of the literature reveals a positivity rate of only 1.6%. Despite the low incidence of SLN positivity, these patients commonly develop systemic metastases. Because of the low incidence of SLN positivity, the authors raise a valid question: Should we perform SLN biopsies in patients with DM? Currently available information suggests that the yield is so low that it does not seem justifiable to add to the cost of care or to subject the patient to the risks and morbidity associated with the procedure.

P. G. Lang, Jr, MD

Sentinel Lymph Node Mapping for Thick (≥4-mm) Melanoma: Should We Be Doing It?
Carlson GW, Murray DR, Hestley A, et al (Emory Univ, Atlanta, Ga)
Ann Surg Oncol 10:408-415, 2003   17–41

Background.—Patients with thick (4 mm or greater) primary melanoma are believed to have a worse prognosis than patients with thinner lesions, and elective lymph node dissection has not been proven to improve survival. Most studies attesting to the utility of sentinel lymph node (SLN) biopsy in patients with melanoma have included patients whose tumors were less than 4-mm thick. Whether SLN biopsy can improve survival in patients with thick primary melanoma was examined.

Methods.—The medical records of 114 patients (75 men, 39 women; mean age, 57 years) with thick (4 mm or greater) primary melanoma who underwent successful lymphatic mapping and SLN biopsy between January 1994 and December 1999 were reviewed. During lymphatic mapping, a radiotracer was injected preoperatively around the circumference of the tumor and activity was read intraoperatively with a handheld gamma probe. SLNs were excised and examined by routine hematoxylin and eosin staining and immunohistochemistry. Overall survival and relapse-free survival were determined over a mean follow-up period of 37.8 months.

Results.—Tumor thickness ranged from 4 to 17 mm (mean, 6.3 mm), and tumors were present on the trunk (44 patients, or 38.6%), extremities (41 patients, or 36%), and the head and neck (29 patients, or 25.4%). Forty tumors (35.1%) were ulcerated. SLN biopsy findings were positive for disease in 37 patients (32.5%). One node was positive in 18 patients (48.7%), 2 nodes were positive in 11 patients (29.7%), and 3 or more nodes were positive in 8 patients (21.6%).

Patients with ulcerated tumors had significantly worse 3-year overall survival (57% vs 82%) and relapse-free survival (38% vs 68%) than patients whose tumors were not ulcerated. Patients with positive SLN findings also had significantly worse 3-year overall survival (57% vs 82%) and relapse-free survival (31% vs 71%) than patients without SLN metastasis. In multivariate Cox regression analyses, SLN status was a significant independent predictor of relapse-free survival (relative hazard, 3.66) and overall survival (relative hazard, 2.13). Ulceration was also a significant independent predictor of both relapse-free and overall survival (relative hazards, 1.89 and 1.92, respectively).

Conclusion.—Not all patients with thick primary melanomas have a poor prognosis. In fact, 3-year overall survival was 88% among the 56 patients with nonulcerated tumors and negative SLN findings. In contrast, 3-year overall survival was only 53% among patients with both ulcerated lesions and positive SLN findings. In patients with thick melanomas, the pathologic status of the SLN is a predictor of survival, and lymphatic mapping and SLN biopsy should be routinely performed in this population.

▶ This is yet another study demonstrating that patients with thick melanomas (more than 4 mm) do not have a uniformly poor prognosis and that SLN biopsy serves as a significant prognostic indicator for these patients. In this study, patients with thick melanomas that were ulcerated or who had a positive SLN biopsy specimen had a significantly worse prognosis than those patients without ulceration or who had a negative SLN biopsy specimen. This observation could be of great significance when effective adjuvant therapy becomes available. The question that remains unanswered is whether those patients with a positive SLN biopsy specimen should be subjected to a complete node dissection; ie, will it improve their relapse-free or overall survival?

P. G. Lang, Jr, MD

Sentinel Node Biopsy in Patients With In-Transit Recurrence of Malignant Melanoma
Dewar DJ, Powell BWEM (St George's Hosp, London)
Br J Plast Surg 56:415-417, 2003   17–42

Background.—In-transit recurrence of malignant melanoma is typically treated with wide local excision followed by restaging. In-transit recurrence indicates active systemic disease, however, and treatments to achieve local control may not be sufficient. The utility of sentinel lymph node biopsy (SLNB) in staging 5 patients with in-transit recurrence was described.

> *Case Reports.*—Five patients (3 men, 2 women; age range, 29-61 years) had in-transit melanoma develop from 18 months to 10 years after undergoing wide excision of a primary melanoma. Four patients underwent CT scan, which revealed no evidence of distant metastases. All 5 patients underwent lymphoscintigraphy with a gamma probe to identify the SLNB, followed by wide local excision of the in-transit tumor and removal of the SLN.

In the first patient, the radiotracer was injected into the in-transit deposit; 1 node was identified but was proven to be negative for disease. However, 9 weeks later the patient was seen with a palpable lymph node that was confirmed to harbor disease, and complete lymph node dissection revealed many positive lymph nodes. This patient died of widespread metastatic disease. Thus, in the second patient, the radiotracer was injected into the primary tumor site rather than the in-transit mass. One node was identified and was proven positive for disease, but complete lymph node dissection confirmed the absence of occult disease in the lymph node basin.

The courses of patients 3 to 5 were similar: colloid was injected into the primary tumor, a sentinel lymph node positive for disease was identified, and subsequent lymph node dissection ruled out further disease. One of the last 4 patients has remained disease free for 7 months, 2 subsequently had another in-transit recurrence, and had a distant cutaneous metastasis. These recurrences were excised, and the patients have remained disease free for 8 months to 2.5 years.

Conclusion.—SLNB can accurately stage lymph nodes in patients with in-transit recurrence of malignant melanoma. The lymph node draining the primary site more accurately reflects nodal status than the lymph node draining the in-transit recurrence. Thus, radiotracer should be injected at the primary site rather than at the site of recurrence.

▶ Satellite lesions and in-transit metastases of melanoma are associated with a significant risk for recurrence and with regional and distant metastases. In-transit metastases portend a poor prognosis with a 5-year survival rate of 53%. If there are also regional node metastases, the 5-year survival rate decreases to 26%.[1]

Although based on limited data, several conclusions can be drawn from this article. First, when performing an SLNB in a patient with in-transit satellites, the radioactive colloid and blue dye should be injected around the site of the primary tumor, not around the satellite lesion(s). Second, an SLNB specimen has a high probability of being positive in a patient with in-transit metastases. The question that remains is whether the procedure is justified in this setting. Although, from a prognostic standpoint, it adds considerable information, it is unclear whether SLN removal or a subsequent complete node dissection alters prognosis or disease-free interval.

Although 4 of the 5 patients reported here were still alive, 3 of the 4 developed recurrent disease. Although these 3 patients subsequently appeared to do well, the duration of follow-up was relatively brief.

P. G. Lang, Jr, MD

Reference

1. Balch CM, Buzaid AC, Soong S, et al: Final version of the American Joint Committee on Cancer staging system for cutaneous melanoma. *J Clin Oncol* 19:3635-3648, 2001.

Complications Associated With Sentinel Lymph Node Biopsy for Melanoma

Wrightson WR, for the Sunbelt Melanoma Trial Study Group (Univ of Louisville, Ky; et al)
Ann Surg 10:676-680, 2003   17–43

Background.—Sentinel lymph node (SLN) biopsy is considered a safe, minimally invasive procedure for staging regional lymph nodes in patients with melanoma. However, little information is available to specifically determine the morbidity associated with this procedure. The morbidity associated with SLN biopsy was compared with that of completion lymph node dissection (CLND).

Methods.—Data were obtained on 2120 patients enrolled in the Sunbelt Melanoma Trial, a prospective, multicenter study of SLN biopsy in melanoma. Participants underwent SLN biopsy and were followed prospectively. Those with evidence of nodal metastasis in the SLN underwent CLND.

Findings.—At a median follow-up period of 16 months, major or minor complications associated with SLN biopsy developed in 4.6% of the patients. Of the 444 patients undergoing SLN biopsy plus CLND, 23.2% had complications (Table 3). No deaths occurred.

Conclusion.—In this large prospective study of patients with melanoma, SLN biopsy was associated with a significantly lower rate of complications

TABLE 3.—Distribution of Nodal Basin Sites in Sentinel Lymph Node Biopsy and Completion Lymph Node Dissection

Location	SLN Complications, n (%)	CLND Complications, n (%)	P Value*
Neck	9/370 (2.4)	5/50 (10.0)	.008
Axilla			
Total complications	63/1426 (4.4)	52/262 (19.9)	<.0001
Lymphedema	4/1426 (.3)	12/262 (4.6)	<.0001
Groin			
Total complications	53/657 (8.1)	65/127 (51.2)	<.0001
Lymphedema	10/657 (1.5)	40/127 (31.5)	<.0001

*χ-square.
Abbreviations: SLN, Sentinel lymph node; *CLND*, completion lymph node dissection.
(Courtesy of Wrightson WR, for the Sunbelt Melanoma Trial Study Group: Complications associated with sentinel lymph node biopsy for melanoma. *Ann Surg* 10(6):676-680, 2003.)

than SLN biopsy plus CLND. Most SLN-related complications were minor and easy to manage. In rare cases, SLN biopsy alone produced lymphedema.

▶ This article confirms that SLN biopsy is a much more benign procedure than CLND. Hematoma/seroma formation, wound infection, and occasional lymphedema are the most frequently associated complications. The authors suggest that prophylactic antibiotics, given prior to either procedure, might decrease the incidence of wound infections. Not surprisingly, complications—especially lymphedema—were more commonly seen in association with SLN biopsy and CLND of the inguinal nodal basin. The lack of focal nerve injury in association with SLN biopsy of the parotid gland was reassuring. Notably, the authors did not observe any complications associated with the use of blue dye in their series of more than 2100 cases.[1]

P. G. Lang, Jr, MD

Reference

1. Leong SP, Donegan E, Heffernon W, et al: Adverse reactions to isosulfan blue during selective sentinel lymph node dissection in melanoma. *Ann Surg Oncol* 7:361-366, 2000.

Metastatic Melanoma in Pregnancy: Risk of Transplacental Metastases in the Infant
Alexander A, Samlowski WE, Grossman D, et al (Univ of Utah, Salt Lake City)
J Clin Oncol 21:2179-2186, 2003   17–44

Background.—Melanoma in pregnancy is not uncommon, but metastasis to the fetus via the placenta is quite rare and almost always fatal. The literature regarding metastatic melanoma in pregnancy was reviewed in an effort to provide more information on which to base clinical recommendations in this high-risk population.

Methods.—Cases of placental and/or fetal melanoma metastasis were identified via a MEDLINE search and by screening of references, analysis of 4 comprehensive literature reviews on the subject, and by communication with authors of previously published reports.

Results.—Since the first case report in 1866, there have been 87 cases of placental and/or fetal metastasis published; 27 of these cases (31%) were attributable to melanoma. Among the entire group of 87 cases of metastasis, 72 cases (83%) had placental involvement only, 10 (11%) had fetal metastasis without placental examination, and 5 (6%) had both placental and fetal involvement. Of the 15 cases of fetal involvement, data on sex were available in 12 cases and showed a predilection for males (9 of 12 cases, or 75%). Age at presentation with metastasis ranged from 0 to 20 months (mean, 4.5 months). Three infants survived; 2 underwent chemotherapy and bone marrow transplantation and 1 (with melanoma metastasis) had spontaneous regression.

Among the 27 cases of melanoma metastasis, 24 cases (100% of those examined microscopically) had placental involvement and 6 cases (22%) also had fetal involvement. Only 1 of the 6 fetuses with melanoma metastasis survived. Among these 27 cases, only 3 infants were born at term. Overall, 18 infants (67%) were healthy and unaffected, while 9 infants (33%) died between 0 and 10.25 months after birth.

Among the 16 survivors for whom follow-up information was available (mean, 14.2 months), patients have survived for up to 4 years with no evidence of disease. No treatment guidelines exist, yet recommendations include skin inspection, abdominal US, and screening for melanogens in the infant's urine. Also, 2 attempts with novel immune-based therapies have been unsuccessful.

Conclusion.—About 22% of cases of placental involvement by metastatic melanoma also have fetal involvement, and the survival of fetuses with metastatic melanoma is poor. Because metastasis is not always present at birth, children of mothers with melanoma should be monitored for the development of melanoma for at least 24 months, and the placentas should be closely examined to identify disease. At present, it is unclear whether adjuvant therapy can be useful for infants at risk for maternal melanoma metastasis.

▶ Although melanoma occurs infrequently in pregnancy, it is the most common tumor metastasizing to the placenta and fetus. Based on their review of the literature, the authors conclude that male fetuses appear to be more prone to develop metastatic lesions. Metastasis to the placenta is much more common than metastasis to the fetus, suggesting that the fetus, in many instances, is capable of eliminating circulating melanoma cells. Placental metastasis appears to be associated with an increase in premature births, but not infant mortality. Metastasis to the fetus may not be apparent at birth; consequently, the authors suggest close monitoring (for at least 24 months) of infants born to mothers with metastatic melanoma. The mortality rate in infants with metastasis is quite high.

P. G. Lang, Jr, MD

18 Lymphoproliferative Disorders

Cutaneous Lymphoid Hyperplasia: A Lymphoproliferative Continuum With Lymphomatous Potential
Nihal M, Mikkola D, Horvath N, et al (Univ of Wisconsin, Madison; Case Western Reserve Univ, Cleveland, Ohio; Veterans Affairs Med Ctr, Cleveland, Ohio)
Hum Pathol 34:617-622, 2003   18–1

Introduction.—Cutaneous lymphoid hyperplasia (CLH) may be idiopathic or arise in response to foreign antigens. Most cases appear as a solitary or localized cluster of asymptomatic papules or nodules, usually on the face. The condition is proposed to be the benign end of a continuum of lymphoproliferative disorders, with cutaneous lymphoma at the malignant extreme. "Clonal CLH," a transitional state capable of evolution to cutaneous B-cell lymphoma (CBCL), has been identified. Biopsy samples from patients with CLH were examined to determine the prevalence of dominant clonality and risk of lymphoma among CLH cases.

Methods.—The 44 patients had been referred to a cutaneous lymphoproliferative disorders program from 1991 through 2000. Representative portions of specimens obtained from well-developed lesions were divided for routine histopathology and fresh-frozen immunoperoxidase and molecular analysis. Thirty-eight cases of CLH were typical, with a mixed B-cell/T-cell composition; 6 cases contained at least 90% T cells (T-cell CLH [T-CLH]). An algorithm that incorporates histopathologic, immunopathologic, and molecular biologic data was used to analyze and classify cases. Immunoglobulin heavy chain (IgH) and T-cell receptor (TCR)-gamma gene rearrangements were assessed with polymerase chain reaction assays.

Results.—Thirty-eight patients had solitary or localized lesions (4 were T-CLH) and 6 had regional or generalized lesions (2 were T-CLH). Forty cases were of idiopathic cause. During a median follow-up period of 24 months, progression occurred in only 2 cases which evolved to overt CBCL. All cases contained a mixture of B cells, T cells, macrophages, and dendritic cells. Twenty-seven cases (61%) showed clonal CLH: 12 IgH+ (3 cases of T-CLH); 13 TCR+ (1 case of T-CLH); and 2 IgH+/TCR+ (neither was T-CLH) (Table 1). The lack of detectable clonality in 1 of the 2 cases that

TABLE 1.—Immunoglobulin and T-cell Receptor Gene Rearrangement in CLH Patients

CLH Subtype	Number of Case	IgH+	TCR+	(Dual +) IgH & TCR	Dominant Clonal	Polyclonal
CLH	38	9	12	2	23	15
		FR1/2 = 7	Vγ(1-8) + = 4			
		FR3 = 2	Vγ(9) + = 8			
			Vγ(1-8) + Vγ(9) + = 3			
T-CLH	6	3	1	0	4	2
		FR1/2 = 2	Vγ1-8+ = 1			
		FR3 = 1				
Total	44	12	13	2	27	17

Abbreviations: CLH, Cutaneous lymphoid hyperplasia; *T-CLH*, T-cell CLH; *IgH*, immunoglobulin heavy chain; *TCR*, T-cell receptor.

(Courtesy of Nihal M, Mikkola D, Horvath N, et al: Cutaneous lymphoid hyperplasia: A lymphoproliferative continuum with lymphomatous potential. *Hum Pathol* 34:617-622, 2003.)

evolved to CBCL was probably related to the inability of polymerase chain reaction methods to detect dominant clonality in all cases.

Discussion.—Many cases of CLH are true hyperplasias, but many others represent a clonal proliferative disorder that may progress to overt cutaneous lymphoma. Clonal overgrowth probably involves both B- and T-cell lineages.

▶ Dermatopathologists have struggled with the histopathologic analysis of CLHs. It has been hoped that molecular techniques might untie the Gordian knot in this regard. In the current report approximately 60% of the 44 patients with CLH studied demonstrated clonality; however, only 2 of the 44 patients had overt CBCL develop. Interestingly, one of the patients had no detectable clonality, whereas the other one did. Perhaps longer follow-up of this cohort of CLH patients may give more information on the usefulness of this technique for predicting biologic behavior. Meanwhile, the struggle will go on for dermatopathologists faced with this challenging problem.

J. C. Maize, MD

Lymphomatoid Papulosis Associated With Mycosis Fungoides: A Study of 21 Patients Including Analyses for Clonality
Zackheim HS, Jones C, LeBoit PE, et al (Univ of California, San Francisco; Stanford Univ, Calif)
J Am Acad Dermatol 49:620-623, 2003   18–2

Introduction.—Lymphomatoid papulosis (LyP) is now considered a predominantly CD30+ form of cutaneous T-cell lymphoma (CTCL) and is its least aggressive variety. An association appears to exist between LyP and other lymphomas, including mycosis fungoides (MF). Of the 54 patients with LyP in this study, 21 (39%) had associated MF. The charts of all 21 patients were reviewed, and 7 of the patients had a clonality analysis.

Methods.—The study included 12 men and 9 women (ages 36-74 years) with a duration of LyP ranging from 2 to 34 years and MF ranging from 0.1 to 30 years. Analysis for T-cell receptor-γ gene rearrangements of paraffin-embedded biopsy specimens was performed by heteroduplex analysis of polymerase chain reaction.

Results.—The diagnosis of LyP preceded MF in 14 (67%) patients, MF preceded LyP in 4 (19%), and the disorders appeared concurrently in 3 (14%). Twenty patients had type A LyP, and 1 had type B. Analysis of biopsy specimens of the LyP and MF lesions in 7 patients established the presence of an identical clone in the LyP and MF lesions. In 1 patient, biopsy specimens from 2 different MF lesions showed different sequences.

Conclusion.—The finding of a common clone in the LyP and MF lesions of the same patient strengthens the view that LyP is a form of CTCL, despite different phenotypic expressions and clinical manifestations, and that LyP and MF are related T-cell lymphoproliferative disorders.

▶ The authors concede that the high percentage of patients with LyP who had associated MF may reflect selection bias. The 39% of their patients with the association was even higher than that reported in other university-based studies.

B. H. Thiers, MD

Bexarotene Is a New Treatment Option for Lymphomatoid Papulosis
Krathen RA, Ward S, Duvic M (Univ of Texas, Houston)
Dermatology 206:142-147, 2003   18–3

Introduction.—Lymphomatoid papulosis (LyP) is an eruption that follows a benign course in most patients, but the risk of subsequent systemic lymphoma is increased. The lesions of LyP can be asymptomatic, slightly pruritic or painful, and necrosis or infection may develop. Treatments have included acyclovir, methotrexate, and carmustine (Table 1). Bexarotene, a rexinoid with selectivity for intracellular retinoid X receptors over retinoic acid receptors, has been used to treat cutaneous manifestations of cutaneous T cell lymphoma. In this first case series, 10 patients with chronic symptomatic LyP were treated with oral or topical bexarotene.

Methods.—Three patients with more than 10% body surface area involvement were treated with an oral starting dose of up to 300 mg/m²/d. Oral fenofibrate, atorvastatin, or both were also administered to keep fasting triglyceride levels below 400 mg/dL, and levothyroxine was given to keep free T_4 at normal levels. Seven patients received topical bexarotene gel 1%.

Results.—Treatment duration ranged from 5 to 18 months for patients receiving oral bexarotene and from 3 to 20 months for those given topical bexarotene. Complete responses occurred in 2 patients, 1 who was treated orally and 1 who was treated topically. One patient in the oral therapy group was not evaluable, and the other had a partial response. Among those re-

TABLE 1.—Agents Reported Beneficial in the Treatment of LyP

Agent	Dose	Patients With Benefit	Reference
Acyclovir	200 mg p.o. q.d. × 6 weeks	1 of 4	19
	500 mg i.v. t.i.d. × 5 days	1 of 1	18
Carmustine	10 mg in alcohol q.d. for 4-17 weeks	7 of 7	24
(BCNU)	then 2-4 mg/ml (topical)	3 of 3	25
Tetracycline	Dose not specified	5 of 14	26
	1.5 g p.o. q.d.	0 of 1	9
	1 g p.o. q.d. × 1 month	? 1 of 2	16
Methotrexate	15-25 mg p.o. q.wk.	1 of 1	21
	5-25 mg p.o. q.wk.	3 of 3	22
	2.5-5 mg p.o. q.wk.	8 of 8	23
	10-60 mg p.o. q.wk. induction then 15-20 mg p.o. q.wk.	39 of 45	28
Interferon α-2b	1 MU/lesion 3 ×/week	1 of 1	17
Interferon α-2a,2c	3 MU 2a	4 of 4 on 2a	27
	15 MU 2c	1 of 1 on 2c	
PUVA	51-481 J/cm² total	5 of 5	20

Abbreviation: LyP, Lymphomatoid papulosis.
(Courtesy of Krathen RA, Ward S, Duvic M: Bexarotene is a new treatment option for lymphomatoid papulosis. *Dermatology* 206:142-147, 2003. Reproduced with permission of S. Karger AG, Basel.)

maining patients who were treated topically, there were 4 partial responses, 1 minimal response, and 1 patient with stable disease.

Conclusion.—No curative therapy currently exists for LyP. Initial findings in this small series of patients suggest that bexarotene may be beneficial. The topical gel preparation is more convenient and avoids the side effects of oral therapy.

▶ Both topical and systemic bexarotene are extremely expensive, and the latter is certainly not a benign drug, occasionally causing severe hypertriglyceridemia and hypothyroidism. Thus, the assertion by the authors that bexarotene "may be considered for first-line therapy" of LyP is open to challenge. Moreover, the ability of bexarotene (or any other drug) to prevent progression of LyP to lymphoma is uncertain.

B. H. Thiers, MD

Hypopigmented Mycosis Fungoides in Caucasian Patients: A Clinicopathologic Study of 7 Cases

Ardigó M, Borroni G, Muscardin L, et al (Univ of Graz, Austria; Univ of Pavia, Italy; Istituto Dermatologico SS Maria e Gallicano, Rome)
J Am Acad Dermatol 49:264-270, 2003   18–4

Introduction.—Hypopigmented mycosis fungoides (MF), an uncommon variant of cutaneous T-cell lymphoma, is usually seen in dark-skinned persons, especially children. The clinical, histologic, and molecular features of 7 Caucasian patients with hypopigmented MF were described.

Findings.—The patients included 5 adults (3 men and 2 women) aged 26 to 73 years at disease onset, and 2 children (1 boy and 1 girl) aged 14 and 10 years, respectively, at the time of diagnosis. All but 2 patients had erythematous lesions when evaluated; none had signs of atopy, psoriasis, or other inflammatory skin diseases. Biopsy specimens confirmed MF in all cases. The phenotype of neoplastic lymphocytes was T helper in 4 cases and T suppressor in 3 (including the 2 children). A polymerase chain reaction technique detected monoclonality of the T lymphocytes in the hypopigmented lesions of all patients. Molecular studies after laser-beam microdissection of the epidermis in 4 patients showed the monoclonal population of T lymphocytes to be confined mainly to the epidermis. Follow-up information was available for 6 patients. One was alive with complete remission at 6 months, 1 was alive with progressive disease at 171 months, and 4 were alive with stable disease at 16 to 232 months.

Discussion.—Only 9 of the 106 patients with hypopigmented MF reported in the literature have been Caucasian. Lesions in the 7 cases reported here appeared on the trunk (Fig 6; see color plate XV) and upper extremities, eyebrow (Fig 7; see color plate XVI) and forehead, arms, flanks, and buttocks. Lesions in 3 patients responded to conventional treatments (psoralen ultraviolet A-range, ultraviolet B). Diagnosis may be delayed because of the rarity of the disorder and its prolonged, nonaggressive course. Unusual

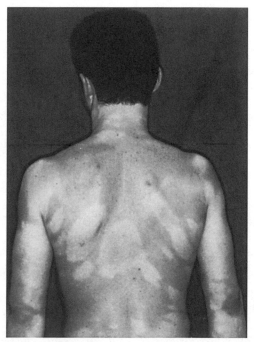

FIGURE 6.—Patient 7. Several confluent hypopigmented lesions on the trunk and upper extremities. (Reprinted by permission of the publisher from Ardigó M, Borroni G, Muscardin L, et al: Hypopigmented mycosis fungoides in Caucasian patients: A clinicopathologic study of 7 cases. *J Am Acad Dermatol* 49:264-270, 2003. Copyright 2003 by Elsevier.)

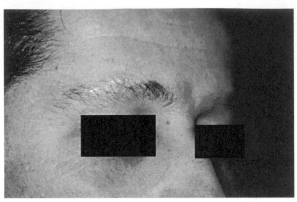

FIGURE 7.—Patient 7. Erythematous lesions with focal area of subtle hypopigmentation and partial alopecia on the eyebrow and forehead, corresponding to follicular mucinosis. (Reprinted by permission of the publisher from Ardigó M, Borroni G, Muscardin L, et al: Hypopigmented mycosis fungoides in Caucasian patients: A clinicopathologic study of 7 cases. *J Am Acad Dermatol* 49:264-270, 2003. Copyright 2003 by Elsevier.)

hypopigmented lesions in Caucasian patients should undergo biopsy to rule out hypopigmented MF.

▶ Hypopigmented MF occurs most commonly in dark-skinned individuals, with onset at a younger age than in more commonly observed variants of the disease. Children are sometimes affected and often show a T suppressor CD8+ phenotype, in contrast to the T helper CD4+ phenotype more often associated with the disease. Ardigó et al present a series of 7 Caucasian patients with hypopigmented MF. The pathogenesis of the hypopigmentation is unclear, but it may result from destruction of melanocytes by T lymphocytes infiltrating into affected skin.

B. H. Thiers, MD

Correlations Between Clinical, Histologic, Blood, and Skin Polymerase Chain Reaction Outcome in Patients Treated for Mycosis Fungoides
Dereure O, Balavoine M, Salles M-T, et al (Univ Hosp of Montpellier, France)
J Invest Dermatol 121:614-617, 2003   18–5

Background.—The relationship between posttreatment clinical, histologic, blood, and skin T-cell receptor–targeted polymerase chain reaction (PCR) data was investigated in patients with mycosis fungoides (MF) who had a dominant gene rearrangement at diagnosis.

Methods.—Twenty-seven patients with MF and dominant gene rearrangement in skin lesions at diagnosis were included in the study. Peripheral blood samples and molecular data in skin and blood obtained before and after treatment were analyzed.

Findings.—Sixteen of 25 patients had a dominant gene rearrangement detected in blood before treatment. In only 8 of 13 patients with complete clinical and histologic responses did the dominant gene rearrangement disappear from cutaneous lesions. Skin PCR findings remained positive in all 10 patients with histologically persistent disease. A dominant gene rearrangement persisted in the blood of 10 of 16 patients after treatment. Blood data in these patients did not correlate with skin molecular response.

Conclusions.—A dominant gene rearrangement is commonly found in the peripheral blood of patients with MF. Even when skin lesions are treated successfully in patients with MF, PCR findings may remain positive in lesional sites.

▶ Dereure et al demonstrate that, despite apparent clinical control of the disease, dominant gene rearrangements frequently persist in either the skin or the blood of patients with MF. Although the clinical relevance of this observation is uncertain, it might provide an explanation for the relapses that are common in MF patients. The key question that needs to be answered is whether it is necessary to achieve molecular clearance to achieve clinical cure.

B. H. Thiers, MD

Long-term Outcome of 525 Patients With Mycosis Fungoides and Sézary Syndrome: Clinical Prognostic Factors and Risk for Disease Progression
Kim YH, Liu HL, Mraz-Gernhard S, et al (Stanford Univ, Calif)
Arch Dermatol 139:857-866, 2003   18–6

Introduction.—Numerous studies have examined clinical factors predictive of survival in patients with mycosis fungoides (MF) and Sézary syndrome (SS), but there are few reports on long-term outcome of these uncommon disorders. Cases from a single academic referral center for cutaneous lymphoma were analyzed retrospectively for patient and disease characteristics associated with disease progression and survival.

Methods.—The 525 patients with MF and SS received their diagnosis and were managed at the Stanford University Cutaneous Lymphoma Clinic from 1958 through 1999. All were examined to determine TNM and B categories and clinical stage; needle aspiration or lymph node biopsy, bone marrow biopsy, and additional imaging studies were performed when indicated. Long-term actuarial overall and disease-specific survivals and disease progression were calculated by the Kaplan-Meier method. Relative risk for survival was calculated from expected survivals in race-, age-, and sex-matched control populations.

Results.—The median age at diagnosis was 57 years. Most patients were seen initially with T1 (30%) or T2 (37%) disease; one third had T3 (18%) or T4 (15%) skin involvement. The median survival of the 525 patients was 11.4 years. Actuarial overall survival rates were 68% at 5 years, 53% at 10 years, and 17% at 30 years. The rates of disease-specific survival at these periods were 81%, 74%, and 64%, respectively. Compared with the general population, the relative risk for death for all patients with MF was 2.4. Survival outcome was worse for those with a more advanced T classification and clinical stage. The overall survival rate was similar for patients with stage IB or IIA disease, but disease-specific survival was significantly worse for those with stage IIA disease. The most important clinical prognostic factors in multivariate analysis were patient age, T classification, and the presence of extracutaneous disease. Twenty-nine of 34 patients with extracutaneous disease at diagnosis died, and 26 of these deaths were from MF.

Conclusion.—The risk for disease progression or death in patients with MF and SS varies according to patient and disease characteristics, the most important of which are age, severity of the initial T classification, and the presence of extracutaneous disease.

▶ The data presented by Kim et al demonstrate significant disease-specific survival differences among the different clinical stages of MF and validate the usefulness of the current clinical staging system of the National Cancer Institute. Patient age at presentation, TNM and B classification, overall clinical stage, and the presence or absence of extracutaneous disease were the most significant univariate clinical prognostic indicators, with the T classification and status of extracutaneous disease being the most important. The authors further noted that the severity of the initial skin presentation determined the risk for disease progression.

B. H. Thiers, MD

Narrowband UVB and Psoralen-UVA in the Treatment of Early-Stage Mycosis Fungoides: A Retrospective Study
Diederen PVMM, van Weelden H, Sanders CJG, et al (Univ Med Ctr Utrecht, The Netherlands)
J Am Acad Dermatol 48:215-219, 2003   18–7

Introduction.—Treatment options for patients with early stage mycosis fungoides (MF) include topical steroids, phototherapy (UVB), photochemotherapy (psoralen plus UVA [PUVA]), topical nitrogen mustard, and total skin electron-beam irradiation. Studies of patients with psoriasis report that broadband UVB is safer than PUVA, and that narrowband UVB is more effective and causes less irritation and erythema than broadband UVB. Patients with MF treated with narrowband UVB or PUVA were retrospectively assessed for response to treatment, relapse-free interval, and irradiation dose.

Methods.—Patients included in the study had stage Ia and Ib MF and were treated between 1982 and 1998. Thirty-five received PUVA and 21 received narrowband UVB (311 nm). More patients were treated with PUVA during the early years of the study period. The 2 treatment groups were similar in age and gender distribution. Narrowband UVB therapy was conducted twice a week for 3 to 66 months (mean, 14 months); PUVA was administered twice a week for 2 to 37 months (mean, 11 months). Biopsy specimens were obtained before and after treatment.

Results.—Among patients treated with narrowband UVB, 17 (81%) achieved complete remission and 4 (19%) achieved partial remission. The rate of complete remission in the PUVA group was 71%; 29% of the patients achieved partial remission. Progressive disease did not occur in either treatment group. The mean relapse-free interval was similar in the 2 groups (24.5 months with UVB and 22.8 months with PUVA). In both groups, relapses were treated with topical steroids, topical nitrogen mustard, narrowband UVB, or PUVA.

Conclusion.—Narrowband UVB is an effective treatment modality for patients with early stage MF. With fewer side effects and excellent remission rates, narrowband UVB may be preferable to PUVA as the initial therapy in early stage MF. Progression or lack of response might then require PUVA or other therapies.

▶ Narrowband UVB offers several practical advantages over PUVA. The results of the study by Diederen et al are highly encouraging. Unfortunately, the patients were not randomized, and it is possible that those with somewhat more extensive disease were more likely to receive PUVA, thus skewing the results. In the treatment of psoriasis, PUVA certainly appears to be the more effective, although more toxic, modality. Such may be the case with MF. Thus, it would seem that in patients with MF in whom phototherapy is being considered, narrowband UVB may offer a more convenient initial strategy, with PUVA being reserved for those who fail to respond.

B. H. Thiers, MD

Topical Bexarotene Therapy for Patients With Refractory or Persistent Early-Stage Cutaneous T-Cell Lymphoma: Results of the Phase III Clinical Trial
Heald P, Mehlmauer M, Martin AG, et al (Yale Univ, New Haven, Conn; Washington Univ, St Louis; Ligand Pharmaceuticals Incorporated, San Diego, Calif)
J Am Acad Dermatol 49:801-815, 2003   18–8

Introduction.—An oral formulation of the synthetic retinoid bexarotene is effective in the treatment of both early and advanced cutaneous T-cell lymphoma (CTCL). The safety and efficacy of topical bexarotene gel was examined in an open-label phase III study of patients with refractory or persistent early stage CTCL.

Methods.—The multicenter multinational study included patients age 18 or older who previously had used at least 1 of 4 qualifying therapies: topical nitrogen mustard, topical carmustine, a phototherapy, or electron beam radiation therapy. After washout periods, patients were to apply bexarotene gel 1% topically to all CTCL lesions. The frequency of application started at every other day, then escalated at 1-week intervals to a maximum of 4 times daily as tolerated. The primary end point was the overall and complete response rate by the higher of 2 measures: the Physician's Global Assessment of Clinical Condition or the Composite Assessment of Index Disease Severity.

Results.—Fifty patients from 25 centers received bexarotene gel. The median age of the group at study entry was 64; 80% of patients were white and 54% were women. Most patients were stage IA (50%) or IB (44%). A complete clinical response (CCR) or a partial response (PR) was seen in 27 (54%) patients; 5 (10%) had a CCR. The earliest time to onset of response ($\geq$50% improvement) was 28 days. The projected median time to response was 142 days. Seven (26%) responding patients relapsed after a median duration of monitoring of 214.5 days. Disease progression occurred in 16 of 50 (32%) patients. Forty-seven patients experienced at least 1 bexarotene-related adverse event, usually an irritant dermatitis. Systemic exposure to bexarotene was low.

Conclusion.—Patients with refractory or persistent early-stage CTCL often experienced improvement with minimal side effects after applying bexarotene gel. This agent has the advantages of a self-administered outpatient therapy with little risk of systemic toxicity.

▶ Cost remains a major obstacle to the widespread adaptation of topical bexarotene gel for the treatment of CTCL. There also appears to be somewhat of an inconsistent approach among the various therapies for early stages of the disease. Should the entire cutaneous surface be treated (as with topical mechloroethamine or phototherapy) or should only the evident CTCL lesions be targeted (as with topical bexarotene)?

B. H. Thiers, MD

Low-Dose Methotrexate to Treat Mycosis Fungoides: A Retrospective Study in 69 Patients

Zachkheim HS, Kashani-Sabet M, McMillan A (Univ of California, San Francisco)
J Am Acad Dermatol 49:873-878, 2003   18–9

Introduction.—Low-dose methotrexate (MTX) is often used in the treatment of cutaneous T-cell lymphoma, but only a few studies have reported outcome in a series of patients. A retrospective study evaluated the long-term results of MTX in the treatment of mycosis fungoides (MF).

Methods.—The 69 patients included in the review received MTX once weekly, either orally or, in a few cases, by subcutaneous injection. The median weekly dose was approximately 25 mg. Patients were evaluated according to response rates and time to treatment failure (TTF). Outcome was classified as complete response (CR), partial response (PR; $\geq$50% improvement), stable disease (<50% improvement and <25% worsening), and progressive disease (>25% worsening). Patients were monitored for periods of up to 201 months.

Results.—Patch/plaque stage T2 disease ($\geq$10% skin involved) was present in 60 patients, all of whom had failed to respond to previous therapy. Twenty responded to MTX, with CR occurring in 7 (12%) patients and PR in 13 (22%). The median TTF in this subgroup of patients was 15 months.

Only 2 patients with stage T1 disease were treated; one had disease progression and discontinued MTX and the other had PR. Only 1 of 7 patients with tumor stage disease (T3) achieved PR; the maximum response in the remaining 6 patients was stable disease. Side effects caused treatment failure in 6 of 69 patients.

Discussion.—A third of patients with stage T2 MF responded to MTX, and a proportion of these patients could be successfully maintained on low-dose MTX for prolonged periods. Because response to MTX is apparent within a few months, not much time is lost if the treatment proves ineffective.

▶ As with all treatments for cutaneous T-cell lymphoma, patients with patch-plaque lesions responded better to low-dose MTX than those with tumors. Interestingly, the same authors have previously reported results with low-dose MTX in erythrodermic patients that were superior to those observed in the current study of patients with patch-plaque disease.[1]

B. H. Thiers, MD

Reference

1. Zackheim HS, Kashani-Sabet M, Hwang ST: Low-dose methotrexate to treat erythrodermic cutaneous T-cell lymphoma: Results in twenty-nine patients. *J Am Acad Dermatol* 34:626-631, 1996.

Analysis of Long-term Outcomes of Combined Modality Therapy for Cutaneous T-cell Lymphoma
Duvic M, Apisarnthanarax N, Cohen DS, et al (Univ of Texas, Houston)
J Am Acad Dermatol 49:35-49, 2003   18–10

Introduction.—Patients with mycosis fungoides, Sézary syndrome, or both often respond to multiple therapies but fail to achieve cure, and remissions, especially in advanced disease, may be short-lived. A multiphased combined modality regimen initiated at the study institution in 1987 was designed to improve treatment efficacy and outcome in mycosis fungoides, the most common manifestation of cutaneous T-cell lymphoma (CTCL). Ninety-four of 95 patients were able to be evaluated for response, response durability, and survival.

Methods.—Fifty of 95 patients who started the regimen had early stage (I-IIa) and 45 had late-stage (IIb-IV) CTCL (Table 1). Treatment consisted of subcutaneous interferon-α and oral isotretinoin, followed by total-skin electron beam therapy and long-term maintenance therapy with topical nitrogen mustard and interferon-α. Patients with late-stage disease also received 6 cycles of chemotherapy before electron beam therapy. The duration of complete response (CR) or disease-free survival was estimated for the 56 patients who achieved CR; overall survival was estimated for all 95 patients.

Results.—The overall response rate to the combined modality therapy was 84%; 56 evaluable patients (60%) achieved CR documented by skin bi-

TABLE 1.—Overall Clinical TNM Staging

Stage	Clinical Description	T	N	M	Median Survival (y)
IA	Limited patch/plaque < 10%	T1	N0	0	N/A*
IB	Generalized patch/plaque > 10%	T2	N0	0	12.8
IIA	Patch/plaque + adenopathy†	T1-2	N1	0	10
IIB	Tumors +/− adenopathy†	T3	N0-1	0	3.2
III	Erythroderma +/− adenopathy†	T4	N0-1	0	4.6
IVA	Histologically + nodes	T1-4	N2-3	0	2.5
IVB	Visceral involvement	T1-4	N0-3	M1	2.5

*Stage 1A survival similar to age-matched control patients.
†Dermatopathic/reactive lymphadenopathy.
(Reprinted by permission of the publisher from Duvic M, Apisarnthanarax N, Cohen DS, et al: Analysis of long-term outcomes of combined modality therapy for cutaneous T-cell lymphoma. *J Am Acad Dermatol* 49:35-49, 2003. Copyright 2003 by Elsevier.)

opsy and staging. There were only 6 cases of disease progression, 5 of which occurred in late-stage groups. Both overall clinical stage and T stage were significantly associated with the rate of CR. Three patients with late-stage mycosis fungoides, however, achieved sustained remissions lasting more than 5 years. The median disease-free survival was 62 months for early stage and 7 months for late-stage disease; the median overall survival times were, respectively, 145 months and 36 months. In multivariate analysis, only age was significantly associated with disease-free survival (hazard ratio 2.9 for age ≥60 years), and only stage with overall survival (hazard ratio 18.2 for late stage).

Conclusion.—Despite the uncontrolled and nonrandomized nature of this study, the findings support the use of a combined modality regimen for patients with early stage CTCL and, to a lesser extent, for those with late-stage disease. Toxicity was moderate but tolerable. Five-year survival did not differ significantly, however, between combined modality therapy and total-skin electron beam therapy alone.

▶ The philosophy behind combined modality therapy is to increase response rates while decreasing the incidence of adverse effects from the individual agents. Very often, lower doses of the component therapies can be used than if either is used alone. Combined modality therapy has been shown to be beneficial in the treatment of psoriasis, and appears to have a role in the treatment of CTCL as well. Duvic et al present data showing that combined modality therapy improves remission durations compared with total-skin electron beam therapy alone. One important caveat to be appreciated is that although disease-free survival is increased, there is no overall change in survival.

B. H. Thiers, MD

Multicenter Study of Pegylated Liposomal Doxorubicin in Patients With Cutaneous T-cell Lymphoma

Wollina U, Dummer R, Brockmeyer NH, et al (Hosp Dresden-Friedrichstadt, Dresden, Germany; Univ of Zürich, Switzerland; Ruhr-Univ, Bochum, Germany; et al)

Cancer 98:993-1001, 2003   18–11

Introduction.—Pegylated liposomal doxorubicin (PEG-DOXO) has been shown to be effective as second-line therapy in single center trials and case reports of patients with cutaneous T-cell lymphoma (CTCL). The safety, efficacy, toxicity, and disease-free survival of single-agent PEG-DOXO as second-line chemotherapy in patients with recurrent or recalcitrant CTCL were assessed retrospectively with use of the first known multicenter data.

Methods.—Of 34 patients evaluated (31 male, 3 female), 27 received PEG-DOXO at 20 mg/m^2, 5 received the chemotherapy at 20 to 30 mg/m^2, and 2 received it at 40 mg/m^2. IV PEG-DOXO was administered every 2 weeks to 6 patients, every 2 to 3 weeks to 4 patients, and every 4 weeks to 23 patients. A single course of PEG-DOXO was administered to 1 patient. Outcomes were assessed and adverse effects were documented.

Results.—A minimum of 1 cycle of PEG-DOXO was administered to 34 patients. Disease was classified as mycosis fungoides in 28 patients, mycosis fungoides with follicular mucinosis in 2 patients, small or medium sized pleomorphic CTCL in 2 patients, Sezary syndrome in 1 patient, and CD30-positive CTCL in 1 patient.

Fifteen patients had a complete response (CR). This included patients who achieved a CR and those who achieved a CR defined by clinical criteria only with no biopsy. Fifteen patients had a partial response (PR). The total response rate (CRs plus PR) was 88.2%. Two patients had to discontinue therapy, 1 after a single PEG-DOXO infusion due to grade 3 capillary leakage syndrome and 1 after 2 cycles due to a suicide attempt not associated with treatment or with CTCL. The remaining patients received at least 4 cycles of PEG-DOXO.

The mean overall survival was 17.8 months for 33 patients, the mean event-free survival was 12.0 months, and the mean disease-free survival was 13.3 months for 16 patients. Adverse effects were observed in 14 of 34 patients (41.2%). These were temporary and generally mild. Six patients had grade 3 or 4 adverse effects.

Conclusion.—The treatment schedule with PEG-DOXO was less toxic than with most of the established chemotherapy regimens. It was effective, indicating that it is a promising second-line alternative treatment. The rate of severe adverse effects was low compared with other chemotherapy protocols for patients with CTCL.

▶ Most systemic therapies for advanced CTCL are only marginally effective and typically do not improve the prognosis of affected patients. The efficacy and safety data presented by Wollina et al, if confirmed, would certainly represent a major advance in the treatment of this notoriously refractory condition.

B. H. Thiers, MD

Systemic Therapy With Cyclophosphamide and Anti-CD20 Antibody (Rituximab) in Relapsed Primary Cutaneous B-cell Lymphoma: A Report of 7 Cases

Fierro MT, Savoia P, Quaglino P, et al (Univ of Turin, Torino, Italy)
J Am Acad Dermatol 49:281-287, 2003   18–12

Introduction.—Rituximab, a chimeric antibody directed against CD20, has proved effective in the treatment of patients with refractory/relapsed low-grade or follicular B-cell non-Hodgkin lymphomas. Seven patients with relapsed primary cutaneous B-cell lymphoma who achieved a high rate of response with IV rituximab treatment have previously been reported. The clinical activity and toxicity of IV rituximab, preceded by single-dose cyclophosphamide, were evaluated in 7 additional patients with this disease.

Methods.—Four men and 3 women with a median age of 68 years were studied. The median time between primary diagnosis and study entry was 4.3 years. Cutaneous lesions appeared on the head, trunk, or limbs; extracutaneous involvement was present in 4 patients (lymph nodes in 3 and kidney in 1). Cyclophosphamide was administered 1 week before the start of IV rituximab, which was given weekly for 4 consecutive weeks. Outcome was classified as complete response, partial response, stable disease, or progressive disease. Patients were also evaluated for toxicity.

Results.—Two patients underwent rituximab therapy after their first relapse, 2 after a second relapse, and 3 after 3 or more relapses after chemotherapy (with local radiotherapy in 3 patients). The overall objective response rate was 85.7%; 5 patients achieved a complete response and 1 had a partial response. Two patients had a cutaneous relapse during a median follow-up period of 13 months. The response durations of the remaining disease-free patients are now 5, 7, 17, and 18 months. Treatment was well tolerated in all patients.

Discussion.—Primary cutaneous B-cell lymphoma has a favorable prognosis, but a subgroup of patients may have recurrent cutaneous relapses or systemic spread. Repeated infusions of chemotherapy can result in persistent systemic toxicity. In these patients who had frequent relapses, the combination of cyclophosphamide and rituximab yielded a high response rate with a favorable toxicity profile.

Cutaneous B-Cell Lymphoma With Loss of CD20 Immunoreactivity After Rituximab Therapy

Clarke LE, Bayerl MG, Ehmann WC, et al (Pennsylvania State Univ, Hershey)
J Cutan Pathol 30:459-462, 2003   18–13

Background.—The antigen CD20 is expressed by approximately 95% of B-cell lymphomas, and reliable anti-CD20 antibodies that react with fixed, paraffin-embedded tissues have been available for more than a decade. In addition to its use as a diagnostic marker, CD20 is now an important therapeutic target. Rituximab is a human-mouse chimeric monoclonal antibody that targets the CD20 antigen and causes rapid depletion of both benign and malignant B cells. Rituximab has demonstrated substantial efficacy in the treatment of B-cell lymphoma, but there have been several reports of loss of CD20 expression after rituximab therapy. A case was described in which a patient with a CD20-positive systemic B-cell lymphoma had a CD20-negative relapse with secondary cutaneous involvement after therapy with rituximab.

Case Report.—Man, 51, was seen in July 2002 with swelling of the left chest and left axillary lymphadenopathy. He had first been seen in 1993 with retroperitoneal lymphadenopathy, which was diagnosed as stage IIIA follicle center lymphoma (follicular lymphoma), mixed large and small cell type. Complete remission was achieved with 6 cycles of cyclophosphamide, doxorubicin, vincristine, and prednisone. However, the patient subsequently suffered several relapses, all of which were treated with rituximab. At the final relapse in July 2002, he was treated with rituximab without benefit. Biopsy of a skin nodule at this time demonstrated an atypical lymphocytic infiltrate that was negative for CD20, CD3, lysozyme, and myeloperoxidase but strongly positive for CD45rb and the B-cell marker CD79a.

Conclusion.—Loss of CD20 expression in cutaneous B-cell lymphoma (both primary and secondary) may occur after rituximab therapy. Immunohistochemistry for CD79a—also a widely expressed B-cell marker—is useful for identification of CD20-negative B cells in these cases. Loss of CD20 expression may become more common as the use of rituximab increases.

▶ This case report illustrates the phenomenon of "antigenic modulation," in which the target antigen of a specific therapy—in this case an anti-CD20 monoclonal antibody for B-cell lymphoma—is lost, allowing treatment-resistant cells devoid of the antigen to proliferate. This may be a key factor in limiting the long-term effectiveness of some of the emerging biological therapies for cancer, which depend on the presence of a specific target antigen.

B. H. Thiers, MD

Sweet Syndrome in Multiple Myeloma: A Series of Six Cases

Bayer-Garner IB, Cottler-Fox M, Smoller BR (Baylor Med College, Houston; Univ of Arkansas, Little Rock)
J Cutan Pathol 30:261-264, 2003   18–14

Introduction.—Sweet syndrome (SS), a neutrophilic dermatosis that responds to treatment with steroids, is idiopathic in most cases but may occur in patients with malignant hematologic disorders. The paraneoplastic syndrome has been reported in acute myelogenous leukemia, lymphoma, and myelodysplastic syndromes and may be related to levels of granulocyte colony stimulating factor (G-CSF). The association of SS with multiple myeloma (MM) was examined in 6 patients.

Methods.—Cases of MM were retrieved from a pathology database. The reports of 2357 patients with MM were reviewed to identify those in whom SS developed. Records of the 6 patients with MM and SS (0.25%) were examined for age and sex, biopsy site, immunoglobulin secretory status, bone marrow Bartl grade, type of transplant, treatment with G-CSF or GM-CSF, and cytogenetics. Biopsy specimens from 5 patients with SS and from 25 patients with SS unrelated to MM underwent syndecan-1 immunohistochemistry.

Results.—Patients with MM and SS were 4 men and 2 women with an average age of 60.2 years. Lesions were located on the trunk, arm, or thigh. Five of the 6 patients secreted an IgG paraprotein. One patient was treated with chemotherapy only (supported with GM-CSF), and 5 had received a peripheral stem cell transplant (supported with G-CSF). Three patients had normal karyotypes, 1 had 3 separate chromosomal deletions in 3 of 20 cells examined, and 2 patients had complex karyotypes. Syndecan-1 immunoreactivity in the 30 cases of SS stained (including 5 with MM) showed scant plasma cells in only 5 cases, none of whom had coexistent MM.

Discussion.—Previous studies have reported elevation of endogenous G-CSF levels during acute exacerbations of SS, and some have reported a link between exogenous administration of G-CSF and the development of SS. No specific cytogenetic anomaly was identified in these patients with MM and SS. In the setting of MM, there may be an increased risk of development of SS among IgG secretors.

▶ Iatrogenic G-CSF–induced SS has previously been described. Dermatologists should be aware of this complication, given the frequent use of this growth factor in patients undergoing chemotherapy.

B. H. Thiers, MD

Imatinib for Systemic Mast-Cell Disease
Pardanani A, Elliott M, Reeder T, et al (Mayo Clinic, Rochester, Minn; Salisbury District Hosp, Wiltshire, England)
Lancet 362:535-537, 2003   18–15

Introduction.—Activating mutations in c-*kit*, the receptor for stem-cell factor (including the common Asp816 to Val [D816V] mutations), have been suspected in the pathogenesis of mast-cell disease. Data from in vitro trials suggest that the tyrosine kinase inhibitor imatinib is a potent inhibitor of wild type and specific mutant c-*kit*, but no reports of it being used to treat patients with mast-cell disease are available. The efficacy of imatinib was assessed in 12 adult patients with systemic mast-cell disease.

Methods.—Patients were treated with a daily dose of 100 mg or 400 mg if no response was noted at lower doses. The primary endpoint was mast-cell cytoreduction, which was monitored via serial bone-marrow biopsies, or clearance of histologically verified mast-cell skin lesions. Secondary objectives were evaluation of drug safety and changes in other disease-associated markers.

Results.—Of 10 patients who were evaluated for response, 5 (50%) had a measurable response to imatinib. Of these, 4 had important mast-cell cytoreduction and 2 had complete clinical and histologic remission. In 5 patients with eosinophilia, 3 experienced complete clinical and hematologic remission. The 2 patients who did not respond to treatment were the only patients with the c-*kit* D816V mutation.

Conclusion.—Imatinib either inhibits the growth-promoting role of wild type c-*kit* or targets an oncogenic kinase.

▶ A larger study will be necessary to better delineate which patients with mast-cell disease are likely to benefit from imatinib treatment and to clarify the optimum doses and duration of therapy.

B. H. Thiers, MD

19 Thromboembolism and Other Lower Extremity Disorders

An Association Between Atherosclerosis and Venous Thrombosis

Prandoni P, Bilora F, Marchiori A, et al (Univ of Padua, Italy; Univ of Amsterdam; Univ of Maastricht, The Netherlands)
N Engl J Med 348:1435-1441, 2003   19–1

Background.—The pathogenesis of venous thromboembolism has not been fully elucidated. Classic risk factors for this disease include cancer, surgery, immobilization, fractures, paralysis, pregnancy, childbirth, and use of estrogens. However, the cause of venous thromboembolism remains unexplained in about one third of patients. Atherosclerosis is associated with activation of both platelets and blood coagulation and an increase in fibrin turnover. Whether atherosclerosis is associated with an increased risk of venous thrombosis was investigated.

Methods.—US of the carotid arteries was performed in 299 unselected patients with deep venous thrombosis of the legs without symptomatic atherosclerosis and in 150 control subjects. The patient group included those with spontaneous thrombosis and those with secondary thrombosis from acquired risk factors. Both patients and control subjects were assessed for the presence of plaques.

Results.—At least one carotid plaque was identified in 72 of 153 patients (47.1%) with spontaneous thrombosis, in 40 of 146 patients (27.4%) with secondary thrombosis, and in 48 of 150 (32%) control subjects. The odds ratios for carotid plaques in patients with spontaneous thrombosis, compared with patients with secondary thrombosis and control subjects, were 2.3 and 1.8, respectively. The strength of this association did not change on multivariate analysis that adjusted for risk factors for atherosclerosis.

Conclusion.—An association was found between atherosclerotic disease and spontaneous venous thrombosis. Atherosclerosis may induce venous thrombosis, or the 2 conditions may have common risk factors.

▶ The authors demonstrate an association between atherosclerosis and spontaneous venous thrombosis. Although the findings did not establish a causative role for atherosclerosis in venous thromboembolism, they do suggest a link between arterial and venous disorders. Future research should investigate the potential role of statins and antiplatelet agents as preventive interventions.

B. H. Thiers, MD

Increased Plasma Levels of Lipoprotein(a) and the Risk of Idiopathic and Recurrent Venous Thromboembolism
Marcucci R, Liotta AA, Cellai AP, et al (Clinica Medica Generale e Cardiologia, Firenze, Italy)
Am J Med 115:601-605, 2003   19–2

Background.—Increased lipoprotein(a) [Lp(a)] concentrations are known to be a risk factor for cardiovascular disease. However, their effects on venous thromboembolism have not been established.

Methods.—The current case-control study included 603 adults with a history of venous thromboembolism and 430 healthy persons. Assessment included measures of Lp(a), homocysteine, and antithrombin levels, factor V Leiden and factor II (prothrombin) polymorphisms, and anticardiolipin antibodies.

Findings.—Twenty-four percent of patients had Lp(a) levels exceeding 300 mg/L compared with 13% of the healthy persons. A multivariate analysis indicated an independent correlation between increased Lp(a) concentrations and venous thromboembolism after adjustment for acquired and hemostasis-related risk factors. These findings were verified in 341 patients with idiopathic venous thromboembolism and in those with recurrent thromboembolism.

Conclusions.—These data suggest that Lp(a) is an independent risk factor for venous thromboembolism in adults. Thus, Lp(a) may be involved in the pathogenesis of idiopathic and recurrent disease.

▶ Clinical evidence links high plasma Lp(a) levels with atherosclerotic disease.[1] The article by Marcucci et al is a methodologically strong study that establishes Lp(a) as an important risk factor for venous thromboembolism.[2] Interestingly, an article abstracted elsewhere in this volume (Abstract 19–1) demonstrates an association between atherosclerosis and venous thrombosis.

B. H. Thiers, MD

References

1. Misirli H, Somay G, Ozbal N, et al: Relation of lipid and Lp(a) to ischemic stroke. *J Clin Neurosci* 2:127-132, 2002.
2. Crowther N: Lipoprotein (a): Another risk factor for venous thrombosis? *Am J Med* 115:667-668, 2003.

Frequency of Venous Thromboembolism in Low to Moderate Risk Long Distance Air Travellers: The New Zealand Air Traveller's Thrombosis (NZATT) Study
Hughes RJ, Hopkins RJ, Hill S, et al (Wellington School of Medicine and Health Sciences, New Zealand; Med Research Inst of New Zealand, Wellington; Auckland School of Medicine, New Zealand; et al)
Lancet 362:2039-2044, 2003   19–3

Background.—Researchers have not yet established the frequency and role of risk factors for venous thromboembolism associated with air travel. The frequency of this disorder and its risk factors were investigated in a group of long-distance air travelers.

Methods.—A prospective study was done that included 878 persons 18 to 70 years old. All were traveling at least 4 hours or more in aircraft, and all had a negative D-dimer before travel. Persons who became D-dimer positive or who had high clinical probability symptoms in the 3 months after traveling were further examined by bilateral compression US and CT pulmonary angiography.

Findings.—All participants traveled at least 10 hours with a mean total time in aircraft of 39 hours. The frequency of venous thromboembolism in the 878 travelers was 1.0%. After travel, 112 persons were examined radiologically. Four persons had pulmonary embolism, and 5 had deep venous thrombosis. Six persons with venous thromboembolism had clinical risk factors before travel, and 2 were subsequently found to have a thrombophilic risk factor. Aspirin use was documented in 5 persons and compression stockings were worn by 4. Two affected persons traveled exclusively in business class.

Conclusions.—Multiple long-distance air flights appear to be associated with venous thromboembolism, even in persons with low to moderate risk. Further study is warranted to determine the role of traditional risk factors and prophylactic measures.

▶ The authors confirm the association between venous thromboembolism and long-distance air travel. The risk extends even to those without previously identified predisposing factors, and it includes travelers of all classes. Thus, they recommend that the term "economy class syndrome" should be avoided, with the disorder being renamed "traveler's thrombosis" or, more specifically, "air travel-related venous thromboembolism."

B. H. Thiers, MD

Comparison of Four Clinical Prediction Scores for the Diagnosis of Lower Limb Deep Venous Thrombosis in Outpatients

Constans J, Boutinet C, Salmi LR, et al (Hôpital Saint-André, Bordeaux, France; Société Régionale de Médecine Vasculaire Aquitaine, France; Université Victor Segalen-Bordeaux II, France)

Am J Med 115:436-440, 2003   19–4

Introduction.—Individual clinical signs and symptoms lack sensitivity and specificity, yet clinical prediction scores for deep venous thrombosis have been developed. The 4-item Kahn score is simple to compute but has not proved useful in medical inpatients; the 9-item Wells index seems useful in outpatients. The 6-item St André score, initially developed for hospitalized patients, was revised for an ambulatory setting.

Methods.—Patients referred for evaluation of suspected deep venous thrombosis were examined by experienced angiologists who recorded unilateral calf pain and completed a form that included all items used in the Wells, Kahn, and St André scores. This information was recorded before patients underwent US. In a sample of 444 outpatients, the Wells, Kahn, and St André hospital scores were compared for their ability to predict deep vein thrombosis. A validation sample of 282 outpatients was used to evaluate the new St André outpatient score.

Results.—In the first sample, 126 (28%) patients had deep venous thrombosis. The Wells score was a better predictor of this diagnosis than were the Kahn and St André scores. With the use of the Wells score, 70% of those with a high probability of deep venous thrombosis actually had a thrombosis. A thrombosis was found in 11% of those with a low Wells score probability. The new St André score (Table 2) assigned a point for 5 predictors and subtracted a point for "other plausible diagnosis." In a validation sample of 282 outpatients, this new score identified 31 patients who had a high probability of deep venous thrombosis; 58% did have a thrombosis. Only 3 (4%) of 70 patients with a low probability score had a thrombosis. This ambulatory

TABLE 2.—Independent Predictors of Deep Vein Thrombosis in the Derivation Sample (444 Patients)

Predictor	Odds Ratio (95% Confidence Interval)	P Value
Male sex	2.0 (1.2-3.3)	0.006
Lower limb paralysis or immobilization	3.7 (1.1-12)	0.04
Confinement to bed >3 days	2.9 (1.1-7.9)	0.04
Lower limb enlargement	4.0 (2.5-6.6)	<0.001
Unilateral pain	5.1 (2.8-9.3)	<0.001
Other diagnosis	0.2 (0.1-0.4)	<0.001

(Reprinted from Constans J, Boutinet C, Salmi LR, et al: Comparison of four clinical prediction scores for the diagnosis of lower limb deep venous thrombosis in outpatients. *Am J Med* 115:436-440, 2003. Copyright 2003, with permission from Excerpta Medica Inc.)

score and the Wells score had similar test operating characteristics in the validation sample.

Conclusion.—The St André hospital score contained items such as cancer and confinement to bed that were less important in an outpatient setting of suspected deep venous thrombosis. The new 6-item St André score, developed by multivariate analysis, had diagnostic power similar to that of the 9-item Wells score.

▶ Other articles reviewed in this YEAR BOOK OF DERMATOLOGY AND DERMATO-LOGIC SURGERY have assessed the utility of the D-dimer test for the diagnosis of venous thromboembolism. The study by Constans et al helps quantify clinical criteria for the prediction of that diagnosis in outpatients.

B. H. Thiers, MD

D-Dimer Levels and Risk of Recurrent Venous Thromboembolism
Eichinger S, Minar E, Bialonczyk C, et al (Univ of Vienna; Wilhelminenspital, Vienna; Hanuschkrankenhaus, Vienna)
JAMA 290:1071-1074, 2003
19–5

Background.—It is now common clinical practice to screen patients with venous thromboembolism (VTE) for thrombophilic risk factors. However, assessment of the risk of recurrence for an individual patient is complex because of the numerous risk factors. There is a need for a laboratory method that measures multifactorial thrombophilia. The relation between recurrent VTE and D-dimer levels, a global marker of coagulation activation and fibrinolysis, was prospectively evaluated.

Methods.—This prospective cohort study included 610 patients over age 18 years who were treated with oral anticoagulants for at least 3 months with a first spontaneous VTE and in whom D-dimer levels were measured shortly before discontinuation of oral anticoagulation. Patients were observed at 3-month intervals in the first year after discontinuation of oral anticoagulants and every 6 months thereafter from July 1992 to October 2002. The primary outcome measure was objectively documented symptomatic recurrent VTE.

Results.—Seventy-nine patients (13%) had recurrent VTE with a mean observation time of 38 months. Patients with recurrence had significantly higher D-dimer levels compared with patients without recurrence. Compared with patients with D-dimer levels of 740 ng/mL or higher, the relative risk of recurrence was 0.6, 0.6, and 0.3 in patients with D-dimer levels of 500 to 749 ng/mL, 250 to 499 ng/mL, and less than 250 ng/mL, respectively. The cumulative probability of recurrent VTE at 2 years was 3.7% among patients with D-dimer levels of less than 250 ng/mL, compared with 11.5% among patients with higher levels. The relative risk of recurrence in patients with D-dimer levels of less than 250 ng/mL was 60% lower than in patients with higher levels.

Conclusion.—Patients with a first spontaneous VTE and a D-dimer level of less than 250 ng/mL after discontinuation of oral anticoagulation have a low risk of recurrence of VTE.

▶ D-dimer levels are a global indicator of coagulation activation and fibrinolysis, and high D-dimer levels may be associated with an increased risk for first VTE and an increased risk of recurrence. Eichinger et al demonstrate the value of determining D-dimer levels in a specific clinical situation. For example, in this study, the investigators found that patients with a first spontaneous VTE and a D-dimer level less than 250 ng/mL after withdrawal of oral anticoagulant therapy had a low risk of recurrence. Unfortunately, the conclusions drawn in this subset of patients cannot necessarily be extrapolated to other patients experiencing VTE, as the utility of the D-dimer test may vary depending on the clinical setting.[1]

B. H. Thiers, MD

Reference

1. Schutgens RE, Esseboom EU, Haas FJ, et al: Usefulness of a semiquantitative D-dimer test for the exclusion of deep venous thrombosis in outpatients. *Am J Med* 112:617-621, 2002.

A Diagnostic Strategy Involving a Quantitative Latex D-Dimer Assay Reliably Excludes Deep Venous Thrombosis
Bates SM, Kearon C, Crowther M, et al (McMaster Univ, Hamilton, Ont, Canada)
Ann Intern Med 138:787-794, 2003   19–6

Background.—Clinical diagnosis of deep venous thrombosis (DVT) can be inaccurate. Thus, objective testing is usually considered mandatory in patients with suspected DVT. Whether a negative finding on a quantitative latex D-dimer assay obviates the need for further testing in patients with a low or moderate pretest probability of DVT was determined.

Methods.—Five hundred fifty-six consecutive outpatients with suspected first DVT seen at 3 Canadian hospitals were enrolled in the prospective study. Before D-dimer testing, patients were classified as having low, moderate, or high pretest probability of DVT (Table 1). Those with low or moderate pretest probability and a negative D-dimer result did not receive further testing or anticoagulant treatment. All other patients underwent serial compression ultrasonography. Patients who did not receive a diagnosis of DVT were followed for symptomatic venous thromboembolism.

Findings.—Fifty-one percent of the patients had low or moderate pretest probability and a negative D-dimer test. One of these patients subsequently received a diagnosis of DVT. Overall, the negative likelihood ratio of the D-dimer test was 0.03.

Conclusions.—A negative finding on a quantitative latex D-dimer assay obviates the need for additional evaluation in patients with a low or moder-

TABLE 1.—Standardized Model Used to Assess Pretest Probability*

Attribute	Score
Active cancer (treatment ongoing or within previous 6 months, or palliative treatment)	1
Paralysis, paresis, or recent plaster immobilization of the lower extremities	1
Major surgery or bedridden for >3 days within 4 weeks	1
Localized tenderness along the distribution of the deep venous system	1
Calf and thigh swollen	1
Calf swelling >3 cm compared with asymptomatic leg (measured 10 cm below tibial tuberosity)	1
Pitting edema (greater in the symptomatic leg)	1
Nonvaricose collateral superficial veins	1
Alternative diagnosis at least as likely as deep venous thrombosis	−2

*In patients with bilateral symptoms, the more symptomatic leg is used. A score <0 indicates low pretest probability, a score of 1 or 2 indicates moderate pretest probability, and a score of >2 indicates high pretest probability. (Adapted from Wells PS, Anderson DR, Bormanis J, et al: Value of assessment of pretest probability of deep-vein thrombosis in clinical management. *Lancet* 350:1795-1798, 1997, with permission from Elsevier. Courtesy of Bates SM, Kearon C, Crowther M, et al: A diagnostic strategy involving a quantitative latex D-dimer assay reliably excludes deep venous thrombosis. *Ann Intern Med* 138:787-794, 2003.)

ate pretest probability of DVT. Patients with an abnormal finding on D-dimer testing can be assessed safely with serial compression ultrasonography.

▶ The results suggest that in patients with a low or moderate pretest probability of their first DVT, a negative D-dimer test result effectively rules out that diagnosis. Similar studies should be done on other difficult-to-diagnose patient populations such as those suspected of having recurrent DVT, pulmonary embolism, or upper-extremity DVT.

B. H. Thiers, MD

Limitations of D-dimer Testing in Unselected Inpatients With Suspected Venous Thromboembolism

Brotman DJ, Segal JB, Jani JT, et al (Johns Hopkins Hosp, Baltimore, Md)
Am J Med 114:276-282, 2003   19–7

Background.—The absence of elevated D-dimer levels can safely exclude venous thromboembolism in outpatients. Whether D-dimer testing is similarly useful in unselected hospitalized patients was examined.

Methods.—The subjects were 203 unselected hospitalized patients undergoing radiologic evaluation for possible deep venous thrombosis (DVT) or pulmonary embolism (PE). D-dimer levels were assessed in fresh whole blood (SimpliRED assay) and in thawed citrated plasma (using a D-dimer enzyme-linked immunosorbent assay [ELISA], a D-Di plasma agglutination assay, and an immunoturbidimetric assay). C-reactive protein (CRP) levels were also measured to evaluate inflammation.

Results.—Radiography identified proximal DVT or PE in 45 of these 203 patients (22%). The D-dimer ELISA identified 43 of these patients, for a sensitivity of 96% and a specificity of 23%. The other 3 tests generally had higher specificity (13%-59%), but their sensitivity was less than 70%. Of the 45 patients with thrombosis, 19 (42%) had a false-negative test with 1 or more D-dimer assay. Specificity of the D-dimer methods was significantly lower in patients more than 60 years old, patients hospitalized for 4 days or more, and patients whose CRP level was in the highest quartile.

Conclusion.—Venous thromboembolism is rather common in hospitalized patients, and the low specificity of D-dimer testing limits its utility in this population, particularly in older patients, those with a longer hospital stay, and those with a high CRP level. It is unlikely that D-dimer testing will spare unselected inpatients the inconvenience and cost of radiology work-up.

▶ The D-dimer test measures the degradation products of cross-linked fibrin. It is most useful for its high sensitivity and negative predictive value in the exclusion of DVT. However, it is frequently positive, making ultrasonography necessary for many patients suspected of having DVT. Thus, a patient with a negative D-dimer test and a negative US examination can be presumed not to have a DVT. Limitations of the D-dimer tests were discussed in an article reviewed in the 2003 YEAR BOOK OF DERMATOLOGY AND DERMATOLOGIC SURGERY.[1]

B. H. Thiers, MD

Reference

1. Schutgens REG, Esseboom EU, Haas FJLM, et al: Usefulness of a semiquantitative D-dimer test for the exclusion of deep venous thrombosis in outpatients. *Am J Med* 112:617-621, 2002. (2003 YEAR BOOK OF DERMATOLOGY AND DERMATOLOGIC SURGERY, pp 357-358.)

Outpatient Therapy With Low Molecular Weight Heparin for the Treatment of Venous Thromboembolism: A Review of Efficacy, Safety, and Costs
Segal JB, Bolger DT, Jenckes MW, et al (Johns Hopkins Univ, Baltimore, Md)
Am J Med 115:298-308, 2003   19–8

Introduction.—High-quality systematic reviews have reported that low molecular weight heparin, administered subcutaneously, is as efficacious as IV unfractionated heparin in the treatment of deep vein thrombosis without increasing the likelihood of major hemorrhagic complications. Most trials compared the 2 agents in an inpatient setting. The evidence concerning the efficacy and safety of treating deep venous thrombosis was examined in an outpatient versus an inpatient setting. The cost effectiveness of treatment with low molecular weight heparin or unfractionated heparin, regardless of the setting, was also assessed.

Methods.—A literature search was performed through March 2002 for trials comparing outpatient and inpatient treatment of venous thromboembolism with low molecular weight heparin or unfractionated heparin and for trials addressing the costs of low molecular weight heparin use in any setting. Trials with comparison groups or decision analyses were included.

Results.—Eight trials (3 randomized trials and 5 cohort investigations) compared outpatient use of low molecular weight heparin with inpatient use of unfractionated heparin by 3762 patients. The rate of recurrent venous thrombosis was similar for the 2 groups (median, 4%; range, 0%-7% vs median, 6%; range, 0%-9%) as was major bleeding (median, 0.5%; range, 0%-2% vs median, 1%; range, 0%-2%). The use of low molecular weight heparin was linked with shorter hospitalization (median, 2.7 days; range, 0.03-5.1 days vs median, 6.5 days; range, 4-9.6 days) and lower costs (median difference, $1600).

Comparisons of outpatient and in-hospital use of low molecular weight heparin showed no difference in outcomes, although there were savings in hospital costs. Low molecular weight heparin was more cost saving and cost effective, compared with unfractionated heparin (savings, 0% to 64%; median, 57%).

Conclusion.—Outpatient treatment of deep venous thrombosis with low molecular weight heparin is likely to be efficacious, safe, and cost-effective.

▶ Segal et al declare that low molecular weight heparin appears to be a safe, efficacious, and cost-effective agent for the outpatient treatment of deep venous thrombosis. Less clear, however, is whether outpatient treatment with low molecular weight heparin is safe and feasible for patients at high risk of adverse events or who are unable to fully comply with therapy. Moreover, it remains uncertain whether low molecular weight heparin is a good alternative for patients with pulmonary embolism.[1]

B. H. Thiers, MD

Reference

1. Koopman MMW, Bossuit PMM: Low molecular weight heparin for outpatient treatment of venous thromboembolism: Safe, effective, and cost reducing? *Am J Med* 115:324-325, 2003.

Long-term, Low-Intensity Warfarin Therapy for the Prevention of Recurrent Venous Thromboembolism
Ridker PM, for the PREVENT Investigators (Harvard Med School, Boston; et al)
N Engl J Med 348:1425-1434, 2003   19–9

Background.—The treatment of patients with idiopathic venous thromboembolism usually includes a 5- to 10-day course of heparin followed by 3 to 12 months of oral anticoagulation therapy with full-dose warfarin, with adjustment of the dose to an international normalized ratio between 2.0 and 3.0. However, recurrent venous thromboembolism is a major clinical problem after cessation of anticoagulation therapy, with an estimated incidence of 6% to 9% each year. No therapeutic agent has been shown to provide an acceptable benefit-to-risk ratio for the long-term management of venous thromboembolism. The Prevention of Recurrent Venous Thromboembolism (PREVENT) trial was conducted to test the hypothesis that long-term, low-intensity warfarin therapy could safely and effectively reduce the risk of recurrent venous thromboembolism in patients with a previous idiopathic venous thrombosis.

Methods.—The study enrolled patients with idiopathic venous thromboembolism who had received full-dose anticoagulation therapy for a median of 6.5 months. The patients were randomly assigned to placebo or low-intensity warfarin with a target international normalized ratio of 1.5 to 2.0. Participants were monitored for recurrent venous thromboembolism, major hemorrhage, and death.

Results.—The intention was to enroll 750 patients, but the study was terminated early after randomization of 508 patients, who were followed for up to 4.3 years. Of the 253 patients assigned to placebo, 37 had recurrent venous thromboembolism (7.2/100 person-years) compared with 14 of 255 patients assigned to low-intensity warfarin (2.6/100 person-years). This represented a risk reduction of 64%. The risk reductions were similar for all subgroups, including patients with and without inherited thrombophilia. Major hemorrhage occurred in 2 patients assigned to placebo and 5 patients assigned to low-intensity warfarin. There were twice as many deaths in the placebo group (8 patients) as in the low-intensity warfarin group (4 patients). Low-intensity warfarin was associated with a 48% reduction in the composite end point of recurrent venous thromboembolism, major hemorrhage, or death and a reduction of 76% to 81% in the risk of recurrent venous thromboembolism on per-protocol and as-treated analyses.

Conclusion.—Long-term, low-intensity warfarin therapy is highly effective for the prevention of recurrent venous thromboembolism.

▶ Dermatologists commonly see patients with venous insufficiency, many of whom suffer from recurrent venous thromboembolism. Previous studies have shown that short-term use of full-dose warfarin is highly effective after a first episode of venous thrombosis, and many patients receive such therapy for 12 months or longer to prevent recurrence. However, a target international normalized ratio between 2 and 3 is associated with a high incidence of major bleeding episodes, raising concern regarding the net clinical benefit of long-term warfarin treatment. Ridker et al demonstrate that long-term, low-intensity warfarin therapy is a highly effective strategy to prevent recurrent venous thromboembolism. The authors are to be complimented for investigating an agent whose generic status provides little financial incentive for investigation by the major drug makers. Interestingly, another trial found that low-intensity warfarin treatment was significantly less effective than conventional-intensity warfarin treatment for the prevention of venous thromboembolism, with no significant difference in the rate of bleeding complications.[1] These divergent findings are difficult to reconcile. The "tightrope" of anticoagulant dosing was discussed in an editorial that accompanied the article by Ridker et al.[2]

B. H. Thiers, MD

References

1. Kearon C, Ginsberg JS, Kovacs M, et al: Low-intensity (INR 1.5-1.9) versus conventional-intensity (INR 2.0-3.0) anticoagulation for extended treatment of unprovoked VTE: A randomized double blind trial. *Blood* 100:150a, 2002. abstract.
2. Schafer AI: Warfarin for venous thromboembolism—walking the dosing tightrope. *N Engl J Med* 348:1478-1480, 2003.

Comparison of Low-Intensity Warfarin Therapy With Conventional-Intensity Warfarin Therapy for Long-term Prevention of Recurrent Venous Thromboembolism

Kearon C, for the Extended Low-Intensity Anticoagulation for Thrombo-Embolism Investigators (McMaster Univ, Hamilton, Ont, Canada; et al)

N Engl J Med 349:631-639, 2003   19–10

Background.—Warfarin is effective in the prevention of recurrent venous thromboembolism but also is associated with a significant risk of bleeding. Previous studies have suggested that after 3 months of conventional warfarin therapy, a lower dose of anticoagulant medication may result in less bleeding and still prevent recurrent venous thromboembolism. This hypothesis was tested in a randomized double-blind trial in which patients with unprovoked venous thromboembolism maintained warfarin therapy with a target international normalized ratio (INR) of 1.5 to 1.9 (low-intensity therapy) or warfarin therapy with a target INR of 2.0 to 3.0 (conventional-intensity therapy).

Methods.—The trial enrolled 738 patients who had completed 3 or more months of warfarin therapy for unprovoked venous thromboembolism. The patients were randomly assigned to continuation of warfarin with either low-intensity or conventional-intensity therapy. The patients were followed for an average of 2.4 years.

Results.—Of the 369 patients assigned to low-intensity therapy, 16 had recurrent venous thromboembolism, compared with 6 of 369 patients assigned to conventional-intensity therapy. An episode of major bleeding occurred in 9 patients in the low-intensity therapy group and 8 patients in the conventional-intensity therapy group. There was no significant difference in the frequency of overall bleeding between the 2 groups.

Conclusion.—These findings indicate that in patients being treated for recurrent venous thromboembolism, conventional-intensity warfarin therapy (INR of 2.0 to 3.0) is more effective than low-intensity therapy (INR of 1.5 to 1.9) for the prevention of recurrent venous thromboembolism and that the low-intensity regimen does not reduce the risk of clinically significant bleeding.

▶ The results of this study and other similar trials suggest that low-intensity anticoagulant therapy reduces the risk of recurrent thrombosis by about 75% and that conventional-intensity therapy reduces the risk by more than 90%. As the risk of bleeding appears to be similar in the 2 groups, the authors argue that the intensity of anticoagulant therapy for patients who have had unprovoked venous thromboembolism should not be reduced after the first 3 months of treatment. Thus, the data do not support the use of low-intensity warfarin therapy in this clinical setting and, as stated in an accompanying editorial, indicate that the target INR should be in the 2.0-3.0 range.[1]

B. H. Thiers, MD

Reference

1. Büller HR, Prins MH: Secondary prophylaxis with warfarin for venous thromboembolism. *N Engl J Med* 349:702-704, 2003.

Clinical Impact of Bleeding in Patients Taking Oral Anticoagulant Therapy for Venous Thromboembolism: A Meta-analysis

Linkins L-A, Choi PT, Douketis JD (McMaster Univ, Hamilton, Ont, Canada; Univ of British Columbia, Vancouver, Canada)
Ann Intern Med 139:893-900, 2003   19–11

Background.—When deciding how long to continue anticoagulant treatment in patients with venous thromboembolism, physicians need to consider the clinical impact of anticoagulant-related bleeding. Estimates of the clinical effects of such bleeding, defined as the case-fatality rate of major bleeding and risk for intracranial bleeding, were provided.

Methods.—In this literature review, 2 independent reviewers extracted data from randomized, controlled trials and prospective cohort studies of patients with venous thromboembolism receiving oral anticoagulant therapy for at least 3 months. In addition, all studies reviewed reported major bleeding and death as primary outcomes. Thirty-three studies, involving a total of 4374 patient-years of oral anticoagulant treatment, met study criteria.

Findings.—The case-fatality rate of major bleeding for all patients was 13.4%. That of intracranial bleeding was 1.15 per 100 patient-years. Patients given anticoagulant treatment for more than 3 months had a 9.1% case-fatality rate of major bleeding and an intracranial bleeding rate of 0.65 per 100 patient-years after the first 3 months of therapy.

Conclusions.—The clinical impact of anticoagulant-related major bleeding is considerable in patients with venous thromboembolism. Clinicians need to consider this when deciding whether to continue long-term oral anticoagulant treatment in an individual patient.

▶ The authors summarize evidence from prospective studies involving patients with thromboembolism receiving anticoagulation with a coumarin derivative for at least 3 months. The target international normalized ratio was 2.0 to 3.0. The data show a significant incidence of major and intracranial bleeding. Clinicians must take this into account when assessing the benefits and risks of long-term oral anticoagulant therapy.

B. H. Thiers, MD

Subcutaneous Fondaparinux Versus Intravenous Unfractionated Heparin in the Initial Treatment of Pulmonary Embolism

Büller HR, for the Matisse Investigators (Academic Med Ctr, Amsterdam; et al)
N Engl J Med 349:1695-1702, 2003   19–12

Background.—IV unfractionated heparin, the standard initial treatment for hemodynamically stable patients with pulmonary embolism, requires laboratory monitoring and hospitalization. The safety and efficacy of the synthetic antithrombotic agent fondaparinux were compared with those of unfractionated heparin in a large series of patients with acute symptomatic pulmonary embolism.

Methods.—A randomized open-label study was done that included 2213 patients who received fondaparinux subcutaneously once a day or a continuous IV infusion of unfractionated heparin. The fondaparinux dosage was 5, 7.5, or 10 mg for patients weighing less than 50 kg, 50 to 100 kg, or more than 100 kg, respectively. Both agents were administered for at least 5 days and until the use of vitamin K antagonists yielded an international normalized ratio (INR) exceeding 2.0.

Findings.—Of the 1103 patients assigned to fondaparinux, 3.8% had recurrent thromboembolic events, compared with 5% of the 1110 given heparin. Major bleeding was documented in 1.3% and 1.1%, respectively. At 3 months, mortality rates in the 2 groups were similar. Fondaparinux was given partly on an outpatient basis in 14.5% of the patients assigned to that group.

Conclusions.—In the initial treatment of hemodynamically stable patients with pulmonary embolism, fondaparinux given subcutaneously once a day without monitoring is at least as effective as adjusted-dose, IV unfractionated heparin. Fondaparinux also appears to be as safe as unfractionated heparin.

Comparison of Ximelagatran With Warfarin for the Prevention of Venous Thromboembolism After Total Knee Replacement

Francis CW, for the EXULT Study Group (Univ of Rochester, NY; et al)
N Engl J Med 349:1703-1712, 2003   19–13

Background.—Ximelagatran is an oral direct thrombin inhibitor that does not need monitoring of coagulation or dose adjustment. Previous research on preventing venous thromboembolism after total knee replacement found that the efficacy of ximelagatran, 24 mg twice daily, is similar to that of warfarin. Whether a higher ximelagatran dose is superior to warfarin was determined in a randomized double-blind study.

Methods.—The study included 1851 patients. The efficacy of a regimen of 7 to 12 days of oral ximelagatran, 24 or 36 mg twice daily, beginning the morning after surgery, was compared with that of a regimen of warfarin started in the evening of the day of surgery.

Findings.—Oral ximelagatran, 36 mg twice daily, was superior to warfarin in the primary composite end point of venous thromboembolism and death from all causes, occurring in 20.3% and 27.6% of the ximelagatran and warfarin groups, respectively. The 2 groups did not differ significantly in major bleeding, perioperative indicators of bleeding, wound characteristics, or the composite secondary end point of proximal deep-vein thrombosis, pulmonary embolism, and death.

Conclusions.—Oral ximelagatran given the morning after total knee replacement appears to be better than warfarin in preventing venous thromboembolism. The drugs had similar rates of hemorrhagic complications.

Secondary Prevention of Venous Thromboembolism With the Oral Direct Thrombin Inhibitor Ximelagatran
Schulman S, for the THRIVE III Investigators (Karolinska Hosp, Stockholm; et al)
N Engl J Med 349:1713-1721, 2003   19–14

Background.—Because the risk of major bleeding may outweigh the risk of recurrence, secondary prevention with vitamin K antagonists is not given for more than 6 months in many patients with venous thromboembolism. The long-term efficacy and safety of treatment with fixed-dose oral ximelagatran beginning after 6 months of standard anticoagulant treatment for venous thromboembolism were assessed.

Methods.—The double-blind multicenter study included 1233 patients with venous thromboembolism who had undergone 6 months of anticoagulant treatment. By random assignment, patients received extended secondary prevention with the oral direct thrombin inhibitor ximelagatran, 24 mg, or placebo twice daily for 18 months. Coagulation was not monitored. Bilateral US of the legs and perfusion lung scanning were done at baseline.

Findings.—Symptomatic recurrent venous thromboembolism was confirmed in 12 (2.0%) of 612 patients in the ximelagatran group and in 71 (11.6%) of 611 patients in the placebo group (hazard ratio = 0.16). Six patients in the ximelagatran group and 7 in the placebo group died from any cause. Bleeding was documented in 134 (21.9%) and 111 (18.1%) patients, respectively (hazard ratio = 1.19). The incidence of major bleeding was low. None of the patients died of hemorrhage. The cumulative risks of a transient increase in the alanine aminotransferase concentrations to more than 3 times the upper limit of normal was 6.4% and 1.2% in the ximelagatran and placebo groups, respectively.

Conclusions.—These data suggest that oral ximelagatran is superior to placebo for the extended prevention of venous thromboembolism. The frequency of bleeding complications is not significantly increased with ximelagatran, but the number of patients with transient increases in alanine aminotransferase concentrations is higher than with placebo.

▶ As observed by Shapiro in an accompanying editorial, the first decade of the 21st century has been a time of great advances in the treatment of thrombotic disorders.[1] Biological therapies appear to be next: early trials are underway of agents that inhibit the tissue factor-dependent initiation of hemostasis.[2]

B. H. Thiers, MD

References

1. Shapiro SS: Treating thrombosis in the 21st century (editorial). *N Engl J Med* 349:1762-1764, 2003.
2. Moons AH, Peters RJ, Bijsterveld NR, et al: Recombinant nematode anticoagulant protein c2, an inhibitor of the tissue factor/factor VIIa complex, in patients undergoing elective coronary angioplasty. *J Am Coll Cardiol* 41:2147-2153, 2003.

Migration of Human Keratinocytes in Plasma and Serum and Wound Reepithelialisation

Henry G, Li W, Garner W, et al (Univ of Southern California, Los Angeles)
Lancet 361:574-576, 2003   19–15

Background.—When skin is wounded, what triggers human keratinocytes at the wound edge to migrate and resurface the wound? Because these keratinocytes are surrounded for the first time by serum rather than plasma, some substance in serum may promote this migration. This hypothesis was tested in colloidal gold migration assays.

Methods.—In vitro human keratinocyte migration assays were performed with cells attached to polylysine (control) or a collagen matrix with no growth factor, with serum, or with plasma. Keratinocyte polarization, p38 mitogen-activated protein kinase (p38MAPK; essential for migration of human keratinocytes) activation, and matrix metalloproteinase 9 (MMP-9; promotes keratinocyte migration) production were also measured in the presence of serum or plasma.

Results.—The migration index (MI) was 2% in the control condition and only 11% to 12% in the presence of collagen alone or collagen with plasma. However, the MI was 28% in the presence of collagen and serum. Keratinocytes exposed to plasma were rounded and nonpolarized, whereas those exposed to serum were elongated and polarized. P38MAPK was moderately activated in the presence of collagen alone or collagen with plasma, but it was markedly increased in the presence of collagen with serum. Results were similar for MMP-9.

Conclusion.—Serum promotes the migration of keratinocytes over a collagen matrix in a manner analogous to current knowledge of human skin healing. The mobility of keratinocytes is greatly enhanced in the presence of serum, probably because of the activation of p38MAPK and the induction of MMP-9. It is hoped that research into which serum and matrix components are involved in keratinocyte migration will provide insights into how wounded skin re-epithelializes.

▶ The authors test the hypothesis that serum and plasma have different effects on the ability of human keratinocytes to migrate. Their observation that serum, but not plasma, promotes human keratinocyte migration over a collagen matrix may lead to new therapeutic strategies to enhance wound healing.

B. H. Thiers, MD

Diabetic Neuropathic Foot Ulcers: Predicting Which Ones Will Not Heal
Margolis DJ, Allen-Taylor L, Hoffstad O, et al (Univ of Pennsylvania, Philadelphia)
Am J Med 115:627-631, 2003   19–16

Background.—Diabetes can be complicated by neuropathic foot ulcers, a serious condition. A clinically useful prognostic model for identifying ulcers that are unlikely to heal was developed.

Methods.—A cohort study of 27,630 patients with a diabetic neuropathic foot ulcer was designed by using an administrative and medical records database from a large wound care system. Clinicians adhered to a standard algorithm of good wound care, debridement, and offloading. The outcome was healing by the twentieth week of treatment. The wound labeled as "primary" was the one investigated in patients with more than 1 wound. Several prognostic models of varying mathematical complexity were assessed.

Findings.—Forty-seven percent of the cohort had healing by week 20 of treatment. In the simplest model, 1 point each was counted if the wound was older than 2 months, larger than 2 cm^2, or had a grade of 3 or greater on a 6-point scale. In the validation dataset, the likelihood of a wound not healing was 0.35 for a count of 0, 0.47 for a count of 1, 0.66 for a count of 2, and 0.81 for a count of 3.

Conclusions.—Prognostic factors that are already part of the wound care evaluation can be used to create a simple prognostic model to predict which diabetic neuropathic foot ulcers are unlikely to heal. The model may be used to determine who will benefit from standard care and to design clinical trials.

▶ The authors have devised a simple prognostic model to help predict the treatment responsiveness of diabetic neuropathic foot ulcers. Such a model could help improve the design of clinical trials to assess various therapeutic approaches for this condition.

B. H. Thiers, MD

The Role of Hyperbaric Oxygen Therapy in Ischaemic Diabetic Lower Extremity Ulcers: A Double-blind Randomised-controlled Trial
Abidia A, Laden G, Kuhan G, et al (Univ of Hull, England; BUPA Hosp, Hull, England)
Eur J Vasc Endovasc Surg 25:513-518, 2003   19–17

Introduction.—Lower-extremity ulcers in patients with diabetes are a source of major concern because bacterial infection can lead to limb-threatening complications. Hyperbaric oxygen therapy is of potential benefit in cases of diabetic lower-extremity ulcers, but a lack of supporting research and relatively high costs have limited its use as an adjunctive treatment. The role of hyperbaric oxygen therapy in patients with peripheral arterial disease (PAD) and diabetic lower-extremity ulcers was examined in a double-blind trial.

Methods.—The 18 patients recruited to the study were randomly assigned to receive 100% oxygen (treatment group) or air (control group), administered at 2.4 atmospheres of absolute pressure for 90 minutes daily, 5 days per week, for a total of 30 sessions. Wound care and use of antibiotics were standardized. The primary outcome was reduction in ulcer size at 6 weeks after the end of treatment.

Results.—Five of 8 ulcers in the treatment group, but only 1 of 8 ulcers in the control group, were healed with complete epithelialization at 6-week follow-up. The median decrease in wound area was 100% in the treatment group and 52% in the control group at 6 weeks. At 6 months, the 2 groups had a similar reduction in ulcer size (100% and 95%, respectively). Visits for dressing of the study ulcers were far more frequent in the control group; thus, the mean total cost per patient per year for ulcer dressing was £1972 in the treatment group versus £7946 in the control group. Adjunctive hyperbaric oxygen therapy was expensive (£3000 per patient), but it reduced the average cost of treatment to £2960 per patient.

Discussion.—Among patients with PAD and nonhealing lower-extremity ulcers, hyperbaric oxygen treatment enhanced healing. The therapy may be a cost-effective, valuable adjunct when patients are unable to undergo reconstructive surgery.

Hyperbaric Oxygen for Treating Wounds: A Systematic Review of the Literature
Wang C, Schwaitzberg S, Berliner E, et al (Tufts-New England Med Ctr, Boston; Agency for Healthcare Research and Quality, Rockville, Md)
Arch Surg 138:272-279, 2003   19–18

Introduction.—Because wounds often have a reduced oxygen supply, healing might be enhanced by improving oxygenation of the area surrounding the wound. The use of adjunctive hyperbaric oxygen (HBO) therapy has been reported for necrotizing infections and a variety of other disorders.

Available literature on the benefits of HBO in treating wounds was reviewed for study quality, outcomes, and adverse events.

Methods.—A MEDLINE search included articles published in English between mid 1998 and August 2001 and reporting clinical outcome in human subjects with 10 specific categories of wounds. Randomized controlled trials (RCTs), nonrandomized comparison studies, and case series were considered, but conference reports and review articles were excluded.

Results.—Fifty-seven studies involving 2700 patients were assessed; 7 were RCTs, 16 were nonrandomized studies, and 34 were case series. No study required wound tissue hypoxia for patient eligibility, and none included patients with acute peripheral arterial insufficiency. The number of HBO sessions ranged from 4 to 44. Conditions for which HBO may be beneficial were soft tissue radionecrosis, compromised skin grafts, osteoradionecrosis, gas gangrene, and chronic nonhealing diabetic wounds. A number of studies, primarily those on gas gangrene, reported HBO-related adverse events, including seizures and pressure-related traumas. A few deaths were associated with these adverse events.

Discussion.—The overall quality of reports assessing HBO therapy for treatment of wounds was poor, with inadequate or no controls in most studies. HBO may be helpful for some wounds, but current evidence is insufficient to determine when and in what patients therapy should be initiated. The adverse events associated with HBO require further investigation before the therapy can be widely recommended.

▶ Abidia et al (Abstract 19–17) freely admit that a large multicenter trial is needed to confirm their preliminary results suggesting that hyperbaric oxygen therapy may be a useful adjunct in the management of ischemic lower-extremity ulcers in diabetics. Wang et al (Abstract 19–18) reviewed the literature to assess the efficacy of hyperbaric oxygen for treating wounds. They found that most published studies were of poor quality with inadequate controls. Thus, there seems to be insufficient evidence to determine the appropriate time to initiate therapy and to establish criteria to determine which patients would most benefit from such therapy.

B. H. Thiers, MD

Topical Treatment of Pressure Ulcers With Nerve Growth Factor: A Randomized Clinical Trial
Landi F, Aloe L, Russo A, et al (Catholic Univ of the Sacred Heart, Rome; Natl Research Council, Rome; Wake Forest Univ, Winston-Salem, NC; et al)
Ann Intern Med 139:635-641, 2003   19–19

Introduction.—Pressure ulcers of the foot are a major cause of morbidity in older persons and an important health care challenge in nursing home residents. A pressure sore dramatically raises the cost of medical and nursing care. Management includes local wound care and surgical repair. The topical application of growth factors is the most recent treatment option. The efficacy of topical application of nerve growth factor was compared with that of conventional topical treatment in 36 patients with severe noninfected pressure ulcers of the foot.

Methods.—Eighteen patients received growth factor treatment and 18 received conventional topical treatment in a randomized, double-blind, placebo-controlled trial. Treatment response was assessed by tracing the perimeter of the wound onto sterile, transparent block paper and determining the stage.

Results.—At baseline, treatment and control groups were similar in demographic variables, clinical characteristics, and functional measures. The mean ulcer area was 1012 mm² in both the treatment and control groups ($P <$ .02). The average decrease in pressure ulcer area at 6 weeks was statistically greater in the treatment group (738 vs 485 mm²; $P = .034$).

Conclusion.—The topical application of nerve growth factor may be effective in the treatment of patients with severe pressure ulcers of the foot. The combined findings that keratocytes and fibroblasts produce nerve growth factor, that epithelial cells bear nerve growth factor receptors and respond to nerve growth factors, and that nerve growth factor accelerates wound healing in mouse skin are consistent with the hypothesis that nerve growth factor may have a direct action on the epithelium and is implicated in functional activity in wound healing.

▶ Pressure ulcers, especially of the foot, are a common problem in elderly debilitated patients. They respond poorly to therapy and can be a source of considerable morbidity. Landi et al found that daily topical application of nerve growth factor produced statistically significant acceleration in ulcer healing compared with standard therapy. Unfortunately, patients most at risk for pressure ulcers, ie, individuals with diabetes and peripheral vascular disease, were excluded from the current investigation. Future trials should compare topical nerve growth factor with other proven treatment methods, such as hydrocolloid dressings, and also investigate the use of topical nerve growth factor in other clinical settings, such as truncal pressure ulcers.[1]

B. H. Thiers, MD

Reference

1. Thomas DR: The promise of topical growth factors in healing pressure ulcers. *Ann Intern Med* 139:694-695, 2003.

20 Miscellaneous Topics in Dermatologic Surgery and Cutaneous Oncology

Lidocaine Iontophoresis for Topical Anesthesia Before Dermatologic Procedures in Children: A Randomized Controlled Trial
Zempsky WT, Parkinson TM (Univ of Connecticut; Connecticut Children's Med Ctr, Hartford; Iomed, Inc, Salt Lake City, Utah)
Pediatr Dermatol 20:364-368, 2003   20–1

Background.—Dermatologic procedures in children are often painful. In the topical anesthesia method of lidocaine iontophoresis, lidocaine is driven into the skin under the influence of electric current. The effects of iontophoresis of 2% lidocaine with 1:100,000 epinephrine were compared with those of 1:100,000 epinephrine plus saline (placebo).

Methods.—The double-blind placebo-controlled study included 60 children scheduled for dermatologic procedures. Fifty children were undergoing shave biopsy; 7, curettage; 2, injection; and 1, punch biopsy.

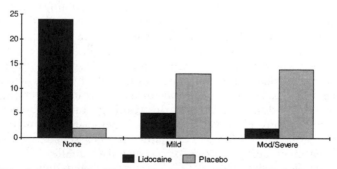

FIGURE 1.—Patient pain ratings (Oucher scale). (Courtesy of Zempsky WT, Parkinson TM: Lidocaine iontophoresis for topical anesthesia before dermatologic procedures in children: A randomized controlled trial. *Pediatr Dermatol* 20:364-368, 2003. Reprinted by permission of Blackwell Publishing.)

Findings.—No supplemental anesthesia was needed in 29 (93.5%) of 31 lidocaine recipients, compared with 2 (6.9%) of 29 placebo recipients. After the procedure, patient-reported pain using the Oucher scale was significantly less in the lidocaine group than in the placebo group (Fig 1). Parents and investigators also judged pain to be less in the lidocaine group. Blanching or erythema or both were noted in 58 of 60 patients. However, these effects resolved within 1 hour in all patients. No other adverse events occurred.

Conclusions.—Lidocaine iontophoresis is an effective and safe method of topical anesthesia before dermatologic procedures in children. The patients tolerated lidocaine iontophoresis well.

▶ Lidocaine iontophoresis seems to be an effective method of delivery of local anesthesia to young children who are fearful of needles. The apparent need for a special formulation of lidocaine and the personnel time required to administer iontophoresis may limit its usefulness in the average practitioner's office.

S. Raimer, MD

Hemangiomas of Infancy: Clinical Characteristics, Morphologic Subtypes, and Their Relationship to Race, Ethnicity, and Sex
Chiller KG, Passaro D, Frieden IJ (Univ of California, San Francisco; Univ of Illinois, Chicago; Emory Univ, Atlanta, Ga)
Arch Dermatol 138:1567-1576, 2002   20–2

Background.—The most common benign tumors in children are hemangiomas of infancy, which vary greatly in appearance, size, and depth of cutaneous involvement. The relationship of hemangioma subtype and anatomical location with demographic factors, complications, and other anomalies was investigated.

Methods and Findings.—The charts of 327 patients with 472 hemangiomas of infancy seen between 1997 and 2000 at 1 center were reviewed. Seventy-two percent of the hemangiomas were localized, 18% were segmental, 8% were indeterminate, and 3% were multifocal. Segmental lesions were larger and more often correlated with developmental abnormalities. These lesions also required more intensive and prolonged treatment. More complications and a poorer overall outcome were associated with segmental lesions. In Hispanic children, lesions were more likely to involve mucous membranes, to be segmental, and to be associated with abnormalities, such as PHACE syndrome (Posterior fossa brain malformations, hemangiomas, arterial anomalies, coarctation of the aorta and cardiac defects, and eye abnormalities). In addition, lesions in this ethnic group were associated with more complications. However, an increased incidence of segmental hemangiomas was the only variable in Hispanic infants associated with more extensive treatment, complications, or associated anomalies.

Conclusions.—On the basis of clinical features, hemangiomas of infancy may be classified as localized, segmental, indeterminate, or multifocal. A greater frequency of complications and associated abnormalities are associated with segmental lesions. This type of hemangioma appears to be more frequent in Hispanic infants.

▶ This study adds new knowledge about hemangiomas by documenting that there is increased morbidity, a less favorable outcome, and that there are more associated anomalies associated with segmental compared with localized lesions. It also is apparent that structural defects may occur in association with segmental hemangiomas at any anatomical site. The authors observe that there seems to be an increased incidence of segmental hemangiomas in Hispanic infants.

S. Raimer, MD

Carbon Dioxide Laser Dermabrasion for Giant Congenital Melanocytic Nevi
Reynolds N, Kenealy J, Mercer N (Frenchay Hosp, Bristol, England)
Plast Reconstr Surg 111:2209-2214, 2003   20–3

Background.—Clinicians continue to disagree on the management of giant congenital melanocytic nevi. The results of 7 patients treated with carbon dioxide laser dermabrasion were discussed.

Patients and Outcomes.—The patients were 5 girls and 2 boys, 1½ months to 8 years old. Five children were younger than 1 year. All were treated with the same type of carbon dioxide laser, a Coherent UltraPulse 5000C, under general anesthesia. The 350 or 500 mJ setting was typically used. Multiple passes were made, with residual debris wiped away between passes. The number of passes depended on the lesion depth and clinical judgment of how deeply the treatment could be applied before a risk of scarring might occur. In some children, a second treatment was needed. Localized areas of deeper pigmentation were treated with a 3-mm collimated handpiece. Preferred aftercare included a hydrocellular dressing, applied immediately after the procedure. The length of recovery depended on the amount of fluid lost. The follow-up time ranged from 1.5 to 6 years. The outcomes were encouraging, and the cosmetic appearance was considerably improved, with far less scarring and disfigurement than with nonlaser dermabrasion or excision and grafting.

Conclusions.—This technique provides a more controlled method of dermabrasion than has been available previously, enabling the margins of the lesions to be treated adequately. Improvement in cosmetic appearance was marked, a result that will be of benefit in the psychosocial development of these children.

▶ Reynolds et al report their experience in managing large congenital nevi; 7 children were treated using an ultrapulsed carbon dioxide laser. The authors noted significant cosmetic improvement in the lesions; however, the results of only 2 cases are illustrated, and in 1 of these, there appears to be significant scarring. The authors provide a good review of the literature on large congenital nevi; unfortunately, there are some problems with their approach. First, laser resurfacing of nonfacial areas is risky and carries with it a significant risk of scarring. Second, only the most superficially located melanocytes are destroyed, thus leaving behind the deeper melanocytes that may serve as a precursor to melanoma. Finally, does the performance of more than 3 passes improve the therapeutic results or simply increase the risk of scarring and textural change?

P. G. Lang, Jr, MD

Treatment of Keloids by Surgical Excision and Immediate Postoperative Single-Fraction Radiotherapy

Ragoowansi R, Cornes PG, Moss AL, et al (St George's Hosp, London; Royal Marsden Hosp, Surrey, England)

Plast Reconstr Surg 111:1853-1859, 2003   20–4

Introduction.—Keloids, in contrast to hypertrophic scars, extend beyond the wound and remain thick and raised for years. Recurrence rates are high for keloids treated by surgery alone, but the addition of postoperative radiotherapy appears to reduce the rate of relapse. At the study institution, high-risk keloids have been treated for the past 10 years by extralesional excision with single-fraction radiotherapy administered within 24 hours. Eighty cases were reviewed to assess the outcome of this method.

Methods.—Eighty patients with 80 keloid scars had failed all other forms of treatment. Initiating events for the scars included injury, infection, burns, iatrogenic response, and spontaneous occurrence. After excision, the operative scars were covered with topical lignocaine hydrochloride 2% and chlorhexidine 0.25% in a sterile lubricant gel. A nonopaque, semiocclusive polyurethane dressing was then placed over the entire site. Patients received a 10-Gy dose of superficial 60-kV (for all sites except the earlobe) or 100-kV (for the earlobe) photon irradiation. Patients were followed at 4 weeks, 3 months, 6 months, and then yearly.

Results.—All keloid scars were controlled at 4 weeks. Treatment failure had occurred at 1 year in 6 of 64 patients with follow-up, and an additional 4 of 54 patients monitored at 5 years had relapsed. There were no cases of serious toxicity, but hyperpigmentation occurred in many nonwhite patients and sometimes lasted for months or years before fading.

Conclusion.—Excision with immediate adjuvant single-fraction radiotherapy was effective in controlling keloids in the majority of these patients, all of whom had failed previous therapies. When early relapse was signaled by itching or scar pain, other treatments such as topical silicone gel or intralesional steroids were used. This salvage therapy was successful in several cases. Patients must be informed of the potential risk of cancer induction, and radiotherapy is not recommended for children with keloids.

▶ There is no ideal treatment for the management of keloids, and recurrence after surgical excision is not uncommon. In this study, the authors report their experience with surgical excision, followed by a single fraction radiotherapy. Considering that these patients had failed prior treatment, the results appear to be quite good (84% control of keloids at 5 years). However, the study has several flaws that might have impacted the results. For example, by 5 years 25% of the patients had been lost to follow-up. What if the majority of these patients had suffered a recurrence? Patients who chose to have their ears pierced again and who developed a keloid were considered treatment failures. This could result in a falsely high-recurrence rate. This would also explain why the control of chest keloids was better than that for keloids of the earlobes. The inclusion of patients without clinical evidence of recurrence other than itching and pain at the site could also have skewed the results. The authors rightly emphasize the importance of giving the radiation within 24 hours of excising the lesion to ensure maximum benefit. The authors also suggest that control may be more effective if their protocol is used for previously untreated lesions as opposed to recurrent lesions.[1] Although surgical excision followed by radiation therapy is an approach worth considering, this reviewer's experience has not been as favorable as the authors', even with primary lesions, and especially for keloids located on the chest and back.

P. G. Lang, Jr, MD

Reference

1. Kovalic JJ, Perez CA: Radiation therapy following keloidectomy: A 20 year experience. *Int J Radiat Oncol Biol Phys* 17:77, 1989.

Subject Index

Author Index

VISIT OUR HOME PAGE!
www.us.elsevierhealth.com/periodicals

ELSEVIER
MOSBY